Vaccines and Vaccination: Feature Papers

Vaccines and Vaccination: Feature Papers

Guest Editor

Pedro Plans-Rubió

MDPI

Basel • Beijing • Wuhan • Barcelona • Belgrade • Novi Sad • Cluj • Manchester

Guest Editor
Pedro Plans-Rubió
College of Physicians
of Barcelona
Barcelona
Spain

Editorial Office
MDPI AG
Grosspeteranlage 5
4052 Basel, Switzerland

This is a reprint of the Special Issue, published open access by the journal *Vaccines* (ISSN 2076-393X), freely accessible at: https://www.mdpi.com/journal/vaccines/special_issues/182PRES5LH.

For citation purposes, cite each article independently as indicated on the article page online and as indicated below:

Lastname, A.A.; Lastname, B.B. Article Title. *Journal Name* **Year**, *Volume Number*, Page Range.

ISBN 978-3-7258-5967-2 (Hbk)
ISBN 978-3-7258-5968-9 (PDF)
https://doi.org/10.3390/books978-3-7258-5968-9

Contents

About the Editor

Pedro Plans-Rubió

Pedro Plans-Rubió is a member of the College of Physicians of Barcelona, Spain. Responsible for Health Registries at the Public Health Agency, Department of Health of Catalonia, Spain (until 2025). Expert of the European Commission for assessing public health and health economics projects. Member of the Group of Prioritization of Treatments (GIP), Heath Emergency Preparedness and Response (HERA), European Commission. Member of the Non-communicable diseases risk factor Collaboration (NCD-RisC) research group. Member of the CIBER of Epidemiology and Public Health (CIBERESP), Instituto de Salud Carlos III, Madrid, Spain (until 2025). Currently, Editor-in-Chief of Section "Vaccine Advancement, Efficacy and Safety" of the *Vaccines* journal and Editor of the journal *PharmacoEconomics Open*. He has served as Guest Editor for the *Vaccines* journal's Special Issue on "Strategies to Increase Vaccination Coverage and Vaccine Confidence" and "Efficacy, Immunogenicity and Safety of COVID-19 Vaccines and COVID-19 Vaccination Strategies". He has developed and participated in epidemiological and seroepidemiological studies of vaccine-preventable infectious diseases. including measles, pertussis, mumps, rubella, tetanus, diphtheria, polio, hepatitis A, hepatitis B, tuberculosis, COVID-19 and influenza. Dr. Plans-Rubió has authored and co-authored peer-reviewed publications on epidemiology of infectious diseases, evaluation of vaccination programs, epidemiology of factors of non-communicable diseases, economic studies of medicines, and strategies for the prevention, control and eradication of vaccine-preventable diseases.

Preface

Vaccines are among the most effective and cost-effective health interventions, but the development of vaccines and vaccination programs must overcome multiple challenges to achieve their expected outcomes. The aim of this reprint is to present research and review articles on the most recent results and findings in relation to the challenges that must be overcome the development of vaccines and vaccination programs to achieve their expected outcomes. The articles included in this reprint addressed issues related to the analysis of interventions to increase vaccination coverage, the analysis of measles vaccination coverage indicators worldwide and in different in World Health Organization (WHO) regions, the analysis of factors related to vaccine hesitancy and acceptance, the development of new vaccines, the economic analysis of new cancer vaccines, and the clinical characteristics mechanisms and therapeutic potentialities of regulatory T cells in the management of patients with COVID-19.

Pedro Plans-Rubió
Guest Editor

vaccines

MDPI

Editorial

Vaccines and Vaccination: Feature Papers

Pedro Plans-Rubió

College of Physicians of Barcelona, 08017 Barcelona, Spain; pedro.plans@yahoo.es

This Special Issue, entitled "Vaccines and vaccination: Feature Papers", included articles that addressed various issues related to vaccines and vaccination, including studies assessing interventions to increase vaccination coverage [1], studies assessing vaccination coverage indicators in World Health Organization (WHO) regions [2], studies assessing vaccination hesitancy and vaccination acceptance [3–6], economic studies of cancer vaccines [7], reviews regarding the development of new vaccines [8,9], and reviews of vaccine-preventable diseases [10].

The article by Gerin et al. [1] presented the results of a study assessing the effectiveness of a training course for health professionals that aimed to enhance vaccination coverage among people living with HIV (PLHIV) in Brazil. The study found that the training course resulted in greater vaccination coverage for the 13- and 23-valent pneumococcal vaccines, human papilloma virus vaccine, meningococcal C vaccine, measles–mumps–rubella vaccine, and yellow fever vaccine. The training course was effective due to the fact that recommendation by a health professional is one of the factors influencing vaccination acceptance [11,12].

The article by Plans-Rubió [2] assessed the coverage of measles vaccination with zero, one and two doses of vaccine and the anti-measles herd immunity levels in World Health Organization (WHO) regions in 2023; and the variation from 2019 to 2023 for measles vaccination coverage and anti-measles herd immunity-related indicators. To achieve the Immunization Agenda objective of eliminating measles in at least five of the six WHO regions by 2030 (IA2030), it is necessary to increase the two-dose vaccination coverage to ≥95% in all countries and WHO regions, and to reduce the number of children who have not received at least one measles vaccine (zero-dose measles children) by 50% from 2019 to 2030 [13–15]. However, this study found that the global two-dose measles vaccination coverage decreased by 3.7%, the global zero-dose measles vaccination coverage increased by 7.8, and the number of countries with ≥95% two-dose measles vaccination coverage decreased by 39.6% from 2019 to 2023. This study concluded that measles vaccination programs should therefore be improved in all WHO regions in order to eradicate measles worldwide.

Four articles published in this Special Issue were focused on vaccination acceptance and vaccination hesitancy [3–6]. Vaccine hesitance is defined as a delay in the acceptance or refusal of vaccines despite the availability of vaccine services [16,17]. Vaccine hesitancy is a complex issue influenced by factors such as misinformation, complacency, and a lack of confidence in vaccines and vaccination services [18–20]. Christodoulakis et al. [3] developed a scoping review study to assess the hesitancy towards COVID-19 booster doses among healthcare workers worldwide. The study found vaccine hesitancy rates of 19.7% to 66.5% in Asia, 27% to 46.1% in Africa, and 14% to 60.2% in Europe. The vaccine hesitancy rates ranged from 12.8% to 43.7% among physicians, 26% to 37% among nurses, and 26% to 34.6% among pharmacists. The study concluded that future pandemic vaccination programs should develop activities to improve vaccination rates among healthcare workers.

The article by Vicente-Alcaide et al. [4] assessed the acceptance of COVID-19 vaccination among Spanish prisoners and prison workers, finding that 88.72% of prisoners and prison workers agreed to be vaccinated and 89.64% would recommend the vaccine to others. In addition, 89% of prisoners and prison workers believed that the benefits of COVID-19 vaccination were greater than its potential adverse effects.

The article by De Vito [5] presents the results of a narrative review regarding the vaccinations available for adults living with HIV. This study found that vaccinations were strongly recommended among adults living with HIV, although data on immunogenicity, tolerability, and clinical efficacy were limited. This article concluded that clinicians should collect the history of vaccinations in all new patients with HIV and assess their antibody levels against different vaccine-preventable pathogens, especially in patients with low CD4 numbers.

The article by Limbu and Gautam [6] presents the results of a systematic review assessing the relationships between Health Belief Model (HBM) constructs and COVID-19 vaccination intention. This study found that perceived benefits, perceived barriers, and cues to action were the three most frequent predictors for primary and booster COVID-19 vaccination.

One of the articles included in this Special Issue focused on the economic analysis of a new cancer vaccine. Novakova et al. [7] evaluated the financial feasibility of introducing a peptide-based neoantigen cancer vaccine (NCV) for the treatment of patients with triple-negative breast cancer (TNBC). The survival rate at five years for patients with metastatic TNBC is 10%, while that for other metastatic breast cancer subtypes is 30%, and they have limited treatment options [21,22]. The study proposes that a neoantigen cancer vaccine could enhance T-cell responses independently of genetic factors, unlike approved immunotherapies for TNBC. In the UK, the conventional treatment costs per patient with TNBC range from GBP 2200 to GBP 54,000, and the total costs of treating TNBC patients reached GBP 230 million in 2024. The incremental cost-effectiveness ratio in terms of cost per life year for the quality-adjusted life year gained (QALY) of approved TNBC therapies was GBP 52,000 for atezolizumab, GBP 34,000 for pembrolizumab and GBP 38,000 for chemotherapy. The incremental cost-effectiveness ratio for a NCV vaccine (11 doses) was GBP 2200 in the best-case scenario, where the NCV was assumed to be administered at cost with a decentralized approach and zero intermediary supply chain. In contrast, the incremental cost-effectiveness ratio was GBP 55,000 in the worst-case scenario, where the NCV was produced by a laboratory that aimed to recover the research and development costs. The cost-effectiveness ratios of the NCV were lower and greater than the NICE willingness-to pay threshold of GBP 50,000 in the best-case scenario and the worse-case scenario, respectively.

The article by Choi et al. [8] assessed the efficacy of a new vaccine against *Clostridium botulinum* Neurotoxin Types A and B in an animal model (mice). The vaccine was generated by combining the HCC domains of botulinum neurotoxin type A and type B in *Escherichia coli* to produce a recombinant protein (rHCCB-L-HCCArHCcB) that inhibits their receptor binding. This study found that mice immunized with the anti-neurotoxin vaccine had significantly greater levels of antibodies than mice immunized with alum alone, showing that this vaccine was effective in protecting against lethal levels of neurotoxins of type A and type B.

The article by Onnocks et al. [9] presents a review concerning the potential use of attenuated and/or genetically modified oncolytic viruses (OV) for cancer therapy. Tumor antigen-presenting vaccines can be based on peptides, DNA, and dendritic cells as antigen-presenting cells. Oncolytic viruses are non-pathogenic viruses that can initiate post-oncolytic anti-cancer immunity by infecting cancer cells and cause oncolysis [23].

The article by Dhawan et al. [10] presents a review addressing the influence of regulatory T-cells (Tregs) on the prognosis of COVID-19. Decreased levels of Tregs among COVID-19 patients can be associated with lower inflammatory inhibition, which is associated with a worse COVID-19 prognosis. The severity of COVID-19 is also associated with abnormalities in the Tregs phenotype, including a reduction in the expression of FoxP3, IL-10 and TGF-beta [24]. This study shows the need to maintain COVID-19 vaccination among vulnerable populations who are at a greater risk of COVID-19 complications.

The articles published in this Special Issue reveal that the success of vaccination programs can depend on multiple factors, including the development and production of effective and cost-effective vaccines, vaccination acceptance and hesitancy, and the effective and efficient implementation of vaccination programs.

Funding: This editorial did not receive any funding.

Conflicts of Interest: The author declares no conflicts of interest.

References

1. Gerin, L.; Gir, E.; Neves, L.A.d.S.; Passos, L.M.R.; Kfouri, R.d.Á.; Spire, B.; Reis, R.K. Vaccination Coverage of People Living with HIV: Before and after Interventional Action. *Vaccines* **2024**, *12*, 897. [CrossRef] [PubMed]
2. Plans-Rubió, P. Measles Vaccination Coverage and Anti-Measles Herd Immunity Levels in the World and WHO Regions Worsened from 2019 to 2023. *Vaccines* **2025**, *13*, 157. [CrossRef] [PubMed]
3. Christodoulakis, A.; Bouloukaki, I.; Aravantinou-Karlatou, A.; Zografakis-Sfakianakis, M.; Tsiligianni, I. Vaccine Hesitancy and Associated Factors Amongst Health Professionals: A Scoping Review of the Published Literature. *Vaccines* **2024**, *12*, 1411. [CrossRef] [PubMed]
4. Vicente-Alcalde, N.; Sferle, S.M.; Franco-Paredes, C.; Tuells, J. Acceptance of the COVID-19 Vaccine by Prisoners and Staff in Spanish Prisons. *Vaccines* **2023**, *11*, 1547. [CrossRef] [PubMed]
5. De Vito, A.; Colpani, A.; Trunfio, M.; Fiore, V.; Moi, G.; Fois, M.; Leoni, N.; Ruiu, S.; Babudieri, S.; Calcagno, A.; et al. Living with HIV and Getting Vaccinated: A Narrative Review. *Vaccines* **2023**, *11*, 896. [CrossRef] [PubMed]
6. Limbu, Y.B.; Gautam, R.K. How Well the Constructs of Health Belief Model Predict Vaccination Intention: A Systematic Review on COVID-19 Primary Series and Booster Vaccines. *Vaccines* **2023**, *11*, 816. [CrossRef] [PubMed]
7. Novakova, A.; Morris, S.A.; Vaiarelli, L.; Frank, S. Manufacturing and Financial Evaluation of Peptide-Based Neoantigen Cancer Vaccines for Triple-Negative Breast Cancer in the United Kingdom: Opportunities and Challenges. *Vaccines* **2025**, *13*, 144. [CrossRef] [PubMed]
8. Choi, E.-S.; Pyo, S.-W.; Kim, S.-H.; Jeon, J.-H.; Rhie, G.-E.; Yun, M.-R.; Yi, H.; Chung, Y.-S. Development of a Recombinant Fusion Vaccine Candidate Against Lethal *Clostridium botulinum* Neurotoxin Types A and B. *Vaccines* **2025**, *13*, 39. [CrossRef] [PubMed]
9. Onnockx, S.; Baldo, A.; Pauwels, K. Oncolytic Viruses: An Inventory of Shedding Data from Clinical Trials and Elements for the Environmental Risk Assessment. *Vaccines* **2023**, *11*, 1448. [CrossRef] [PubMed]
10. Dhawan, M.; Rabaan, A.A.; Alwarthan, S.; Alhajri, M.; Halwani, M.A.; Alshengeti, A.; Najim, M.A.; Alwashmi, A.S.S.; Alshehri, A.A.; Alshamrani, S.A.; et al. Regulatory T Cells (Tregs) and COVID-19: Unveiling the Mechanisms, and Therapeutic Potentialities with a Special Focus on Long COVID. *Vaccines* **2023**, *11*, 699. [CrossRef] [PubMed]
11. Wennekes, M.D.; Almási, T.; Eilers, R.; Mezei, F.; Petykó, Z.I.; Timen, A.; Vokó, Z.; VITAL Consortium. Effectiveness of educational interventions for healthcare workers on vaccination dialogue with older adults: A systematic review. *Arch. Public Health* **2024**, *82*, 34. [CrossRef] [PubMed]
12. Gallup. Wellcome Global Monitor. 2018. Available online: https://wellcome.org/sites/default/files/wellcome-global-monitor-2018.pdf (accessed on 16 June 2025).
13. WHO/UNICEF. Immunization Agenda 2030: A Global Strategy to Leave No One Behind. Available online: https://www.who.int/publications/m/item/immunization-agenda-2030-a-global-strategy-to-leave-no-one-behind#:~:text=The%20Immunization%20Agenda%202030%20(IA2030,opportunities%20to%20meet%20those%20challenges (accessed on 15 June 2025).
14. WHO-UNICEF. Progress and Challenges with Achieving Universal Immunization Coverage. Available online: https://www.who.int/publications/m/item/progress-and-challenges-with-achievinguniversal-immunization-coverage (accessed on 12 June 2025).

15. World Health Organization (WHO). *Measles and Rubella Strategic Framework 2021–2030*; World Health Organization: Geneva, Switzerland, 2020; Available online: https://www.who.int/publications/i/item/measles-and-rubella-strategic-framework-2021-2030 (accessed on 15 June 2025).
16. Mac Donald, N.E.; SAGE Working Group on Vaccine Hesitancy. Vaccine hesitancy: Definition, scope and determinants. *Vaccine* **2015**, *33*, 4161–4164. [CrossRef] [PubMed]
17. European Centre for Disease Prevention and Control (ECDC). *Catalogue of Interventions Addressing Vaccine Hesitancy*; ECDC: Stockholm, Sweden, 2017.
18. Dubé, E.; Laberge, C.; Guay, M.; Bramadat, P.; Roy, R.; Bettinger, J. Vaccine hesitancy: An overview. *Hum. Vaccines Immunother.* **2013**, *9*, 1763–1773. [CrossRef] [PubMed]
19. Larson, H.J.; Gakidou, E.; Murray, C.J.L. The Vaccine-Hesitant Moment. *N. Engl. J. Med.* **2022**, *387*, 58–65. [CrossRef] [PubMed]
20. The Lancet Child Adolescent Health. Vaccine hesitancy: A generation at risk. *Lancet Child. Adolesc. Health* **2019**, *3*, 281. [CrossRef] [PubMed]
21. Hsu, J.Y.; Chang, C.J.; Cheng, J.S. Survival, treatment regimens and medical costs of women newly diagnosed with metastatic triple-negative breast cancer. *Sci. Rep.* **2022**, *12*, 729. [CrossRef] [PubMed]
22. Dieci, M.V.; Tsvetkova, V.; Orvieto, E.; Piacentini, F.; Ficarra, G.; Griguolo, G.; Miglietta, F.; Giarratano, T.; Omarini, C.; Bonaguro, S.; et al. Immune characterization of breast cancer metastases: Prognostic implications. *Breast Cancer Res.* **2018**, *20*, 62. [CrossRef] [PubMed]
23. Schirrmacher, V. Cancer Vaccines and Oncolytic Viruses Exert Profoundly Lower Side Effects in Cancer Patients than Other Systemic Therapies: A Comparative Analysis. *Biomedicines* **2020**, *8*, 61. [CrossRef] [PubMed]
24. Grau-Expósito, J.; Sánchez-Gaona, N.; Massana, N.; Suppi, M.; Astorga-Gamaza, A.; Perea, D.; Rosado, J.; Falcó, A.; Kirkegaard, C.; Torrella, A.; et al. Peripheral and Lung Resident Memory T Cell Responses against SARS-CoV-2. *Nat. Commun.* **2021**, *12*, 3010. [CrossRef] [PubMed]

vaccines

MDPI

Article

Vaccination Coverage of People Living with HIV: Before and after Interventional Action

Larissa Gerin [1,*], Elucir Gir [2], Lis Aparecida de Souza Neves [1], Luzia Márcia Romanholi Passos [1], Renato de Ávila Kfouri [3], Bruno Spire [4] and Renata Karina Reis [2]

1 Epidemiological Surveillance Division, Ribeirão Preto Municipal Health Department, Ribeirão Preto 14015100, São Paulo, Brazil; lisapneves@yahoo.com.br (L.A.d.S.N.); lmrpassos@rp.ribeiraopreto.sp.gov.br (L.M.R.P.)
2 Ribeirão Preto School of Nursing, University of São Paulo, Ribeirão Preto 14040902, São Paulo, Brazil; egir@eerp.usp.br (E.G.); rkreis@eerp.usp.br (R.K.R.)
3 Brazilian Society of Immunization, São Paulo 01309902, São Paulo, Brazil; renatokfouri@uol.com.br
4 Inserm, IRD, SESSTIM, Sciences Economiques & Sociales de la Santé & Traitement de l'Information Médicale, ISSPAM, Aix Marseille University, 13385 Marseille, France; bruno.spire@inserm.fr
* Correspondence: larissagerin@yahoo.com.br; Tel.: +55-1636247234

Abstract: This is a quasi-experimental study that assessed PLHIV vaccination coverage before and after health professionals participated in a training course on PLHIV immunization. The vaccination coverage of 645 PLHIV was assessed in the pre-intervention phase. The vaccine with the best coverage was diphtheria and tetanus (82.64%) and the one with the lowest rate of adequately vaccinated was measles, mumps, and rubella (38.27%). Individuals aged between 30 and 39 years had a 74.00% (1–0.26) lower chance of having the full vaccination schedule when compared to those aged between 10 and 19 years, and among those over 40 years, the chance was 87.00% (1–0.13) lower. Those who were vaccinated in Specialized Care Services (SCS) were 5.77 times more likely to be adequately vaccinated when compared to those who were vaccinated in other health services. Regarding the entire vaccination schedule evaluated, the number of adequately vaccinated increased from 47 (7.29%) to 76 (11.78%). Interventions targeting health professionals were effective in increasing vaccination coverage among PLHIV; however, the achieved coverage remained below the desired level. It is necessary to act on health professionals' knowledge and other aspects to effectively increase vaccination coverage.

Keywords: vaccination coverage; vaccination; HIV; health professionals

1. Introduction

With advances in immunization and improved hygiene and health conditions, a decrease in the number of infectious diseases has been observed; however, the reduction in vaccination coverage and population displacement in the globalized world pose a risk of the resurgence of diseases that have already been eliminated [1].

People living with HIV (PLHIV) have an increased risk of acquiring infectious diseases and, if they do, have a greater chance of developing into more severe forms [2–7].

On the other hand, with increased survival and reduced mortality due to adequate adherence to Antiretroviral Therapy (ART), they end up exposing themselves more to risk scenarios as they maintain work, travel, and leisure activities that put them in contact with potential pathogenic infectious agents. In addition, these individuals end up being more exposed as they are in frequent contact with health services [3,8–10].

Thus, preventing the occurrence of infectious diseases in PLHIV is a strategy to improve the quality of life and life expectancy. In this regard, immunization stands out, and a special vaccination schedule is recommended for these individuals [1,3,10–12].

In Brazil, the Unified Health System (UHS) offers 12 immunobiological agents to PLHIV free of charge through the National Immunization Program (NPI). The vaccination schedule for this group is broader than that offered to the general population. In addition, it is recommended that the vaccination schedule of household contacts of PLHIV and health professionals who provide care for this population be updated, which constitutes extra protection, especially for those with some contraindications to vaccination for having lower CD4 T-lymphocyte (TL) counts. It is recommended that the vaccination schedule be updated as early as possible before the disease progresses and the immune system becomes deficient [3,4,8,10,13–16].

Despite the importance of immunization, few studies have presented vaccination coverage for PLHIV. The majority of studies focus on the vaccination rate for a single vaccine type [2,6,17,18] or inactivated vaccines indicated for this population [1,5,7,9,12,13,19,20], rather than providing a comprehensive overview of vaccination coverage, including attenuated vaccines [3,15].

In a survey conducted in Germany on PLHIV aged at least 50 years, only 20% of the participants reported a completed schedule for the inactivated vaccines evaluated [9]. In an investigation conducted in Brazil regarding attenuated vaccines, it identified coverage of 14.14% [3]. In a retrospective cohort study conducted in the USA in which the schedule of eight vaccines indicated for PLHIV was evaluated, it was found that 41% of the participants were adequately vaccinated [19].

The data show that vaccination coverage among PLHIV is low and that there is no effective assessment of vaccination status in the services where these individuals are monitored. The main determinants of non-vaccination are failure to receive a recommendation from a health professional, lack of knowledge about the indicated vaccines and their schedules, difficulties in accessing immunizers, or simply forgetting appointment dates [1–7,9,11–13,15,21].

The set of aspects exposed reinforces the essential role of health professionals in the indication of immunizers, deconstruction of false contraindications, expansion of vaccine acceptance, and search for unvaccinated individuals to improve adequately vaccinated rates. In addition, the importance of medical professionals in vaccine indication and prescription is highlighted, which would significantly increase the search of individuals for immunobiological agents [3,4,6,7,9,12,13,21].

Given this scenario, this study aimed to evaluate the effectiveness of an interventional action in the vaccination coverage of PLHIV, considering the vaccines recommended by the Brazilian NIP.

2. Materials and Methods

2.1. Study Design and Site

The study was conducted in a Brazilian municipality with a population of about 711,000 inhabitants and a Human Development Index (HDI) of 0.800, which is considered high relative to the whole country. The municipality has a wide network, with 47 Primary Health Care Units (PHCU) (37 of them with vaccine rooms) and five Specialized Care Services (SCS), for outpatient clinical follow-up of PLHIV [22].

This is a quasi-experimental study conducted in three stages:

- Pre-intervention phase—was developed using data obtained from the Information System for Notifiable Diseases (ISND), which is the national country's HIV case notification system. These cases were then identified in the municipal outpatient follow-up system (Hygiaweb) in order to assess the records of vaccines administered and calculate vaccination coverage.
- Intervention phase—a training course on immunization of PLHIV was offered to health professionals involved in vaccination actions in the public services of the municipality of the study and to SCS health professionals.
- Post-intervention phase—one year after the start date of the training course in the intervention phase, data on vaccines administered to PLHIV were collected again,

updating the information collected in the pre-intervention phase regarding vaccination coverage rates.

2.2. Population and Sample

In the pre-and post-intervention phases, the population consisted of all cases notified in the ISND between 2015 and 2020 of people aged at least 13 years who met the following inclusion criteria: being followed up at the SCS of the municipality with the last medical consultation less than 12 months before the start of data collection, residing in the municipality of the study, and having a diagnosis of HIV status up to 180 days from the date of notification. Individuals who died or were transferred to other services or municipalities were excluded.

In the intervention phase, the population consisted of 77 health professionals (nursing assistants, technicians, and nurses) who were working in the 38 public vaccine rooms of the municipality and the health professionals (nursing assistants, technicians, nurses, and doctors) of the five SCS. The professionals completed an online training course, with four modules and a total workload of 3 h, on issues related to PLHIV immunization.

The course was developed by the researcher, and before it was made available to the research subjects, it underwent a pilot evaluation by six professionals who tested its functionality.

2.3. Data Collection

In the pre-and post-intervention phases, data collection was performed on the REDCap platform using a form developed for this study. The form contained sociodemographic variables (sex, age, pregnancy, skin color, education, occupation, and health district of residence) and clinical-epidemiological variables (date and unit of notification, date of diagnosis of HIV infection, follow-up status, date of first and last medical consultation at the service, number of medical consultations, service that performs the follow-up, exposure category, social vulnerabilities, presence of other diseases, CD4 TL count, viral load quantification, use of ART, registered vaccines, and anti-HAV IgG and anti-HBs serology results), and was validated by four specialists and modified according to suggestions received.

Assessing the vaccination schedule is complex, as it requires verification of each vaccine received throughout life, and the schedules can be different if started before or after the diagnosis of HIV infection. In addition, it is necessary to assess susceptibility status in some cases in order to verify whether immunobiological agents are indicated. To ensure an accurate assessment of each individual's vaccination status, data were collected by a professional with over 20 years of experience in the field.

2.4. Data Analysis

In the pre-and post-intervention phases, data were extracted from the REDCap (https://redcap.eerp.usp.br/, accessed on 26 July 2022) platform using a Microsoft Office Excel v. 2406 spreadsheet. After evaluation and correction of possible typing errors, the data were transported to the IBM® Statistical Package for the Social Sciences (SPSS®) Statistics version 25 and R i386 v.3.4.0 programs where the database was structured [23]. Data analysis was performed using descriptive statistics (mean and standard deviation for continuous variables) and proportions for categorical variables.

The comparison between the pre-and post-intervention phases was evaluated using McNemar's test, with p-values < 0.05 considered statistically significant. A logistic regression model, using the Generalized Estimating Equations (GEE) method, was used to estimate the variables associated with an adequate vaccination schedule in the post-intervention phase, and the crude and adjusted odds ratio was calculated with 95% intervals for each variable and a significance level of 5%.

The outcome variable was the complete vaccination schedule according to the vaccination schedule recommended by the NIP (Table 1).

Table 1. Vaccines included in the evaluation of the complete vaccination schedule according to the recommendations of the National Immunization Program (NIP) at the time of the study.

Vaccine	Recommended Schedule †	Schedule Considered
Adult double (diphtheria/tetanus)	Three doses and boosters every 10 years	Complete or in progress without delays
Hepatitis B	Three doses (before diagnosis) Four doses with double dose (after diagnosis) (for susceptibles)	Complete or in progress without delay
Hepatitis A	Two doses (for susceptible)	Complete or in progress without delay
Viral triple (measles, mumps, rubella)	Two doses	Complete or in progress without delay
Yellow fever	Single dose from 5 years of age or two doses	Complete or in progress without delay
Pneumococcal 23-valent	Two doses	1 dose
Pneumococcal 13-valent	Single dose	1 dose
Meningococcal C	Two doses and booster every 5 years	Complete or in progress without delay
HPV	Three doses (men aged 9–26 and women aged 9–45) ‡	Complete or in progress without delay

† Source: [15]. ‡ The pre-intervention phase started on 1 August 2021, and the vaccination schedule indicated by the NIP until this date was considered in the evaluation, without incorporating subsequent updates.

2.5. Ethical Aspects

The research project was submitted to the Research Project Evaluation Committee (RPEC) of the Municipal Health Department of the studied municipality and later to the Research Ethics Committee (REC) of the Ribeirão Preto Nursing School (RPNS) of the University of São Paulo (USP), obtaining a favorable opinion (REC consolidated opinion No. 4.782.341).

3. Results

In the pre-intervention phase, the records of 1688 PLHIV were evaluated. After analyzing the inclusion and exclusion criteria, the sample consisted of 645 individuals in the pre- and post-intervention phases, most of whom were male (83.41%), white (59.84%), and with education above high school (55.97%). The mean age was 32.06 years (SD ± 11.14), with the minimum age being 14 years and the maximum 72 years. The age group with the highest frequency was 20–29 years (45.89%) (Table 2).

Table 2. Distribution of people living with HIV/AIDS according to sociodemographic variables.

Sociodemographic Variables	Participants	
	n	%
Sex		
Male	538	83.41
Female	107	16.59
Skin color		
White	386	59.84
Black	65	10.08
Yellow	3	0.47
Brown	169	26.20
Ignored	22	3.41
Level of education		
Illiterate or incomplete primary education	13	2.02
Complete primary school	69	10.70
Complete elementary school	97	15.04
Complete high school	278	43.10
Complete higher education	83	12.87
Ignored	105	16.28
Age group (years)		
13 to 19	39	6.05
20 to 29	296	45.89
30 to 39	173	26.82
40 to 49	74	11.47
50 to 59	45	6.98
60 or more	18	2.79

For diphtheria and tetanus, hepatitis B, and hepatitis A vaccines, although the number of adequately vaccinated increased in the post-intervention phase, the increase was not statistically significant. In the pre-intervention phase, 533 (82.64%) PLHIV were adequately vaccinated against diphtheria and tetanus, 445 (75.30% of those with vaccination indications) against hepatitis B, and 143 (42.43% of those with vaccination indications) against hepatitis A. They were adequately vaccinated in the post-intervention phase: 539 (83.57%) against diphtheria and tetanus, 453 (76.65% of those with vaccine indications) against hepatitis B, and 151 (44.81% of those with vaccine indications) against hepatitis A. Individuals who were not susceptible to the disease were not considered for assessment of adequately vaccinated against hepatitis A and B (Table 3, Figure 1).

Table 3. Registered vaccination schedules for people living with HIV/AIDS in the pre- and post-intervention phases.

Study Variables	Number of Participants with an Indication for the Vaccine		Pre-Intervention		Post-Intervention		*p*-Value
	n	%	Complete	Incomplete	Complete	Incomplete	
Adult double vaccine	645	100	533	112	539	106	0.480
Hepatitis B	590	91.47	445	145	453	137	0.341
Hepatitis A	335	51.94	142	193	150	185	0.118
13-valent pneumococcal	645	100	382	263	441	204	**<0.001**
23-valent pneumococcal	645	100	349	296	376	269	**0.040**
Meningococcal C	645	100	451	194	493	452	**<0.001**
HPV	234	36.28	134	100	147	87	**0.002**
MMR	635	98.45	243	392	252	383	**0.016**
Yellow Fever	640	99.22	529	111	539	101	**0.004**
Vaccination schedule	645	100	48	597	75	570	**<0.001**

Adult double vaccine (diphtheria and tetanus); HPV—human papillomavirus; MMR—measles/mumps/rubella. Bolded values are significant at 0.05 level.

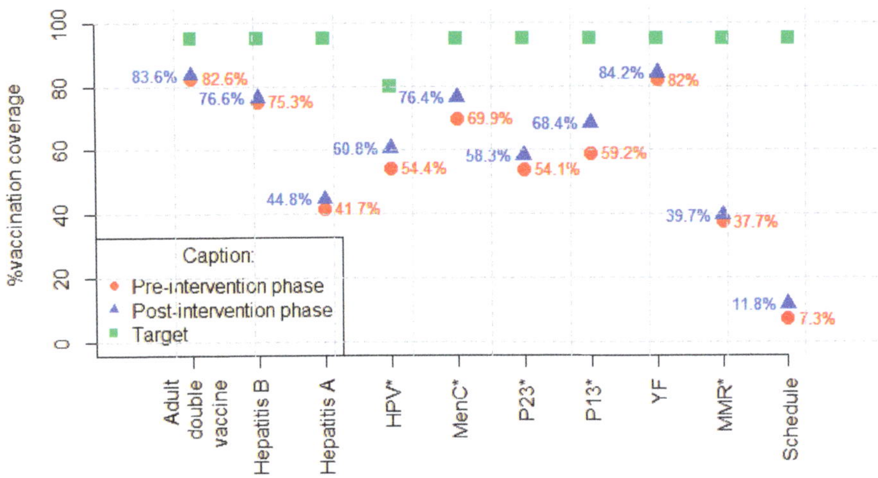

Figure 1. Vaccination coverage by vaccine and schedule were evaluated before and after the intervention. * $p < 0.005$; Adult double vaccine (diphtheria and tetanus); HPV—human papilloma virus; MenC—meningococcal C; P23—23-valent pneumococcal; P13—13-valent pneumococcal; YF—yellow fever; MMR—measles/mumps/rubella.

In the post-intervention evaluation where the information regarding the tests was updated, 471 (73.02%) individuals had reactive anti-HBs serology; however, for 32 (4.96%), there was no result of this test in the electronic medical record, despite being a recommended test for PLHIV. Regarding hepatitis A, 308 (47.75%) had reactive anti-HAV IgG and were, therefore, not susceptible to the disease without an indication for vaccination. For 112 (17.36%), there was no record of this test in the electronic medical record.

As for the 13-valent pneumococcal vaccine, in the post-intervention phase, 59 (22.43%) of the inadequately vaccinated became adequately vaccinated, and the coverage increased from 59.22% to 68.37%. For the 23-valent pneumococcal vaccine, the number of adequately vaccinated increased from 349 (54.11%) to 376 (58.29%). The number of adequately vaccinated with meningococcal C increased from 451 (69.92%) to 493 (76.43%). For the HPV vaccine, among those with an indication for vaccination according to the recommendation at the time of data collection, coverage increased from 57.02% to 62.55% (Table 3, Figure 1).

For attenuated vaccines, which are contraindicated in the presence of severe immunodepression, coverage of the measles/mumps/rubella vaccine (triple viral) increased from 38.27% to 39.69%, and for the yellow fever vaccine, coverage increased from 82.66% to 84.22% (Table 3, Figure 1). Individuals who had a last CD4 LT count of <200 cells/mm^3 were excluded from the analysis in the post-intervention phase because they had contraindications for these vaccines.

Regarding the entire vaccination schedule evaluated according to the study proposal, the number of adequately vaccinated increased from 47 (7.29%) to 76 (11.78%) (Table 3, Figure 1).

In the multivariate analysis of factors associated with vaccination rates, the model results indicate that as age increases, the chance of having a complete vaccination schedule decreases. Individuals aged between 30 and 39 years had a 74.00% lower chance (adjusted OR 0.26 95% CI 0.09–0.74) of having a complete vaccination schedule when compared to those aged between 10 and 19 years, and among those over 40 years, this rate was 87.00% lower (adjusted OR 0.13 95% CI 0.03–0.50) (Table 4).

Table 4. Multivariate analysis of factors associated with vaccination coverage of people living with HIV/AIDS.

Study Variables	Number of Participants		Crude OR (95% CI)	*p*-Value	Adjusted OR (95% CI)	*p*-Value
	n	%				
Sex						
Male	538	83.41	REF †		REF †	
Female	107	16.59	0.16 (0.05–0.55)	**0.004**	0.44 (0.12–1.55)	0.201
Skin color ‡						
White	386	59.84	REF †		REF †	
Black	65	10.08	0.36 (0.1–1.23)	0.103	0.47 (0.14–1.65)	0.241
Mixed race/Asian	172	26.67	0.99 (0.56–1.73)	0.963	1.03 (0.56–1.89)	0.927
Age group (years)						
13 to 19	39	6.05	REF †		REF †	
20 to 29	296	45.89	0.67 (0.31–1.45)	0.307	0.56 (0.23–1.34)	0.193
30 to 39	173	26.82	0.27 (0.11–0.69)	**0.006**	0.26 (0.09–0.74)	**0.011**
40 and over	137	21.24	0.1 (0.003–0.37)	**0.001**	0.13 (0.03–0.51)	**0.003**
Exposure category ‡						
Non-heterosexual	397	61.55	REF †		REF †	
Heterossexual	223	34.57	0.22 (0.1–0.47)	**0.001**	0.53 (0.23–1.22)	0.134

Table 4. *Cont.*

Study Variables	Number of Participants		Crude OR (95% CI)	*p*-Value	Adjusted OR (95% CI)	*p*-Value
	n	%				
Unit where follow-up is carried out						
Specialized Care Service 2 §	190	29.46	REF †		REF †	
Specialized Care Service 1 ‖	124	19.22	0.47 (0.2–1.08)	0.075	0.44(0.19–1.01)	0.052
Specialized Care Service 3 ‖	98	15.20	0.29 (0.11–0.82)	**0.019**	0.33 (0.12–0.91)	**0.033**
Specialized Care Service 4 ‖	109	16.90	1.12 (0.57–2.2)	0.746	1.24 (0.62–2.51)	0.542
Specialized Care Service 5 ¶	124	19.22	0.86 (0.43–1.73)	0.676	1.23 (0.58–2.59)	0.591
CD4 T-lymphocyte count (cells/mm3) ‡						
All > 350	115	17.83	REF †		REF †	
Some < 200	96	14.88	0.34 (0.14–0.78)	**0.011**	0.64 (0.27–1.49)	0.296
Some between 200 and 350 (none < 200)	433	67.13	0.71 (0.33–1.52)	0.373	0.86 (0.41–1.84)	0.704
Use of Antiretroviral Therapy ‡						
No	104	16.2	REF †		REF †	
Yes	539	83.2	7.64 (1.72–34.02)	**0.008**	5.17 (1.17–22.97)	**0.031**
Vaccine room where patients received the last dose of vaccine						
Other units	105	16.28	REF †		REF †	
Specialized Care Service	540	83.72	6.59 (1.92–22.68)	**0.003**	5.77 (1.65–20.19)	**0.006**
Social Vulnerability						
No	489	75.81	REF †		REF †	
Yes	156	24.19	2.3 (1.09–4.85)	**0.029**	2.3 (1.06–4.99)	**0.034**
Complete vaccination schedule						
Pre-intervention phase	47	7.29	REF †		REF †	
Post-intervention phase	76	11.78	1.62 (1.33–1.96)	**0.001**	1.72 (1.39–2.13)	**0.001**

† Reference group; ‡ Data such as "unknown", "examination not available", "no information" were not taken into account for statistical processing; § Specialized Care Service, which had a vaccine room; ‖ Specialized Care Services, which operated in the same facility of basic units with vaccine rooms; ¶ Specialized Care Service, which did not have a vaccine room in the facility. Bolded values are significant at 0.05 level.

Individuals who were followed up at SCS 3 had a 67.00% (adjusted OR 0.32, 95% CI 0.11–0.91) lower chance of being adequately vaccinated when compared to individuals who were followed up at SCS 2. Those with good adherence to ART were 5.17 times (95% CI 1.16–22.97) more likely to have a complete vaccination schedule when compared to individuals who did not have good adherence. Those who were vaccinated in SCS were 5.76 (95% CI 1.65–20.19) times more likely to be adequately vaccinated when compared to those who were vaccinated in other health services (Table 4).

Individuals with some social vulnerability were 2.3 times (95% CI 1.06–4.99) more likely to be adequately vaccinated when compared to those with no identified vulnerability. In the assessment performed after the intervention phase, individuals were 1.72 (95% CI 1.39–2.13) times more likely to have the complete vaccination schedule when compared to the pre-intervention phase. There was no association between the complete vaccination schedule and the variables sex, skin color, CD4 TL count, and exposure category (Table 4).

4. Discussion

In this study, a very small proportion of PLHIV had an appropriate vaccination schedule according to the proposed assessment, both pre- and post-intervention, which reinforces that there is no effective assessment of the vaccination situation in the services that accompany PLHIV [12]. After offering a training course for health professionals from vaccination rooms and health services that accompany PLHIV, there was an improvement in vaccination coverage, but it still remained low.

Studies that analyze predominantly inactivated vaccines in the evaluation of the vaccination schedule of PLHIV present a higher rate of adequately vaccinated individuals [9,12,19]. In a study that included yellow fever and measles-mumps-rubella vaccines among the vaccines evaluated, only 14.1% of PLHIV were adequately vaccinated, a coverage close to that found in the evaluation performed after this study's intervention phase [3].

Despite the risk of exposure to vaccine-preventable diseases, there is fear among both health professionals and PLHIV themselves regarding the safety of vaccine administration and the effectiveness of immunobiological agents in this population [2,24].

The vaccine with the best coverage was diphtheria and tetanus, as in other studies [5,9,12]. This vaccine has been part of the Brazilian immunization schedule for many years, is available in all vaccine rooms, and presents the same vaccination schedule for the entire population, with few contraindications, which perhaps provides teams with greater safety in administrating this immunobiological agent [12].

The hepatitis B vaccine is administered to people who have never been exposed to the virus or have received the vaccine. In our study, around 25% of the individuals eligible to receive the hepatitis B vaccine were not adequately vaccinated. Our findings are similar to the vaccination rates identified in some studies [3,9,15,20], while the number of people adequately immunized with the hepatitis B vaccine was lower in other reports [5,7,12,13,25]. In Brazil, the hepatitis B vaccine has been part of the national calendar since 1998; therefore, because this study population is mostly young, the rate of individuals without any dose of this vaccine was 2.48% in the post-intervention phase.

The increase in the rate of adequately vaccinated for diphtheria/tetanus and hepatitis B vaccines in the post-intervention phase of this study was small and not statistically significant, which can be explained by the fact that most individuals had already received the full course of these vaccines when they were diagnosed with HIV.

Among the inactive vaccines, the hepatitis A vaccine demonstrated the poorest coverage, even in the post-intervention phase, with an increase of only 3% in the number of individuals adequately vaccinated. Some studies have identified better vaccination rates against hepatitis A than our findings [7,9,20]. However, our coverage was higher than that reported in previous studies on PLHIV, in which vaccine hesitancy was identified as one of the factors for non-adherence to vaccination, in addition to low schooling and immunodepression [5,12,25].

Vaccine hesitancy is a complex and dynamic behavioral phenomenon that has been advancing worldwide. It is influenced by confidence in the safety and efficacy of vaccines, the low-risk perception of the population, and because the vaccine is often not available or affordable [26–28].

The vaccination coverage of the 13-valent pneumococcal vaccine was around 68% in the post-intervention phase, while that of the 23-valent was around 58%. Some studies identified higher coverage [9,13,20,29], while others identified lower coverage [3,12,15,25]. A study conducted in Germany revealed that 58.5% of the population had received both the 13-valent and 23-valent pneumococcal vaccines, while 11% had received only the 23-valent vaccine [1].

For the two pneumococcal vaccines indicated for PLHIV, there was a significant increase in the number of adequately vaccinated in the post-intervention phase, with 13-valent showing the greatest increase among the vaccines evaluated.

In an intervention carried out through the implementation of a hospital consultation to assess vaccination status in Spain, the coverage of the 13-valent pneumococcal vaccine increased from 2.9% to 88.0%, and the coverage of the 23-valent pneumococcal vaccine increased from 16.3% to 83.7% [18]. These data reinforce that actions aimed at increasing knowledge and, consequently, confidence in immunizers, targeting both health professionals and patients, have a positive impact on vaccination coverage.

Pneumococcal vaccines and hepatitis A vaccines are not available in vaccination rooms in the studied municipality and need to be requested by filling out a specific form addressed to the Special Immunobiological Agents Reference Center (SIARC). For some months during the study period, pneumococcal vaccines were available in vaccination rooms due to a temporary expansion of indications, which may have contributed to the increase in the number of adequately vaccinated.

The meningococcal C vaccine was the vaccine with a special indication that showed the best coverage in this study, with an increase of 6.51% of adequately vaccinated in the post-intervention phase. One of the factors that contributed to this rate is the fact that the immunobiological agent is available in vaccination rooms. Lower coverage of the meningococcal vaccine has been identified in other studies [9,12]. Vaccine hesitancy and the unavailability of the immunobiological agent in vaccination rooms contribute to low coverage [2,12,16,21,25,29].

Regarding the HPV vaccine, our study exhibited the most comprehensive coverage among the evaluated studies. Given the recent introduction of the vaccine in the medical landscape, vaccination coverage varies considerably across studies, contingent on the timeframe in which they were conducted. The importance of publicizing the necessity of this vaccine for PLHIV has been reinforced by researchers, given that the transmission route of HPV is the same as that of HIV. This publicizing is of particular significance to the population of men who have sex with men (MSM), given their elevated susceptibility to both acquiring the virus and developing persistent infections and malignant lesions [1,14,30–32].

On the other hand, the indication of different schemes for different age groups and constant changes in the vaccination scheme can be a factor that confuses teams and contributes to missed vaccination opportunities. Despite this, in the post-intervention phase, the number of adequately vaccinated showed an increase of about 6.00%, which reinforces that more trained teams regarding the indicated schemes favor the improvement in vaccination rates [6].

In order to assess the indication of attenuated vaccines for PLHIV, it is necessary to evaluate the value of the CD4 TL count since severely immunosuppressed individuals are temporarily contraindicated to receive these vaccines [4,14]. As this is a complex assessment and is not always possible, most studies assessing vaccination coverage do not include the evaluation of attenuated vaccines.

Studies have shown that a large number of PLHIV lack immunity against measles, mumps, and rubella and have reinforced the risk of immunity loss over the years [33–37].

In this study, the measles-mumps-rubella vaccine was the one with the worst coverage among the vaccines evaluated, with a small increase in adequately vaccinated individuals in the post-intervention phase despite the low number of individuals with contraindications. In another study conducted in Brazil, 83.8% of PLHIV had not received any dose of measles, mumps, or rubella vaccine [3]. It is important to ensure a complete vaccination schedule to correct possible vaccine failures and maintain seroconversion.

As the yellow fever vaccine has been part of the vaccination schedule of the studied municipality for many years, due to the fact that it is considered a risk area for the disease, this vaccine coverage was around 84% in the post-intervention phase. Most likely, most of these individuals were already adequately vaccinated before the diagnosis of HIV infection. In addition, the yellow fever vaccination schedule for PLHIV without severe immunodepression does not differ from the schedule indicated for the general population, which is not the case for measles, mumps, and rubella vaccines.

Some authors suggest that vaccination with PLHIV be delayed until the immune system is rebuilt, which would ensure a better response and lower the risk of events supposedly attributable to vaccination or immunization (ESAVI). Although the administration of some vaccines may generate a transient increase in viral load, these events do not present clinical significance, and their risk cannot prevent vaccination [4,9,11,12,15,19,28,38,39].

In this study, individuals with good adherence to ART had a greater chance of being adequately vaccinated, which may indicate better self-care and, in addition, greater confidence on the part of the team in indicating and administering vaccines in this population.

Even if the response to vaccination is reduced for individuals with uncontrolled viral replication or lower CD4 TL counts, it is recommended that the vaccination schedule be updated as soon as possible, taking into account contraindications to attenuated vaccines, without the need for intervals between vaccine administration and test collection [4,9,11,14,38]. A positive approach by the healthcare team in this regard would reduce the number of non-vaccinated [35].

Most of the individuals evaluated in this study were vaccinated in the SCS, which reinforces that having a vaccine room in the services where the individual performs the follow-up facilitates access and increases adherence, and the teams that work in the vaccine rooms of the SCS may be more prepared and safer to administer vaccines to PLHIV [12,15,21].

The assessment of vaccination status and guidance on immunization should be part of the medical consultation, with the prescription of vaccines included in the routine of care, and, in addition, be the practice of various health professionals who assist PLHIV in different services [2,3,6,7,12,13,21,24,40,41].

It is necessary to verify that the individuals referred for vaccination have actually carried out the procedure, and if they do not appear in the vaccination room or delay the completion of the vaccination schedule, it is extremely important to actively search for these individuals.

For PLHIV, the evolution of vaccine-preventable diseases may be more severe, and vaccine immunogenicity may be lower, with shorter protection time when compared to people not living with HIV. For this reason, active surveillance of vaccination status is important. In addition, managers need to know the reasons for non-vaccination and develop strategies to combat vaccine hesitancy and improve vaccination rates [6,16,42–48].

Some limitations should be considered when analyzing these findings, as this study evaluated secondary data through information systems. Without access to individuals, it was not possible to evaluate their vaccination records. Despite the guidance that all vaccination history should be recorded in the system, it is possible that for some individuals, the doses received in other municipalities have not been recorded. The importance of future studies that perform this evaluation with subjects is reinforced. Despite this limitation, this study makes an important contribution to understanding the low vaccination coverage in PLHIV.

5. Conclusions

In recent years, Brazil has experienced a drop in vaccination coverage, the causes of which are multifactorial. Intervening in the knowledge of health professionals regarding issues related to the vaccination of PLHIV has enabled an increase in vaccination coverage among this population, but coverage has still remained low.

This study's findings demonstrate the need to develop measures to improve vaccination rates in populations at a higher risk for vaccine-preventable diseases. Health professionals play a key role in identifying unvaccinated individuals. By recommending vaccination and combating false contraindications, they increase the likelihood that individuals will seek immunization services.

In order to achieve the desired vaccination coverage rates, in addition to the knowledge of health professionals, it is necessary to act on other factors, such as immunobiological agent availability in the services where PLHIV is monitored. It is also necessary for health managers to invest in addressing vaccine hesitancy.

Improvements in the completeness of vaccination schedules would be enhanced by the introduction of an immunization program in the place where clinical follow-up is carried out. This program could adopt an individualized approach, with doctors and nurses assessing vaccination status, providing advice on the vaccines indicated, prescribing the necessary vaccines, and administering them in the same facility.

Author Contributions: Conceptualization, L.G. and R.K.R.; methodology, L.G. and R.K.R.; formal analysis, L.G., E.G., L.A.d.S.N., L.M.R.P., R.d.Á.K., B.S. and R.K.R.; investigation, L.G.; resources, L.G.; data curation, L.G.; writing—original draft preparation L.G., E.G., L.A.d.S.N., L.M.R.P., R.d.Á.K., B.S. and R.K.R.; writing—review and editing, L.G., E.G., L.A.d.S.N., L.M.R.P., R.d.Á.K., B.S. and R.K.R. All authors have read and agreed to the published version of the manuscript.

Funding: This research received no external funding.

Institutional Review Board Statement: The study was conducted in accordance with the Declaration of Helsinki and approved by the Research Ethics Committee (REC) of Ribeirão Preto Nursing School (RPNS) of the USP (REC substantiated opinion no. 4.782.341 approved in 15 June 2021).

Informed Consent Statement: Patient consent was waived because data collection took place in information systems without direct contact with patients and was authorized by the Research Ethics Committee.

Data Availability Statement: Data from this study can be made available upon request.

Acknowledgments: We thank Miyeko Hayashida and Jonas Bodini Alonso for their advice on the statistical analysis.

Conflicts of Interest: The authors declare no conflicts of interest.

References

1. Breitschwerdt, S.; Schwarze-Zander, C.; Tayy, A.A.; Mutevelli, J.; Wasmuth, J.C.; Rockstroh, J.K.; Boesecke, C. Implementation of EACS vaccination recommendations among people living with HIV. *Infection* **2022**, *50*, 1491–1497. [CrossRef] [PubMed]
2. Harrison, N.; Poeppl, W.; Herkner, H.; Tillhof, K.D.; Grabmeier-Pfistershammer, K.; Rieger, A.; Forstner, C.; Burgmann, H.; Lagler, H. Predictors for and coverage of influenza vaccination among HIV-positive patients: A cross-sectional survey. *HIV Med.* **2017**, *18*, 500–506. [CrossRef] [PubMed]
3. Cunha, G.H.; Galvão, M.T.G.; Medeiros, C.M.; Rocha, R.P.; Lima, M.A.C.; Fechine, F.V. Vaccination status of people living with HIV/AIDS in outpatient care in Fortaleza, Ceará, Brazil. *Braz. J. Infect. Dis.* **2016**, *20*, 487–493. [CrossRef] [PubMed]
4. Imaz, A.; Masuet, C. Vaccination coverage for people living with HIV: A key intervention that should be improved. *Enfermedades Infecc. Y Microbiol. Clin.* **2023**, *41*, 141–143. [CrossRef]
5. Jilich, D.; Malý, M.; Fleischhans, L.; Kulířová, V.; Machala, L. Cross-sectional study on vaccination coverage in newly diagnosed HIV-infected persons in the Czech Republic. *Cent. Eur. J. Public Health* **2019**, *27*, 217–222. [CrossRef] [PubMed]
6. Kojic, E.M.; Rana, A.I.; Cu-Uvin, S. Human papillomavirus vaccination in HIV-infected women: Need for increased coverage. *Expert Rev. Vaccines* **2016**, *15*, 105–117. [CrossRef] [PubMed]
7. Valour, F.; Cotte, L.; Voirin, N.; Godinot, M.; Ader, F.; Ferry, T.; Vanhems, P.; Chidiac, C. Vaccination coverage against hepatitis A and B viruses, *Streptococcus pneumoniae*, seasonal flu, and A(H1N1)2009 pandemic influenza in HIV-infected patients. *Vaccine* **2014**, *32*, 4558–4564. [CrossRef] [PubMed]
8. Brasil Ministério da Saúde; Secretaria de Vigilância em Saúde; Departamento de Vigilância, Prevenção e Controle das Infecções Sexualmente Transmissíveis, do HIV/Aids e das Hepatites Virais. Protocolo Clínico e Diretrizes Terapêuticas para Manejo da Infecção pelo HIV em Adultos. Brazil. 2018. Available online: http://www.aids.gov.br/pt-br/pub/2013/protocolo-clinico-e-diretrizes-terapeuticas-para-manejo-da-infeccao-pelo-hiv-em-adultos (accessed on 4 September 2019).
9. Drewes, J.; Langer, P.C.; Ebert, J.; Kleiber, D.; Guys, B. Sociodemographic, HIV-Related Characteristics, and Health Care Factors as Predictors of Self-Reported Vaccination Coverage in a Nationwide Sample of People Aging with HIV in Germany. *Int. J. Environ. Res. Public Health* **2021**, *18*, 4901. [CrossRef] [PubMed]
10. Sociedade Brasileira de Imunizações/Sociedade Brasileira de Infectologia. HIV/AIDS—Guia de Imunização SBIm/SBI. Brazil. 2016. Available online: https://sbim.org.br/publicacoes/guias/567-guia-de-imunizacao-sbim-sbi-hiv-aids-2016-2017 (accessed on 8 July 2022).
11. Chaer, F.; Sahly, H.M. Vaccination in the adult patient infected with HIV: A review of vaccine efficacy and immunogenicity. *Am. J. Med.* **2019**, *132*, 437–446. [CrossRef]
12. Neto, L.F.S.P.; Vieira, J.V.; Ronchi, N.R. Vaccination coverage in a cohort of HIV—Infected patients receiving a care at an AIDS outpatient clinic in Espírito Santo, Brazil. *Braz. J. Infect. Dis.* **2017**, *21*, 515–519. [CrossRef]
13. Boey, L.; Bosmans, E.; Ferreira, L.B.; Heyvaert, N.; Nelen, M.; Smans, L.; Tuerlinckx, H.; Roelants, M.; Claes, K.; Derdelinckx, I.; et al. Vaccination coverage of recommended vaccines and determinants of vaccination in at-risk groups. *Hum. Vaccin. Immunother.* **2020**, *16*, 2136–2143. [CrossRef]
14. Brasil Ministério da Saúde; Secretaria de Vigilância em Saúde. Departamento de Imunização e Doenças Transmissíveis. Manual dos Centros de Referência para Imunobiológicos Especiais. Brazil. 2019. Available online: https://bvsms.saude.gov.br/bvs/publicacoes/manual_centros_imunobiologicos_especiais_5ed.pdf (accessed on 2 May 2018).
15. Ho, Y.L.; Enohata, T.; Lopes, M.H.; Santos, S.S. Vaccination in Brazilian HIV-Infected Adults: A Cross-Sectional Study. *AIDS Patient Care STDs* **2008**, *22*, 65–70. [CrossRef]

16. Crum-Cianflone, N.F.; Wallace, M.R. Vaccination in HIV-infected adults. *AIDS Patient Care STDS* **2014**, *28*, 397–410. [CrossRef] [PubMed]
17. Burns, C.M.; Banks, R.E.; Wilson, B.M.; Carter, R.R.; Jump, R.L.P.; Perez, F. A virtual clinic improves pneumococcal vaccination coverage among patients living with HIV at a Veterans Affairs Medical Center. *AIDS Care* **2018**, *30*, 146–149. [CrossRef]
18. Hernández-García, I.; Román-Calderón, F.; López-Mendoza, H.; Aibar-Remón, C.; Grupo de Trabajo en vacunas HCULB. Evaluación del impacto de una intervención para mejorar las coberturas de vacunación frente a neumococo en pacientes con VIH [Impact of an intervention to improve the vaccination coverage against *Streptococcus pneumoniae* in HIV patients]. *Rev. Esp. Salud Publica* **2019**, *93*, e201912114.
19. Johnson, T.M.; Klepser, D.G.; Bares, S.H.; Scarsi, K.K. Predictors of vaccination rates in people living with HIV followed at a specialty care clinic. *Hum. Vaccin. Immunother.* **2021**, *17*, 791–796. [CrossRef]
20. Tsachouridou, O.; Georgeou, A.; Naoum, S.; Vasdeki, D.; Papagianni, M.; Kotoreni, G.; Forozidou, E.; Tsoukra, P.; Gogou, C.; Chatzidimitriou, D.; et al. Factors associated with poor adherence to vaccination against hepatitis viruses, *Streptococcus pneumoniae* and seasonal influenza in HIV-infected adults. *Hum. Vaccin. Immunother.* **2019**, *15*, 295–304. [CrossRef]
21. Parmejani, P.D.S.S.; Picone, C.M.; Alves, A.P.P.D.S.; Sartori, A.M.C.; Ibrahim, K.Y. Facilitating access to pneumococcal vaccine for people living with HIV: An experience report. *Rev. Esc. Enferm. USP* **2023**, *56*, e20210563. [CrossRef]
22. Preto, R.; Secretaria Municipal da Saúde de Ribeirão Preto. Plano Municipal de Saúde de Ribeirão Preto 2022–2025. Ribeirão Preto, São Paulo, Brazil. 2021. Available online: https://www.ribeiraopreto.sp.gov.br/portal/pdf/saude171202306.pdf (accessed on 6 July 2022).
23. R Core Team. *R: A Language and Environment for Statistical Computing*; R Foundation for Statistical Computing: Vienna, Austria, 2022. Available online: http://www.R-project.org/ (accessed on 23 December 2022).
24. Gerin, L.; Antonini, M.; Santos, K.S.; Gir, E.; Reis, R.K. O conhecimento dos profissionais de saúde sobre vacinação de pessoas vivendo com HIV—Uma revisão integrativa. *Esc. Anna. Nery* **2022**, *26*, e20210210. [CrossRef]
25. Gagneux-Brunon, A.; Fresard, A.; Lucht, F.; Botelho-Nevers, E. Vaccine coverage in PLWH: Disparities and potential impact of vaccine hesitancy. *Hum. Vaccin. Immunother.* **2019**, *15*, 305–306. [CrossRef]
26. Brewer, N.T. What Works to Increase Vaccination Uptake. *Acad. Pediatr.* **2021**, *21*, S9–S16. [CrossRef] [PubMed]
27. Oduwole, E.O.; Pienaar, E.D.; Mahomed, H.; Wiysonge, C.S. Overview of Tools and Measures Investigating Vaccine Hesitancy in a Ten Year Period: A Scoping Review. *Vaccines* **2022**, *10*, 1198. [CrossRef] [PubMed]
28. Sato, A.P.S.S. What is the importance of vaccine hesitancy in the drop of vaccination coverage in Brazil? *Rev. Saúde Pública* **2018**, *52*, 96. [CrossRef] [PubMed]
29. Kopp, A.; Mangin, O.; Gantzer, L.; Lekens, B.; Simoneau, G.; Ravelomanantsoa, M.; Evans, J.; Bergmann, J.F.; Sellier, P. Pneumococcal vaccination coverage in France by general practitioners in adults with a high risk of pneumococcal disease. *Hum. Vaccin. Immunother.* **2021**, *17*, 162–169. [CrossRef] [PubMed]
30. McClung, N.; Burnett, J.; Wejnert, C.; Markowitz, L.E.; Meites, E.; Study Group NHBS. Human papillomavirus vaccination coverage among men who have sex with men-National HIV Behavioral Surveillance, United States, 2017. *Vaccine* **2020**, *38*, 7417–7421. [CrossRef] [PubMed]
31. Pimenta, P.C.; Bani, G.M.A.C.; Júlio, R.S. Cobertura Vacinal de HPV em Pessoas Vivendo com HIV/Aids. 2020. Trabalho de Conclusão de Curso (Biomedicina)—Centro Universitário do Sul de Minas, Varginha, Minas Gerais, Brazil. 2020. Available online: http://repositorio.unis.edu.br/bitstream/prefix/1438/1/poliana.pdf (accessed on 30 July 2022).
32. Santos, J.G.C.; Dias, J.M.G. Vacinação pública contra o papilomavírus humano no Brasil. *Rev. Med. Minas Gerais* **2018**, *28*, e-1982. [CrossRef]
33. Crum, N.F.; Ahmad, A. Immunity against measles in people with HIV: The need for more research and surveillance. *AIDS* **2022**, *36*, 1305–1306. [CrossRef] [PubMed]
34. Dauby, N.; Martin, C.; Hainaut, M.; Grammens, T.; Van den Wijngaert, S.; Delforge, M.; De Wilt, S. Prevalence and risk factors of measles seronegativity in a cohort of HIV-positive subjects: A retrospective study. *HIV Med.* **2018**, *19*, 426–429. [CrossRef]
35. Grabmeier-Pfistershammer, K.; Poeppl, W.; Herkner, H.; Touzeau-Roemer, V.; Huschka, E.; Rieger, A.; Burgmann, H. High need for MMR vaccination in HIV infected adults in Austria. *Vaccine* **2014**, *32*, 6020–6023. [CrossRef] [PubMed]
36. Lefebvre, M.; Secher, S.; Bouchez, S.; Vandamme, Y.M.; Fialaire, P.; Leautez, S.; Blanchi, S.; Michau, C.; Coste-Burel, M.; Brunet-Cartier, C.; et al. Measles seroprevalence in human immunodeficiency virus-infected adults born in the era of measles vaccination. *AIDS* **2022**, *36*, 1273–1278. [CrossRef]
37. Rearigh, L.; O'Neill, J.; Kubat, M.; Sayles, H.; Swindells, S.; Bares, S.H. Surprisingly Low Levels of Measles Immunity in Persons With HIV: A Seroprevalence Survey in a United States HIV Clinic. *Open Forum Infect. Dis.* **2020**, *7*, ofaa428. [CrossRef] [PubMed]
38. Frésard, A.; Gagneux-Brunon, A.; Lucht, F.; Botelho-Nevers, E.; Launay, O. Immunization of HIV-infected adult patients—French recommendations. *Hum. Vaccin. Immunother.* **2016**, *12*, 2729–2741. [CrossRef] [PubMed]
39. Sweileh, W.M. Bibliometric analysis of global scientific literature on vaccine hesitancy in peer-reviewed journals (1990–2019). *BMC Public Health* **2020**, *20*, 1252. [CrossRef] [PubMed]
40. Blackwell, C.W. Knowledge of Vaccination Needs of HIV-Infected Men Who Have Sex with Men in a National Sample of "Gay Friendly" Health care Providers. *Public Health Nurs.* **2016**, *33*, 403–411. [CrossRef] [PubMed]

41. Grace, D.; Gaspar, M.; Paquette, R.; Rosenes, R.; Burchell, A.N.; Grennan, T.; Salit, I.E. HIV-positive gay men's knowledge and perceptions of Human Papillomavirus (HPV) and HPV vaccination: A qualitative study. *PLoS ONE* **2018**, *13*, e0207953. [CrossRef] [PubMed]
42. Bertolini, D.V.; Costa, L.S.; Heijden, I.M.; Sato, H.K.; Marques, H.S. Immunogenicity of a meningococcal serogroup C conjugate vaccine in HIV-infected children, adolescents, and young adults. *Vaccine* **2012**, *30*, 5482–5486. [CrossRef] [PubMed]
43. Dubey, H.; Oster, P.; Fazeli, M.S.; Guedes, S.; Serafini, P.; Leung, L.; Amiche, A. Risk Factors for Contracting Invasive Meningococcal Disease and Related Mortality: A Systematic Literature Review and Meta-analysis. *Int. J. Infect. Dis.* **2022**, *119*, 1–9. [CrossRef] [PubMed]
44. Nichols, J.; Eppes, S. Meningococcal Vaccination: An Update on Meningococcal Vaccine Recommendations for the Primary Care Physician. *Dela J. Public Health* **2022**, *8*, 76–78. [CrossRef] [PubMed]
45. Nolte, F.; Pacchiotti, A.; Castellano, V.; Lamy, P.; Gentile, A. Reticencia a la vacunación: Abordaje de su complejidad. *Rev. Hosp. Niños B Aires* **2018**, *60*, 16–22. Available online: https://pesquisa.bvsalud.org/portal/resource/pt/biblio-1103478 (accessed on 15 January 2021).
46. Thornton, A.C.; Jose, S.; Bhagani, S.; Chadwick, D.; Dunn, D.; Gilson, R.; Main, J.; Nelson, M.; Rodger, A.; Taylor, C.; et al. Hepatitis B, hepatitis C, and mortality among HIV-positive individuals. *AIDS* **2017**, *31*, 2525–2532. [CrossRef]
47. Umutesi, J.; Simmons, B.; Makuza, J.D.; Dushimiyimana, D.; Mbituyumuremyi, A.; Uwimana, J.M.; Ford, N.; Mills, E.J.; Nsanzimana, S. Prevalence of hepatitis B and C infection in persons living with HIV enrolled in care in Rwanda. *BMC Infect. Dis.* **2017**, *17*, 315. [CrossRef] [PubMed]
48. Vargas, J.I.; Jensen, D.; Martínez, F.; Sarmiento, V.; Peirano, F.; Acuña, P.; Provoste, F.; Bustos, V.; Cornejo, F.; Fuster, A.; et al. Comparative Efficacy of a High-Dose vs Standard-Dose Hepatitis B Revaccination Schedule Among Patients WITH HIV: A Randomized Clinical Trial. *JAMA Netw. Open* **2021**, *4*, e2120929. [CrossRef] [PubMed]

vaccines

MDPI

Article

Measles Vaccination Coverage and Anti-Measles Herd Immunity Levels in the World and WHO Regions Worsened from 2019 to 2023

Pedro Plans-Rubió

College of Physicians of Barcelona, 08017 Barcelona, Spain; pedro.plans@yahoo.es

Abstract: Objectives: The objectives of this study were as follows: to determine mean percentages of measles vaccination coverage with zero, one and two doses of vaccine and anti-measles herd immunity levels in World Health Organization (WHO) regions in 2023; to assess variations in measles vaccination coverage and anti-measles herd immunity-related indicators from 2019 to 2023; and to assess whether zero-dose measles vaccination coverage indicators were on track to achieve the Immunization Agenda 2030 objective. Methods: Mean percentages of vaccination coverage with two, one and zero doses of measles vaccine in WHO regions in 2023 were calculated using data from the WHO/UNICEF global and regional immunization information system. Results: In 2023, the global mean two-dose measles vaccination coverage was 65.3%, and mean two-dose vaccination coverage was lower than 95% in all WHO regions; the mean prevalence of measles-protected individuals in the target vaccination population was 87.6%, and anti-measles herd immunity levels in the target vaccination population were sufficient to block the transmission of measles viruses with greater transmissibility ($R_o \geq 15$) only in the Western Pacific and European WHO regions. The global mean two-dose measles vaccination coverage decreased by 3.7% from 2019 to 2023. In 2023, the mean zero-dose measles coverage and number of zero-dose measles children were, respectively, 36.7% and 40.6% greater than the values required to be on track to achieve the 2030 objective. Conclusion: This study found that all measles-vaccination-coverage-related indicators worsened from 2019 to 2023, and the zero-dose measles vaccination coverage and number of zero-dose measles children in 2023 were not on track to achieve the AI2030 objective. Interventions to increase routine two-dose measles vaccination coverage should be developed in all WHO regions.

Keywords: measles vaccination; measles elimination and eradication; WHO regions; two-dose measles coverage; MCV1; MCV2; measles zero-dose coverage; anti-measles herd immunity; measles prevention strategies

1. Introduction

In 2020, the 73rd World Health Assembly endorsed the Immunization Agenda 2030 (IA2030), envisioning "a world where everyone, everywhere, at every age, fully benefits from vaccines for good health and well-being" [1]. In 2011, the Global Vaccine Action Plan was proposed to eliminate measles in at least five WHO regions by 2020 [2]. The IA2030 agenda has committed to eliminating measles in at least five of the six WHO regions by 2030 [1,2].

Measles can be eliminated in all WHO regions and eradicated in the world because measles has only human reservoir, effective measles vaccines are available, and intensive epidemiological surveillance using highly sensitive and specific diagnostic tests can detect all new measles cases [3]. In fact, measles was eliminated in the Americas region in 2016 [4]. Unfortunately, measles re-emerged in Brazil and Venezuela in 2018, the Americas region lost its elimination status in 2019, and measles cases and outbreaks occurred in all WHO regions during the 2019−2023 period [4–8]. In the European region, a total of 9010 measles cases, 4259 hospitalizations and 2 deaths due to measles were reported by European countries to the WHO's centralized information system for infectious diseases (CISID) in 2023 [6–8]. Since 2019, measles elimination has not been verified in any WHO region [2,5].

The WHO considers that achieving and maintaining percentages of routine vaccination coverage of at least 95% with two doses of the measles-containing vaccine (MCV) is the key intervention to achieve measles elimination and eradication [9–12]. Routine measles vaccination includes two doses of measles–mumps–rubella (MMR) vaccine, which must be administered to all children aged 12–15 months and 3–15 years [9,12–15]. High percentages of routine measles vaccination can generate both individual measles protection and sufficient population herd immunity to block measles transmission in the community [9–12,16].

A study carried out in 2019 [10] found that only 14.4% of countries worldwide had a two-dose measles vaccination coverage $\geq$ 95%, and anti-measles herd immunity levels in the target vaccination population were not sufficient against measles viruses with basic reproduction numbers (R_o) $\geq$ 10 in the African and Eastern Mediterranean regions, measles viruses with $R_o \geq 11$ in the Western Pacific region and measles viruses with $R_o \geq 13$ in the Americas, European and South-East Asia regions [10].

The objectives of this study were as follows: (1) to determine the vaccination coverage for zero, one and two doses of measles vaccine and anti-measles herd immunity levels in countries and WHO regions in 2023; (2) to assess variations in measles vaccination coverage and anti-measles herd immunity-related indicators in WHO regions from 2019 to 2023; and (3) to assess whether zero-dose and measles vaccination coverage indicators were on track to achieve the Immunization Agenda 2030 objective.

2. Methods

2.1. Mean Vaccination Coverage with Zero, One and Two Doses of Measles Vaccine in the WHO Regions in 2023

The mean percentages of vaccination coverage for the first and second dose of measles-containing vaccine (MCV1, MCV2) were determined for different regions of the WHO using the information from the WHO/UNICEF global and regional immunization information system [17]. WHO considers six regions: African region, Americas region, Eastern Mediterranean region, European region, South-East Asia region and Western Pacific region (WPR) [2,17]. WHO and UNICEF estimate coverage with the first and second measles-containing vaccine (MCV1 and MCV2) doses delivered by routine immunization services for all countries using annual administrative estimates and vaccination coverage surveys [18]. Percentages of vaccination coverage for the MCV1 vaccine in different countries were estimated among children aged 1 year or among children aged 2 years, when the MCV1 was given to children aged $\geq$ 1 year [18]. Percentages of vaccination coverage for the MCV2 vaccine in different countries were estimated among children at the recommended age, according to national immunization schedules [18].

2.2. Anti-Measles Herd Immunity Levels in the Target Vaccination Population in the WHO Regions in 2023

Anti-measles herd immunity levels in the target vaccination populations were determined in different WHO regions in 2023 from the country-based mean vaccination coverage with one and two doses of measles vaccine, and the effectiveness for one and two doses of measles vaccine [10]. In this study, values of effectiveness in preventing measles cases of 92% and 95% were assumed for one and two doses of the measles vaccine [19].

Herd immunity against measles viruses with R_0 values of 10, 11, 12, 13, 14, 15, 16, 17, 18, 19 and 20 was considered established in the world and in different WHO regions when the mean prevalence of individuals with vaccine-induced measles protection was higher than 90%, 90.9%, 91.7%, 92.3%, 92.9%, 93.3%, 93.8%, 94.1%, 94.4%, 94.7% and 95%, respectively [10,11].

The percentage of countries in different WHO regions with sufficient herd immunity against measles viruses with R_0 values equal to or lower than 10, 12, 15, 18, 19 and 20 were assessed by counting the number of countries in each region with a prevalence of individuals with vaccine-induced measles protection in the target vaccination population higher than 90%, 91.7%, 93.3%, 94.4%, 94.7% and 95%, respectively [10,11].

2.3. Assessment of Whether Zero-Dose Measles Vaccination Indicators in 2023 Were on Track to Achieve the Immunization Agenda 2030 Objective

In this study, tracks required from 2019 to 2030 to achieve a 50% reduction by 2030 were determined for three zero-dose measles coverage indicators: (1) estimated number of children who did not receive the first dose of measles-containing vaccine (MCV1) [20]; (2) mean MCV1-based zero dose coverage; and (3) mean zero dose coverage determined from one and two doses of measles vaccine coverage [10].

Immunization Agenda 2030 proposes a 50% reduction in the number of zero-dose children observed in 2019 by 2030 [20]. For operational purposes, WHO/UNICEF defines zero-dose children for measles vaccination as those who lack the MCV1 vaccine [20]. The track required from 2019 to 2030 to achieve the AI2030 objective of number of zero-dose children was determined by considering the WHO/UNICEF estimated number of children who did not receive the MCV1 vaccine in 2019 (22.2 million) [20], and a 50% lower number (9.65 million) in 2030. To assess whether the number of zero-dose children was on track to achieve the 2030 goal, the estimated number of zero-dose children in 2023 was compared with the number required to be on track.

The track required from 2019 to 2030 for mean MCV1-based zero-dose measles coverage to achieve a 50% reduction by 2030 was determined by considering the mean MCV1-based zero-dose coverage (12.4%) observed in 2019 [10] and a 50% lower coverage (6.2%) in 2030. This analysis can be considered similar to the analysis based on the number of zero-dose measles children because WHO/UNICEF estimates the number of zero-dose children from 100−MCV1 coverage [4,20]. To assess whether the zero-dose measles coverage in 2023 was on track to achieve the 2030 goal, the coverage in 2023 was compared with the coverage required to be on track.

The track required to achieve a 50% reduction from 2019 to 2030 for zero-dose measles coverage (from two-dose and one-dose coverage) was determined by considering the mean zero-dose coverage obtained in 2019 (12.4%) [10] and a 50% lower level in 2030 (6.2%). To assess whether the mean zero-dose measles coverage in 2023 was on track to achieve the 2030 goal, the coverage in 2023 was compared with the mean two-dose coverage required to be on track.

2.4. Statistical Analysis

Microsoft Excel (Microsoft Corporation, Redmond, WA, USA) was used to calculate the following: (1) the mean percentage of vaccination coverage with the MCV1 and MCV2 vaccines in 2023 in different WHO regions; (2) the percentages of vaccination coverage with zero, one and two doses of measles vaccine in different countries of the world; (3) the mean percentages of vaccination coverage with zero, one and two doses of measles vaccine in regions of the WHO; (4) the prevalence of vaccine-induced measles protection in individuals in the target measles vaccination population in different countries of the world on 2023; and (5) the mean prevalence of vaccine-induced measles-protected individuals in the target measles vaccination population in regions of the WHO. Microsoft Excel (Microsoft Corporation, Redmond, WA, USA) was used to assess the establishment of herd immunity against measles viruses in countries of the world and regions of the WHO in 2023.

3. Results

3.1. Mean Percentages of Routine Measles Vaccination Coverage in Countries of the World and Regions of the WHO in 2023

In 2023, the worldwide mean vaccination coverage with the MCV1 and MCV2 measles vaccines were 85.2 and 77.1%, respectively (Table 1). The mean MCV1 vaccination coverage was lower than 95% in all WHO regions, except the Western Pacific region (97%) (Table 1). The mean MCV2 vaccination coverage was lower than 95% in all WHO regions, except the Western Pacific region (95.5%) (Table 1).

Table 1. Mean percentages of vaccination coverage for the MCV1 and MCV2 vaccines in 2023 and the MCV1 vaccine in 2021 in the world and WHO regions.

	MCV1 Vaccine 2023	MCV2 Vaccine 2023	MCV1 Vaccine 2021	*n*
	%	%	%	
World	85.2	77.1	83.3	195
African region (AFR)	71.5	62.0	65.0	47
Americas region (AMR)	93.0	83.0	87.5	35
Eastern Mediterranean region (EMR)	91.5	86.5	80.0	22
European region (EUR)	90.5	92.5	93.0	53
South-East Asia region (SEAR)	62.5	54.5	98.0	11
Western Pacific region (WPR)	97.0	95.5	97.5	27

n: number of countries with vaccine in national routine vaccination programs; MCV1: first dose of measles-containing vaccine; MCV2: second dose of measles-containing vaccine.

3.2. Mean Percentages of Vaccination Coverage with Zero, One and Two Doses of Measles Vaccines in the World and Regions of the WHO in 2023

The worldwide mean percentages of vaccination coverage for zero, one and two doses of measles vaccine were 65.3%, 27.8% and 6.9%, respectively (Table 2). The global mean two-dose measles vaccination coverage found in this study (65.3%) was 31% lower than the 95% objective proposed by the WHO.

The highest mean two-dose measles vaccination coverage was found in the Western Pacific region (93.2%) and the lowest one in the African region (48.1%) (Table 2). The highest mean one-dose measles vaccination coverage was found in the South-East Asia region (46.5%) and the lowest one in the Western Pacific region (6.7%) (Table 2). The highest mean zero-dose measles vaccination coverage was found in the African region (21.1%), while mean percentages of zero-dose coverage lower than 1% were found in the Western Pacific, South-East Asia and European regions (Table 2).

The two-dose measles vaccination coverage was ≥95% in only 17 (8.7%) countries of the world, and it was ≥ 90% in 41 (21%) countries (Table 2).

In the African region, 0% of the countries had a two-dose measles vaccination coverage higher than or equal to 90%, while in the Eastern Mediterranean region, 22.7% and 40.9% of the countries had a two-dose measles vaccination coverage higher than or equal to 95% and 90%, respectively (Table 2).

Table 2. Mean vaccination coverage with zero, one and two doses of measles vaccines, mean prevalence of individuals in the target vaccination population with vaccine-induced measles protection, percentage of countries with anti-measles herd immunity established in the target population vaccination, and percentage of countries with other measles vaccination indicators in regions of the WHO in 2023.

	World	African Region	Americas Region	Eastern Mediterranean Region	European Region	South-East Asia Region	Western Pacific Region
No. of countries	195	47	35	22	53	11	27
Routine measles vaccination-related indicators							
Mean vaccination coverage (%) with two, one and zero doses of measles vaccine							
2 doses	65.3	48.1	72.5	69.1	86.0	53.0	93.2
1 dose	27.8	30.7	25.5	28.2	13.5	46.5	6.7
0 doses	6.9	21.1	2.0	2.6	0.5	0.5	0.2
Percentage of countries with two-dose measles vaccination coverage $\geq$ 95% and $\geq$90%							
$\geq$95%	8.7	0	2.9	22.7	9.4	18.2	14.8
$\geq$90%	21.0	0	8.6	40.9	30.2	36.4	33.3
Percentage of countries where all children had received one or two doses of measles vaccine (0% of zero-dose children)							
	9.7	0	5.7	22.7	9.4	18.2	18.5
Anti-measles herd immunity-related indicators							
Mean prevalence (%) of individuals in the target vaccination population with vaccine-induced measles immunity							
Measles immunity	87.6	74.0	92.3	91.6	94.1	93.1	94.6
Percentage of countries with herd immunity against measles viruses with R_o from 10 to $\geq$20							
$R_o \leq 10$	66.1	40.4	62.9	68.2	92.4	72.7	59.3
$R_o \leq 12$	59.0	27.6	54.3	59.1	88.7	63.6	59.3
$R_o \leq 15$	41.5	10.6	25.7	50.0	66.0	63.6	51.8
$R_o \leq 18$	23.1	0	8.6	45.4	35.8	36.4	33.3
$R_o \leq 19$	0	0	5.7	31.8	13.2	27.3	22.2
$R_o \geq 20$	0	0	0	0	0	0	0

3.3. Anti-Measles Herd Immunity Levels in Countries of the World and Regions of the WHO in 2023

The worldwide mean prevalence of vaccine-induced measles protection found in this study was 87.6% (Table 2). Worldwide measles protection levels were not sufficient to block the transmission of measles viruses with R_o values equal to or greater than 10, as herd immunity against these viruses can be established with a 90% prevalence (Table 2).

The mean (per country) prevalence of measles protection ranged from 74% in African region to 94.1 in the European region and 94.6% in the Western Pacific region (Table 2). Based on the regional mean prevalence of vaccine-induced measles protection, anti-measles herd immunity levels (target vaccination population) were sufficient to block the transmission of measles viruses with greater transmissibility ($R_o \geq 15$) only in the Western Pacific and European WHO regions (Table 2). Anti-measles herd immunity was established against measles viruses with $R_o \leq 18$ (94.4% required) in the Western Pacific region; against viruses with $R_o \leq 16$ (93.8% required) in the European region; against viruses with $R_o \leq 14$ (92.9% required) in the South-East Asia region; against viruses with $R_o \leq 12$ (91.7% required) in the Americas region; and against viruses with $R_o \leq 11$ (90.9% required in the Eastern Mediterranean region (Table 2). Anti-measles herd immunity was not established against measles viruses with $R_o \geq 19$ in any WHO region because the mean prevalence of vaccine-induced immune protection was lower than 94.7% in all regions (Table 2). In the African region, anti-measles herd immunity was not established against viruses with $R_o \geq 10$ because its mean prevalence of vaccine-induced immune protection as lower than 90% (Table 2).

The percentage of countries with sufficient herd immunity against measles viruses with R_o values equal to or lower than 15 was 41.5%, while 23.1% of the countries had sufficient herd immunity against measles viruses with R_o values equal to or lower than 18 (Table 2).

The Eastern Mediterranean, Europe, South-East Asia and Western Pacific regions had the best country-based anti-measles herd immunity profiles, while the African region had the worst profile (Table 2).

3.4. *Variation for Routine Measles Vaccination-Related Indicators in Countries of the World and Regions of the WHO from 2019 to 2023*

The study found that five measles vaccination coverage-related indicators worsened and one indicator improved from 2019 to 2023 (Table 3).

Table 3. Variation for measles vaccination and anti-measles herd immunity indicators in different regions of the WHO between 2019 and 2023.

	World	African Region	Americas Region	Eastern Mediterranean Region	European Region	South-East Asia Region	Western Pacific Region
No. of countries	195	47	35	22	53	11	27
Routine measles vaccination-related indicators							
Mean vaccination coverage (%) with two. one and zero doses of measles vaccine							
2 doses	−3.7	24.0	−1.0	−3.2	2.5	−35.0	30.9
1 dose	7.8	−30.7	5.8	27.6	−11.2	171.9	−71.0
0 doses	7.8	24.9	−25.9	−60.0	−44.4	−64.3	−96.5
Percentage of countries with two-dose measles vaccination coverage ≥ 95% and ≥90%							
≥95%	−39.6	−100.0	−79.7	−4.6	−37.7	−33.3	−33.3
≥90%	−18.6	−100.0	−62.4	7.3	−15.6	0.0	−10.0
Percentage of countries where all children had received one or two doses of measles vaccine (0% of zero-dose children)							
	−24.8	−100.0	−60.1	−20.6	0.0	−33.3	0.0
Anti-measles herd immunity-related indicators							
Mean prevalence (%) of individuals in the target vaccination population with vaccine-induced measles immunity							
Measles immunity	−0.6	−4.6	0.5	3.9	0.4	−0.1	6.5
Percentage of countries with herd immunity against measles viruses with R_o from 10 to ≥20							
$R_o \leq 10$	−6.4	0.0	−15.3	2.2	−2.0	−11.1	−15.8
$R_o \leq 12$	−7.7	−7.4	−17.4	−4.5	−2.1	−12.5	−11.1
$R_o \leq 15$	−19.4	−28.9	−43.8	−4.6	−18.6	16.7	−17.8
$R_o \leq 18$	−28.9	−100.0	−62.4	19.2	−13.7	−33.2	−18.2
$R_o \leq 19$	−100.0	−100.0	−66.7	11.2	−22.4	0.0	0.0
$R_o \geq 20$	0.0	0.0	0.0	0.0	0.0	0.0	0.0

The mean global two-dose measles vaccination coverage decreased by 3.7% and the mean global zero-dose measles vaccination coverage increased by 7.8% from 2019 to 2023

(Table 3). The mean global one-dose vaccination coverage improved by 7.8% from 2019 to 2023 (Table 3).

The percentage of countries with two-dose measles vaccination coverage ≥ 95% and ≥90% decreased by 39.6% and 18.6%, respectively, from 2019 to 2023 (Table 3). The percentage of countries where all children had received at least one dose of measles vaccine (without zero-dose children) decreased by 24.8% from 2019 to 2023 (Table 3).

The global mean two-dose measles vaccination coverage decreased from 2019 to 2023 in the South-East Asia, Eastern Mediterranean and Americas regions, while it improved in the other regions (Table 3). The variation for this indicator ranged from −35% in the South-East Asia region to 30.9% in the Western Pacific region (Table 3).

The mean zero-dose measles vaccination coverage decreased from 2019 to 2023 in all WHO regions except in the African region (Table 3). The variation for this indicator ranged from −96.5% in the Western Pacific region to 24.9% in the African region (Table 3).

The percentage of countries with two-dose measles vaccination coverage ≥ 95% decreased between 2019 and 2023 in all WHO regions (Table 3). The variation for this indicator ranged from −4.6% in the Eastern Mediterranean region to −100% in the African region (Table 3).

The percentage of countries with two-dose measles vaccination coverage ≥ 90% decreased between 2019 and 2023 in all WHO regions, except in the Eastern Mediterranean and South-East Asia regions (Table 3). The variation for this indicator between 2019 and 2023 ranged from 7.3% in the Eastern Mediterranean region to −100% in the African region (Table 3).

The percentage of countries without zero-dose measles vaccination children because all children had received one or two doses of measles vaccine decreased from 2019 to 2023 in all WHO regions, except in the European and Western Pacific regions (Table 3). The variation for this indicator between 2019 and 2023 ranged from 0% in the European and Western Pacific regions to −100% in the African region (Table 3).

3.5. Variation for Anti-Measles Herd Immunity-Related Indicators in Countries of the World and Regions of the WHO from 2019 to 2023

The study found that all anti-measles herd immunity-related indicators assessed in this study worsened in the world from 2019 and 2023 (Table 3). The mean prevalence of individuals with vaccine-induced measles immunity decreased by 0.6%, and the percentage of countries with herd immunity against measles viruses with R_o values ≤ 19 decreased by 100% from 2019 to 2023 (Table 3).

The mean prevalence of individuals in the target vaccination population with vaccine-induced measles immunity increased in the Western Pacific, Eastern Mediterranean, European and Americas regions, while it decreased in the Africa and South-East Asia regions between 2019 and 2023 (Table 3). The variation for this indicator between 2019 and 2023 ranged from 6.5% in the Western Mediterranean region to −4.6% in the African region (Table 3).

3.6. Assessment of Whether Zero-Dose Measles Vaccination Indicators in 2023 Were on Track to Achieve the IA2030 Objective Reduction by 2030

In 2023, the three indicators of zero-dose measles coverage assessed in this study were not on track to achieve a 50% reduction in their 2019 values by 2030. The number of zero-dose measles children estimated by the WHO/UNICEF, the mean MCV1-based zero-dose coverage and the two-dose measles coverage were 40.6%, 46,5% and 36.7% greater than the values required to be on track to achieve the 2030 objective (Figures 1 and 2).

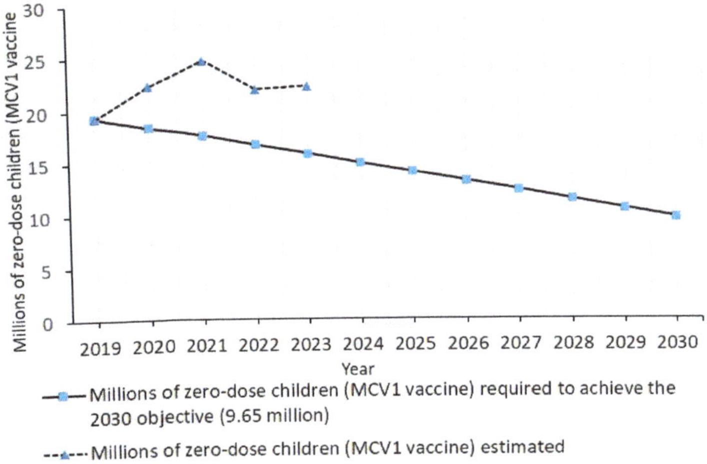

Figure 1. Number of zero-dose measles children (did not receive the MCV1 vaccine) estimated from 2019 and 2023, and number of zero-dose children required from 2019 to 2030 to achieve the IA 2030 objective (9.65 million).

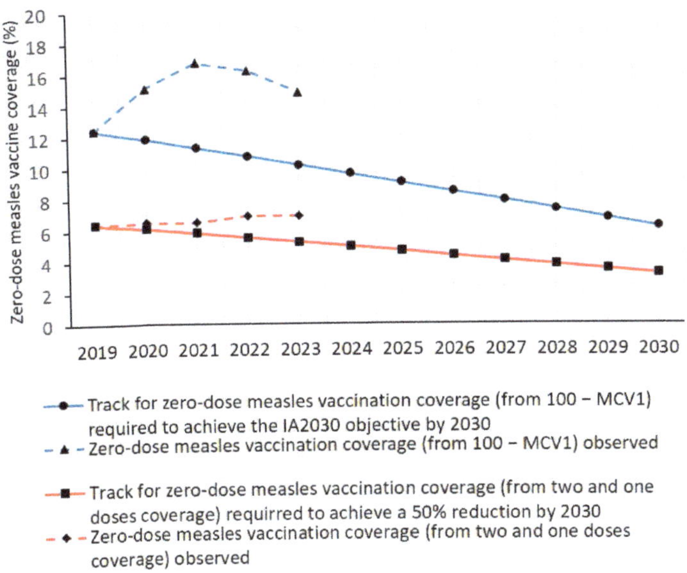

Figure 2. Track to achieve a 50% reduction from 2019 to 2030 for mean MCV1-based zero-dose measles vaccination coverage, and MCV1-based zero-dose coverage observed from 2019 to 2023. Track to achieve a 50% reduction from 2019 to 2030 for mean zero-dose measles vaccination coverage determined from two and one doses of measles vaccination, and zero-dose coverage observed in this study for 2023.

The number of zero-dose measles children estimated by WHO/UNICEF in 2023 (22.2 million) [20] was not on track to achieve the 2030 objective of 9.65 million (Figure 1). To be on track, the number of zero-dose measles children should be reduced by 877,273 per year from 2019 to 2030 (Figure 1). The number of zero-dose measles children estimated in 2023 was 40.6% greater than the number required (15.8 million) to be on track. The number of zero-dose measles children estimated by WHO/UNICEF for 2020 (22.3 million), 2021

(24.7 million) and 2022 (21.9 million) [4,20,21] were also out of track to achieve the IA2030 objective (Figure 1).

In 2023, the mean zero-dose measles vaccination coverage determined from the mean MCV1 coverage (14.8%) was not on track to achieve the 2030 objective of 6.2% (Figure 2). To be on track, the MCV1-based zero-dose coverage should be reduced by 0.56% per year from 2019 to 2030. In 2023, the mean MCV1-based zero-dose coverage was 46.5% greater than the coverage required (10.1%) to be on track to achieve the 2030 objective (Figure 2). The mean MCV1-based zero-dose coverage in 2020, 2021 and 2022 were also off track (Figure 2).

In 2023, the mean zero-dose measles vaccination coverage determined from the coverage for two and one doses of measles vaccine (6.9%) was not on track to achieve the 2030 objective of 3.2% (Figure 2). To be on track, the zero-dose coverage should be reduced by 0.29% per year from 2019 to 2030. In 2023, the mean zero-dose coverage was 36.7% greater than the coverage required (5.2%) to be on track to achieve 2030 (Figure 2). The mean zero-dose coverages in 2020, 2021 and 2022 were also off track (Figure 2).

4. Discussion

This study found four key results for 2023: (1) The global means for two-dose, one-dose and zero-dose measles vaccination coverage were 65.3%, 27.8% and 6.9%, respectively. (2) Mean percentages of two-dose measles vaccination coverage were lower than ≥95% in all WHO regions. (3) The mean prevalence of measles-protected individuals in the target vaccination population was 87.6%. (4) Anti-measles herd immunity levels in the target vaccination population was sufficient to block the transmission of measles viruses with greater transmissibility ($R_o \geq 15$) only in the Western Pacific and European WHO regions.

In addition, this study found that measles vaccination coverage and anti-measles herd immunity-related indicators worsened from 2019 to 2023. The mean measles vaccination coverage increased by 7.8%. The percentage of countries with two-dose measles vaccination coverage ≥ 95% decreased by 39.6%. The mean prevalence of measles-protected individuals in the target vaccination population decreased by 0.6%. The mean MCV1 coverage and the number of zero-dose measles vaccine children in 2023 were not on track to achieve the AI2030 objective of zero-dose measles vaccination coverage.

The global mean zero-dose measles vaccination coverage found in this study in 2023 was 6.9%, and it increased by 7.8% from 2019 to 2023. The worldwide mean zero-dose measles coverage found in 2023 can be explained by the high mean zero-dose coverage in countries in the African region (21.1%), which contrasted with the <3% mean zero-dose coverage in the other WHO regions. The 7.8% increase in this indicator between 2019 and 2023 can be explained by the 24.9% increase in the African region. In fact, the mean zero-dose measles coverage improved in all WHO regions from 2019 to 2023, except in the African region.

In addition, the study found that the percentage of countries without zero-dose measles children because all children had received at least one dose of measles vaccine was only 9.7%. However, the variation for this indicator from 0% in the African region to 22% in the Eastern Mediterranean region shows that reducing the zero-dose measles vaccine children must be a priority in all countries and WHO regions.

Measles meets the criteria for disease eradication, but the results found in this study for 2023 showed that routine measles vaccination programs had not recovered from COVID-19 pandemic disruptions, and progress toward measles elimination in most countries and in all WHO regions had slowed. A similar result was found by WHO/UNICEF [20], and inadequate progress toward measles eradication was found in prior evaluations carried out in 2016 [22], 2019 [10], 2021 [21] and 2022 [4]. The midterm evaluation of the Global Measles Strategic Plan 2012–2020 carried out in 2016 [22] considered that progress toward measles eradication was inadequate in 2016 due to a lack of political will as well as country ownership, reflected in insufficient resources.

The IA2030 agenda has committed to eliminating measles in at least five of the six WHO regions by 2030, and one of the key IA2030 objectives is to reduce the number of children who have not received at least one measles vaccine (zero-dose measles children) by 50% from 2019 to 2030 [1,20]. However, this study found that the three indicators of zero-dose measles coverage assessed were not on track for achieving a 50% reduction from 2019 to 2030. In 2023, the number of zero-dose measles children estimated by the WHO/UNICEF and the mean MCV1-based zero-dose coverage and the two-dose measles coverage were 40.6%, 46.5% and 36.7% greater than their values required to be on track to achieve the 2030 objective.

The priority prevention strategy to eliminate measles in different WHO regions is to achieve and maintain percentages of two-dose measles vaccination coverage equal to or greater than 95% for three reasons. Firstly, achieving and maintaining a routine measles vaccination coverage $\geq$ 95% can generate sufficient population immunity to establish anti-measles herd immunity in the community [10,11,23]. Secondly, it is a critical strategy in the path toward measles elimination because it can be achieved only in countries with strong measles vaccination programs and strong primary healthcare services [20,24]. Thirdly, the strategy to increase measles vaccination coverage with SIAs has limitations that make it insufficient for achieving and maintaining measles elimination [10,11,25].

In each country and WHO region, a routine measles vaccination coverage with two doses of measles vaccine coverage of at least 95% should be achieved in every birth cohort and in different areas and communities to ensure sufficient population immunity to establish anti-measles herd immunity against measles viruses [1–3,10,11,25]. Based on the results of this study, three measles prevention strategies should be developed depending on the two-dose routine measles vaccination coverage and anti-measles vaccine-induced herd immunity levels achieved in 2023. In the European and Western Pacific regions, the main objective should be to increase their mean two-dose measles vaccination coverage from 86–93% to $\geq$95% to avoid cases and outbreaks generated by viruses imported from endemic countries.

In the Eastern Mediterranean, Americas and South-East Asia regions, the main objective should be to increase their 53–72% mean two-dose measles vaccination coverage to $\geq$95% and to increase anti-measles herd immunity levels to block transmission of measles viruses with greater transmissibility.

In the African region, great efforts and international support are necessary to increase the two-dose measles vaccination coverage in the African region from 48% to $\geq$95%, reduce the number of zero-dose measles vaccine children and increase anti-measles herd immunity levels. This study found that insufficient global mean levels for measles vaccination-related and anti-measles herd immunity-related indicators depended greatly on the situation in the African region. Therefore, the global measles eradication objective depends greatly on improving the measles situation in the African region.

The following interventions can be used to increase routine two-dose measles vaccination coverage to $\geq$95% and to increase anti-measles herd immunity levels in all countries and WHO regions: (1) implement advanced vaccination programs [26,27]; (2) increase routine two-dose measles vaccination coverage from 95% to 97% [11]; (3) develop measles screening and vaccination programs to reach susceptible individuals and populations with low measles immunity levels [10,11,25,28,29]; (4) develop supplementary vaccination activities [20,30,31]; (5) implement interventions to increase measles vaccination access and vaccine provision [32]; (6) implement interventions to reduce measles vaccination hesitancy [33–36]; (7) implement interventions to increase healthcare provider engagement [37]; and (8) implement compulsory measles vaccination [38,39].

Screening and vaccination programs can be developed to reach susceptible individuals and populations with low levels of measles protection. This strategy can achieve and maintain herd immunity levels against measles viruses with greater transmissibility by (i) immunizing all susceptible individuals in the population or (2) immunizing susceptible individuals in areas and population groups with low measles protection levels [10,11,25,28,40]. However, seroprevalence studies in representative samples of the population must be developed to detect the areas and population groups with insufficient measles protection levels [25].

Supplementary immunization activities (SIAs) can be developed to reach populations and areas with low percentages of vaccination coverage. SIAs based on catch-up and follow-up vaccination campaigns are currently implemented in countries with inadequate first and/or second measles vaccine dose coverage [20]. In 2022, 115 million people received measles vaccines through SIAs in 44 countries [4]. Catch-up SIAs include children aged 9 months−14 years and follow-up SIAs include children aged 9−59 months. SIAs are implemented to provide a second vaccination opportunity to an entire cohort with low measles vaccination coverage, and to protect children who are susceptible to measles due to primary MCV1 failure [2,20]. However, the strategy to increase measles vaccination coverage with SIAs has important economic and logistic limitations that make it insufficient for achieving and maintain measles elimination, such as their inability to detect and vaccinate all susceptible children [10,11,25]. A recent study [41] assessing the quality and results achieved with SIAs implemented since 2020 found a mean SIA coverage among previously measles-zero-dose children was 58.3%, although only 23% of the 66 countries with a national-level SIA had a post-campaign coverage survey report available, and 50% of the reports included the coverage achieved among previously measles-zero-dose children [41]. The analysis of a high-quality anonymized database from an SIA carried out in Somalia in 2022 found that 94.6% of the children included in SIAs had been previously vaccinated with either one or 2+ measles doses, 5.4% of the children had received previously zero doses of measles vaccine, and the SIA coverage was 92% among previously vaccinated children and only 37.2% among zero-dose children [41].

Parental attitudes and beliefs toward measles vaccination are of great importance in influencing measles vaccination [42,43]. Parental hesitancy to vaccinate their children can be attributed to concerns about vaccine efficacy and safety, measles susceptibility, measles severity, vaccine accessibility and mistrust in experts [33–35]. Health education activities and national vaccination information campaigns can be developed to fight against measles vaccination hesitancy to reduce misinformation about measles vaccine efficacy and safety and to improve trust in vaccines, health providers and vaccination programs. In the United States of America, National Immunization Awareness Month is an annual observance held in August to highlight the importance of vaccination for people of all ages [36]. These interventions can help raise awareness about the importance of vaccination and encourage people to talk to a healthcare provider they trust about staying up to date on their vaccinations.

Delaying measles elimination in countries and WHO regions makes it more difficult to achieve and maintain measles elimination and eradication in the world [44]. The widening measles vaccination coverage and measles immunity gaps among countries and WHO regions found in this study for the 2019−2023 period shows that the risk of measles outbreaks has increased in all countries and the probability of re-establishing measles transmission in countries where measles had been eliminated is now greater than in 2019.

This study has several limitations. Firstly, the analysis carried out in this study used the information on routine vaccination of the WHO/UNICEF global and regional immunization systems. However, the information reported by the WHO/UNICEF global and regional immunization systems is validated periodically by the World Health Organization [17,18,45]. Secondly, herd immunity levels against measles viruses in different WHO regions were assessed by comparing the mean prevalence of individuals with vaccine-induced measles protection and the critical prevalence blocking the transmission of measles viruses in the population. Measles protection levels would be greater assuming greater levels for measles vaccination effectiveness. However, values of measles vaccination effectiveness of 95% and 92% for two and one doses of measles vaccines, respectively, have been found in studies assessing measles vaccination effectiveness [19]. Thirdly, anti-measles herd immunity levels in different WHO regions were assessed against measles viruses with R_0 values from 10 to 20. However, this range of R_0 values has been obtained in studies assessing the transmissibility of measles viruses [10,46].

5. Conclusions

The study found that worldwide percentages of two-dose measles vaccination coverage were lower than ≥95% and anti-measles herd immunity levels in the target vaccination population were sufficient to block the transmission of measles viruses with greater transmissibility (Ro ≥ 15) only in the Western Pacific and European WHO regions. All measles vaccination coverage-related and anti-measles herd immunity-related indicators worsened from 2019 to 2023. The zero-dose measles coverage and number of zero-dose measles children found in 2023 were not on track to achieve the AI2030 objective. Interventions to increase routine two-dose measles vaccination coverage should be developed in all WHO regions to meet the goal of eradicating measles worldwide.

Funding: This research received no external funding.

Institutional Review Board Statement: The study did not require ethical approval.

Informed Consent Statement: Not applicable.

Data Availability Statement: The original contributions presented in this study are included in the article. Further inquiries can be directed to the corresponding author.

Acknowledgments: Mean percentages of measles routine vaccination coverage in regions of the WHO were calculated using the information of the WHO on "WHO/UNICEF estimates of routine vaccines": https://www.who.int/news-room/questions-and-answers/item/who-unicef-estimates-of-national-immunization-coverage.

Conflicts of Interest: The author declares no conflicts of interest.

References

1. World Health Organization (WHO). *Global Vaccine Action Plan*; WHO: Geneve, Switzerland, 2020. Available online: https://www.who.int/publications/i/item/global-vaccine-action-plan-2011-2020 (accessed on 15 October 2024).
2. WHO/UNICEF. Immunization Agenda 2030. A Global Strategy to Leave No One Behind. Available online: https://cdn.who.int/media/docs/default-source/immunization/strategy/ia2030/ia2030-draft-4-wha_b8850379-1fce-4847-bfd1-5d2c9d9e32f8.pdf?sfvrsn=5389656e_69&download=true (accessed on 15 October 2024).
3. WHO. *Eliminating Measles and Rubella in the WHO European Region*; Integrated Guidance for Surveillance, Outbreak Response and Verification of Elimination; WHO Regional Office for Europe: Copenhagen, Denmark, 2024. Available online: https://iris.who.int/bitstream/handle/10665/375923/9789289060783-eng.pdf?sequence=1 (accessed on 20 December 2024).
4. Minta, A.A.; Ferrari, M.; Antoni, S.; Portnoy, A.; Sbarra, A.; Lambert, B.; Hatcher, C.; Hsu, C.H.; Ho, L.L.; Steulet, C.; et al. Progress Toward Measles Elimination—Worldwide, 2000–2022. *MMWR Morb. Mortal. Wkly. Rep.* **2023**, *72*, 1262–1268. [CrossRef]
5. O'Connor, P.; Masresha, B.; Pastor, D.; Musa, N.; Hagan, J.; Khanal, S.; Lee, C.-W.; Crowcroft, N. Global Status Report for the Verification of Measles and Rubella Elimination, 2022. *Vaccines* **2024**, *12*, 947. [CrossRef]

6. WHO. Centralized Information System for Infectious Diseases (CISID). Measles-Number of Cases, 2015–2023. Available online: http://data.euro.who.int/cisid/?TabID=523870 (accessed on 7 October 2024).
7. WHO. Centralized Information System for Infectious Diseases (CISID). Measles-Number of Hospitalizations. 2023. Available online: http://data.euro.who.int/cisid/?TabID=523869 (accessed on 7 September 2024).
8. WHO. Centralized Information System for Infectious Diseases (CISID). Measles-Number of Deaths. 2023. Available online: http://data.euro.who.int/cisid/?TabID=523871 (accessed on 7 October 2024).
9. World Health Organization (WHO). *Measles and Rubella Strategic Framework 2021–2030*; World Health Organization: Geneva, Switzerland, 2020. Available online: https://www.immunizationagenda2030.org/images/documents/measles_rubella_initiative_Digital3.pdf (accessed on 7 October 2024).
10. Plans-Rubió, P. Vaccination Coverage for Routine Vaccines and Herd Immunity Levels against Measles and Pertussis in the World in 2019. *Vaccines* **2021**, *9*, 256. [CrossRef] [PubMed]
11. Plans-Rubió, P. Are the Objectives Proposed by the WHO for Routine Measles Vaccination Coverage and Population Measles Immunity Sufficient to Achieve Measles Elimination from Europe? *Vaccines* **2020**, *8*, 218. [CrossRef]
12. World Health Organization (WHO). *Strategic Plan for Measles and Congenital Rubella Infection in the WHO European Region*; WHO Regional Office for Europe: Copenhagen, Denmark, 2003. Available online: https://iris.who.int/handle/10665/107526 (accessed on 7 October 2024).
13. European Centre for Disease Prevention and Control (ECDC). Measles: Recommended Vaccination. Available online: https://vaccine-schedule.ecdc.europa.eu/Scheduler/ByDisease?SelectedDiseaseId=8&SelectedCountryIdByDisease=-1 (accessed on 2 December 2024).
14. Vanderslott, S.; Dathui, S.; Spooner, F.; Roser, M. Our World in Data. Vaccination. Available online: https://ourworldindata.org/vaccination (accessed on 2 December 2024).
15. Rosenthal, S.R.; Clements, C.J. Two-dose measles vaccination schedules. *Bull. World Health Organ.* **1993**, *71*, 421–428. [PubMed]
16. Gay, N.J. The theory of measles elimination: Implications for the design of elimination strategies. *J. Infect. Dis.* **2004**, *189* (Suppl. 1), S27–S35. [PubMed]
17. UNICEF. WHO/UNICEF Estimates of Routine Vaccination Coverage. 2023. Available online: https://data.unicef.org/topic/child-health/immunization/ (accessed on 9 September 2024).
18. Burton, A.; Monasch, R.; Lautenbach, B.; Gacic-Dobo, M.; Maryanne, N.; Karimov, R.; Wolfson, L.; Jones, G.; Birmingham, M. WHO and UNICEF estimates of national infant immunization coverage: Methods and processes. *Bull. World Health Organ.* **2009**, *87*, 535–541. [CrossRef]
19. Demicheli, V.; Rivetti, A.; Debalini, M.G.; Di Pietrantonj, C. Vaccines for Measles, Mumps and Rubella in Children. *Cochrane Database Syst. Rev.* **2021**, *8*, 2076–2238. [CrossRef]
20. WHO-UNICEF. Progress and Challenges with Achieving Universal Immunization Coverage. Available online: https://cdn.who.int/media/docs/default-source/immunization/wuenic-progress-and-challenges.pdf?sfvrsn=b5eb9141_12&download=true (accessed on 10 December 2024).
21. Minta, A.A.; Ferrari, M.; Antoni, S.; Portnoy, A.; Sbarra, A.; Lambert, B.; Hauryski, S.; Hatcher, C.; Nedelec, Y.; Datta, D.; et al. Progress Toward Regional Measles Elimination—Worldwide, 2000–2021. *MMWR Morb. Mortal. Wkly. Rep.* **2022**, *71*, 1489–1495. [CrossRef] [PubMed]
22. Orenstein, W.A.; Cairns, L.; Hinman, A.; Nkowane, B.; Olivé, J.M.; Reingold, A.L. Measles and Rubella Global Strategic Plan 2012–2020 midterm review report: Background and summary. *Vaccine* **2018**, *36* (Suppl. 1), A35–A42. [CrossRef]
23. World Health Organization (WHO). Measles vaccines: Position paper—April 2017. *Wkly. Epidemiol. Rep.* **2017**, *92*, 205–227.
24. Winter, A.K.; Moss, W.J. Possible Paths to Measles Eradication: Conceptual Frameworks, Strategies, and Tactics. *Vaccines* **2024**, *12*, 814. [CrossRef] [PubMed]
25. Plans, P. New preventive strategy to eliminate measles, mumps and rubella from Europe based on the serological assessment of herd immunity levels is the population. *Eur. J. Clin. Microbiol. Infect. Dis.* **2013**, *32*, 961–996. [CrossRef] [PubMed]
26. Pavia, G.; Branda, F.; Ciccozzi, A.; Romano, C.; Locci, C.; Azzena, I.; Pascale, N.; Marascio, N.; Quirino, A.; Matera, G.; et al. Integrating digital health solutions with immunization strategies: Improving immunization coverage and monitoring in the post-COVID-19 era. *Vaccines* **2024**, *12*, 847. [CrossRef] [PubMed]
27. Stockwell, M.S.; Fiks, A.G. Utilizing health information technology to improve vaccine communication and coverage. *Hum. Vaccin. Immunother.* **2013**, *9*, 1802–1811. [CrossRef] [PubMed]
28. Rabil, M.J.; Tunc, S.; Bish, D.R.; Bish, E.K. Benefits of integrated screening and vaccination for infection control. *PLoS ONE* **2022**, *17*, e0267388. [CrossRef]
29. Rachlin, A.; Hampton, L.M.; Rota, P.A.; Mulders, M.N.; Papania, M.; Goodson, J.L.; Krause, L.K.; Hanson, M.; Osborn, J.; Kelly-Cirino, C.; et al. Use of Measles and Rubella Rapid Diagnostic Tests to Improve Case Detection and Targeting of vaccinations. *Vaccines* **2024**, *12*, 823. [CrossRef]

30. Mokdad, A.H.; Gagnier, M.C.; Colson, K.E.; Dansereau, E.; Zuniga-Brenes, P.; Rios-Zertuche, D.; Haakenstad, A.; Johanns, C.K.; Palmisano, E.B.; Hernandez, B.; et al. Missed opportunities for measles, mumps, and rubella (MMR) immunization in Mesoamerica: Potential impact on coverage and days at risk. *PLoS ONE* **2015**, *10*, e0139680. [CrossRef]
31. Ropero Alvarez, A.M.; Jane Kurtis, H.; Vulanovic, L.; Hasan, H.; Ruiz, C.; Thrush, E. The evolution of Vaccination Week in the Americas. *Rev. Panam. Salud Publica* **2017**, *41*, e150. [CrossRef]
32. Szilagyi, P.G.; Schaffer, S.; Shone, L.; Barth, R.; Humiston, S.G.; Sandler, M.; Rodewald, L.E. Reducing geographical, racial, and ethnic disparities in childhood immunization rates by using reminder/recall interventions in urban primary care practices. *Pediatrics* **2002**, *110*, e58. [CrossRef] [PubMed]
33. Kaufman, J.; Rak, A.; Vasiliadis, S.; Brar, N.; Atif, E.; White, J.; Danchin, M.; Durrheim, D.N. The Case for Assessing the Drivers of Measles Vaccine Uptake. *Vaccines* **2024**, *12*, 692. [CrossRef]
34. Higgins, D.M.; O'Leary, S.T. A World without Measles and Rubella: Addressing the Challenge of Vaccine Hesitancy. *Vaccines* **2024**, *12*, 694. [CrossRef] [PubMed]
35. Wilder-Smith, A.B.; Qureshi, K. Resurgence of measles in Europe: A systematic review on parental attitudes and beliefs of measles vaccine. *J. Epidemiol. Glob. Health* **2020**, *10*, 46–58. [CrossRef]
36. Center for Disease Control (CDC). National Immunization Awareness Month. Available online: https://www.cdc.gov/vaccines/events/niam/index.html (accessed on 3 November 2024).
37. Poland, C.M.; Ratishvili, T. Vaccine hesitancy and health care providers: Using the preferred cognitive styles and decision-making model and empathy tool to make progress. *Vaccine X* **2022**, *11*, 100174. [CrossRef]
38. Salmon, D.A.; Teret, S.P.; Macintyre, C.R.; Salisbury, D.; Burgess, M.A.; Halsey, N.A. Compulsory vaccination and conscientious or philosophical exemptions: Past, present, and future. *Lancet* **2006**, *367*, 436–442. [CrossRef]
39. Haverkate, M.; D'Ancona, F.; Giambi, C.; Lopalco, P.L.; Cozza, V.; Appelgren, E. Mandatory and recommended vaccination in the EU, Iceland and Norway: Results of the VENICE 2010 survey on the ways of implementing national vaccination programs. *Euro Surveill.* **2012**, *17*, 20183. [CrossRef] [PubMed]
40. Pannuti, C.S.; Morello, R.J.; De Moraes, J.C.; Curti, S.P.; Afonso, A.M.S.; Camargo, M.C.C.; De Souza, V.A.U.F. Identification of primary and secondary measles vaccine failures by measurement of immunoglobulin G avidity in measles cases during the 1997 São Paulo Epidemic. *Clin. Diagn. Lab. Immunol.* **2004**, *11*, 119–122. [CrossRef] [PubMed]
41. Danovaro-Holliday, M.C.; Koh, M.; Steulet, C.; Rhoda, D.A.; Trimner, M.K. Lessons from Recent Measles Post-Campaign Coverage Surveys Worldwide. *Vaccines* **2024**, *12*, 1257. [CrossRef]
42. O'Leary, S.T.; Opel, D.J.; Cataldi, J.R.; Hackell, J.M.; Committee on Infectious Diseases; Committee on Practice and Ambulatory Medicine; Committee on Bioethics. Strategies for Improving Vaccine Communication and Uptake. *Pediatrics* **2024**, *153*, e2023065483. [CrossRef]
43. European Centre for Disease Prevention and Control (ECDC). *Catalogue of Interventions Addressing Vaccine Hesitancy*; ECDC: Stockholm, Sweden, 2017.
44. Crowcroft, N.S.; Minta, A.A.; Bolotin, S.; Cernuschi, T.; Ariyarajah, A.; Antoni, S.; Mulders, M.N.; Bose, A.S.; O'Connor, P.M. The Problem with Delaying Measles Elimination. *Vaccines* **2024**, *12*, 813. [CrossRef] [PubMed]
45. WHO-UNICEF. WHO UNICEF Immunization Coverage Estimates 2023 Revision (Released 15 July 2024). Available online: https://www.who.int/publications/m/item/WUENIC_notes (accessed on 29 November 2024).
46. Guerra, F.; Bolotin, S.; Lim, G.; Heffernan, J.; Deeks, S.L.; Li, Y.; Crowcroft, N.S. The basic reproduction number (Ro) of measles: A systematic review. *Lancet Infect. Dis.* **2017**, *17*, e420–e428. [CrossRef]

vaccines

MDPI

Review

Vaccine Hesitancy and Associated Factors Amongst Health Professionals: A Scoping Review of the Published Literature

Antonios Christodoulakis [1,2,†], Izolde Bouloukaki [1,*,†], Antonia Aravantinou-Karlatou [1], Michail Zografakis-Sfakianakis [2] and Ioanna Tsiligianni [1]

[1] Department of Social Medicine, School of Medicine, University of Crete, 71500 Heraklion, Greece; christodoulakisa@uoc.gr (A.C.); medp2012149@med.uoc.gr (A.A.-K.); i.tsiligianni@uoc.gr (I.T.)
[2] Department of Nursing, School of Health Sciences, Hellenic Mediterranean University, 71410 Heraklion, Greece; mzografakis@hmu.gr
* Correspondence: izolthi@gmail.com; Tel.: +30-28-1-039-4607
† These authors contributed equally to this work.

Abstract: Background/Objectives: Healthcare professionals (HCPs) hold significant influence over public attitudes toward vaccinations. Studies suggest that HCPs are hesitant towards the coronavirus disease 2019 (COVID-19) vaccines. This hesitancy could lead to lower vaccination rates in the community. Therefore, this scoping review aimed to assess the extent of hesitancy towards COVID-19 booster doses among HCPs and identify the associated factors. **Methods:** A comprehensive search was conducted in the PubMed and Scopus databases from April to August 2024, using keywords related to COVID-19, vaccine hesitancy, HCPs, and booster vaccination. Studies that had been peer-reviewed, published in English after 2022, and focused on the hesitancy of the COVID-19 booster dose hesitancy among HCPs were included. Out of the 6703 studies screened, 24 studies were included. **Results:** Most of the HCPs have received their initial series of COVID-19 vaccinations. However, there is a lower rate of uptake for booster doses, with hesitancy rates ranging from 12% to 66.5%. Hesitancy rates varied significantly across continents, with Asia, Africa, and Europe ranging from 19.7% to 66.5%, 27% to 46.1%, 14% to 60.2%, respectively. Hesitancy was reported to be influenced by various factors, including concerns about vaccine safety, necessity, and effectiveness of these vaccines. In addition, the hesitancy regarding booster doses was also found to be influenced by factors like age, gender, profession, and previous COVID-19. Physicians, nurses, and pharmacists exhibited vaccine hesitancy rates ranging from 12.8% to 43.7%, 26% to 37%, and 26% to 34.6%, respectively. **Conclusions:** Our review underscores the hesitancy among HCPs towards receiving booster doses across countries around the world and explores the underlying factors. These findings provide valuable insights for the design of future pandemic vaccination programs.

Keywords: vaccination hesitancy; booster dose; healthcare professionals; COVID-19; reasons; factors; review

1. Introduction

The outbreak of the coronavirus disease 2019 (COVID-19) has caused a worldwide emergency situation, affecting various aspects of human life [1]. The unprecedented onset of the COVID-19 pandemic has also imposed a significant burden on healthcare systems worldwide [1]. Measures like social distancing, wearing face masks in public, lockdowns, and quarantines have helped to initially control the transmission of the virus [2,3]. However, to return to normal life, long-term solutions such as universal vaccination were needed [2,4,5]. In this context, the development of COVID-19 vaccines has been suggested to combat the pandemic, by reducing the severity of illness and lowering the spread of the virus [6,7]. Nevertheless, even though the pandemic has been effectively controlled, the virus is still spreading, due to the emergence of new strains of COVID-19 and the declining effectiveness of primary doses of the COVID-19 vaccines [8–10]. This has prompted the World Health Organization (WHO) to consistently update its recommendations for COVID-19 vaccination. These updates emphasize the importance of vaccinating both the general public and healthcare professionals (HCPs) [11].

HCPs are frequently considered a target population for vaccination initiatives, as they possess characteristics typically associated with vaccine acceptance. These include a high level of education, clinical experience, and affiliation with professional organizations that advocate for vaccination [12]. Moreover, HCPs were prioritized for the COVID-19 vaccine due to their occupational exposure and frequent interaction with infected individuals [13]. However, their willingness to get vaccinated varied and often fell short of expectations [14]. Encouraging positive attitudes towards vaccination among HCPs was proposed not only for ensuring their personal safety, as well as the safety of their families and patients, but also to promote its acceptance among others [15]. The reason behind this is that HCPs act as facilitators and communicators for vaccines to patients and the general public [16–18]. More specifically, during both the initial and subsequent COVID-19 vaccination campaigns, HCPs had the role of addressing concerns and misunderstandings about COVID-19 vaccination, and supporting the benefits of getting vaccinated [19,20]. Several studies have reported resistance to receiving COVID-19 booster doses (BDs) which could potentially negatively impact trust in vaccines among the general population [17,21,22]. If HCPs exhibit hesitancy or resistance towards receiving the vaccine, it could reflect a similar attitude among patients, influencing public opinion [23].

The European Centre for Disease Prevention and Control defines vaccine hesitancy as the "delay in acceptance or refusal of vaccines despite availability of vaccination services" [24]. The distribution of initial vaccine hesitancy among HCPs appears to vary, with certain characteristics such as age, sex, race/ethnicity, political affiliation, professional role, and healthcare facility type identified as predictors of vaccine uptake [25–30]. Furthermore, the way HCPs perceive their vulnerability to and the seriousness of COVID-19, as well as their past experience testing positive for the virus, greatly impacted their decision to get vaccinated [26,29]. Importantly, HCPs' initial hesitancy towards vaccinations appears to remain when it comes to receiving BDs of the COVID-19 vaccine, although studies indicate varying levels of acceptance and hesitancy towards BDs [31–34]. Based on the initial findings, HCPs viewed BDs as less important and expressed a lack of confidence in them [35]. Recent data on vaccine uptake indicates that the significance of perceiving COVID-19 vaccination as necessary seems to diminish, with a lower number of HCPs receiving BDs compared to those who received the initial two doses [36]. Due to the dynamic nature of the virus, the potential for viral mutations, and the likelihood of declining immunity, understanding HCPs' hesitancy to receive regular COVID-19 vaccines has significant value for guiding vaccination campaigns.

While concerns regarding vaccine hesitancy among HCPs remain, potentially contributing to disparities in BD uptake, few studies have thoroughly examined the differences in characteristics between HCPs who have received COVID-19 BDs and those who have not. Therefore, the aim of this scoping review was to assess the level of COVID-19 vaccine hesitancy among HCPs and identify the underlying factors that contribute to this hesitancy.

2. Materials and Methods

This scoping review followed the JBI guidelines for conducting scoping reviews [37], and the findings were reported using the PRISMA-ScR checklist Supplementary Materials Table S1 [38]. The research protocol was retrospectively registered (protocol number: INPLASY2024100036) on the International Platform of Registered Systematic Review and Meta-analysis Protocols (INPLASY) at https://doi.org/10.37766/inplasy2024.10.0036 in October 2024, accessed on 9 October 2024.

2.1. Eligibility Criteria

This scoping review focused on two key questions: What is the prevalence of COVID-19 hesitancy among HCPs worldwide, and what are the factors that contribute to this hesitancy? Our scope was global, encompassing studies from all geographical locations without any specific focus on a particular population. This inclusivity ensured that our review captured a diverse range of perspectives and settings. Therefore, in order to be included in this review, studies had to meet the following criteria: (1) being peer-reviewed articles published in English, (2) focusing on HCPs, (3) investigating COVID-19 vaccine hesitancy, acceptance on booster vaccination, and (4) being published from January 2022 onwards. The exclusion criteria included articles that were not peer-reviewed, editorials, opinion pieces, and studies that focused on non-healthcare professional populations. The study selection process included two stages: screening titles and abstracts, and then conducting a full-text review. Two reviewers independently performed the screening process. Differences among reviewers were addressed through discussion and by involving a third reviewer to reach consensus. To maintain transparency and reproducibility, we employed a PRISMA flow diagram to document the selection process.

2.2. Information Sources and Search

A comprehensive approach was taken to find relevant literature through a search strategy. To ensure comprehensive coverage of medical and scientific journals, a literature search was performed in two major literature databases, PubMed and Scopus, from April to August 2024. The search terms used were a mix of keywords and Medical Subject Headings (MeSHs) related to COVID-19, vaccine hesitancy, healthcare professionals, and booster vaccinations. Therefore, we employed in both databases the following keyword combinations and Boolean operators (AND, OR): "COVID-19", "vaccine hesitancy", "healthcare professionals", and "booster vaccination". The search method was based on prior systematic reviews which analyzed vaccine hesitancy towards the COVID-19 vaccine in general populations and HCPs [17,31].

2.3. Data Extraction and Analysis

In this scoping review, we analyzed the data regarding regular COVID-19 vaccination hesitancy in HCPs. This entailed the extraction of information about study design, prevalence of COVID-19 vaccination hesitancy, knowledge, attitudes and factors associated with it in HCPs, of full texts and related results of the included studies by two reviewers using a standardized form for data extraction. After removing duplicates, two independent reviewers evaluated each extraction form, and discussed any discrepancies in a thorough appraisal process. In the extracted data, details about the studies, including the author, year, and country, were added. It also provided information about the participants, such as their profession and sample size. The data encompassed the study design, key findings related to vaccine hesitancy and acceptance, any barriers and challenges that were identified, as well as the coping strategies that were utilized. Two independent reviewers performed the data extraction to guarantee accuracy and consistency. All disagreements during the review's inclusion phase were resolved through discussion to reach a consensus. In instances where reviewer consensus was not achieved, a third, independent reviewer was employed for arbitration. We employed thematic analysis in our research to categorize factors associated with vaccine hesitancy [39]. Thematic analysis included identifying, analyzing, and reporting patterns in the data.

3. Results

3.1. Screening and Procedure

A total of 6703 studies were yielded during the first database search for this scoping review. Following the first screening and removal of duplicates, a total of 4303 articles underwent screening based on their titles. Afterwards, 880 titles met the inclusion criteria and were chosen for further assessment, primarily based on their abstracts. Subsequently, a second/further evaluation was conducted on 44 abstracts that satisfied the inclusion criteria, and their full texts were obtained to be further screened. However, 20 studies were excluded in accordance with the criteria for inclusion/exclusion as described in the methodology. Therefore, 24 full-text studies were finally included in this scoping review. The PRISMA flow diagram in Figure 1 shows the process for the literature search.

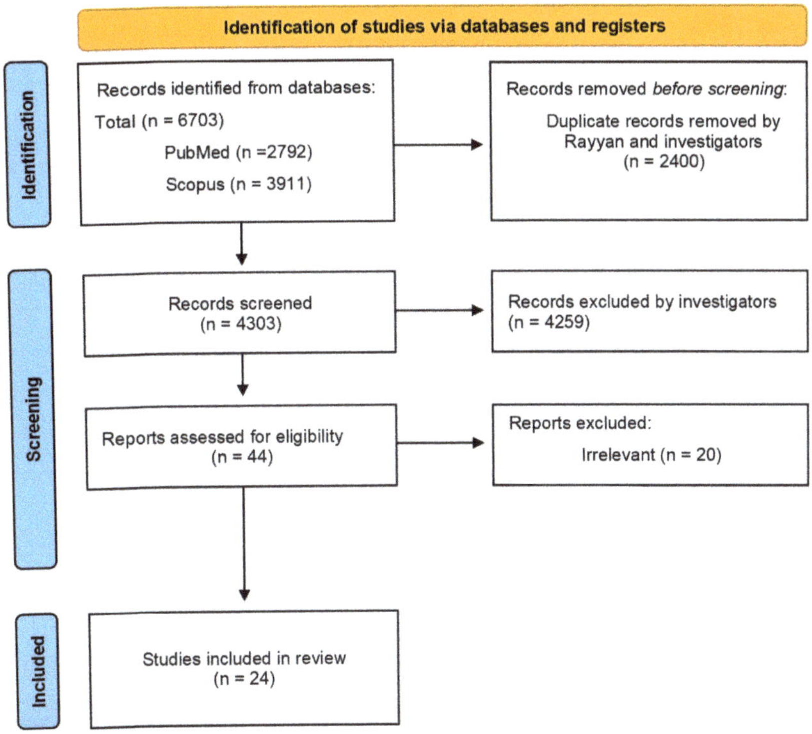

Figure 1. PRISMA 2020 flow diagram for new systematic reviews which included searches of databases and registers only for this scoping review.

3.2. *Overview of Characteristics of the Included Studies*

The characteristics of the 24 included studies [22,40–62] have been outlined in Table 1. All studies were categorized as cross-sectional [22,40–44,46–62], with one of them utilizing a mixed methods approach (combining qualitative and quantitative data) [45]. The included studies were conducted on five out of seven continents, with four studies from the United States of America (USA) [43,55,61,62], two studies from Africa (South Africa and Kongo) [45,58], ten from Asia (China, India, Jordan, Nepal, Israel, Kingdom of Bahrain and Egypt, Palestine, Pakistan, Malaysia) [22,40,46,48–53,59] and eight from Europe (England, Italy, Greece, Belgium, Slovenia) [41,42,44,47,54,56,57,60]. Studies from Asia accounted for 42% of the studies analyzed (10 studies) [22,40,46,48–53,59]. The studies were published from January 2022 to August 2024.

Table 1. Characteristics of included studies (publication year, study type, country of origin, number of participants, vaccine history and hesitancy rates).

Author/Year (Ref.)	Study Type	Country	No of Participants	Vaccination History (%) Number of BDs Received	Vaccine Hesitancy (%)	Hesitancy Among HCPs by Specialty
Arshad et al., 2022 [40]	Quantitative	Pakistan	$n = 1164$	9.9% at least one BD	47.9%	24.4% Medical professionals 23.7% Allied Health Professionals
Dale et al., 2023 [41]	Quantitative	England	$n = 91$	77.1% at least one BD 4.9% 2 BDs 1.2% 3 BDs	Oxford Vaccine hesitancy scale score: 13.56/35.00 (17.1% being above the midpoint).	NR
Della Polla et al., 2022 [42]	Quantitative	Italy	$n = 496$	94.9% at least one BD 48.1% at least 2 BDs	47.4%	NR
Digregorio et al., 2024 [57]	Quantitative	Belgium	$n = 1814$	66.8% 2 BDs 6.3% 3 BDs	14%	NR
Dudley et al., 2023 [43]	Quantitative	USA	$n = 1207$	82% HCPs at least one BD	NR	6.3% Pediatrician 13% Family medicine 26.7% Physician assistant, Nurse Practitioners, and Nurse 26% Pharmacist
Galanis et al., 2023 [44]	Quantitative	Greece	$n = 795$	NR	30.9%	NR
George et al., 2023 [45]	Mixed-Methods	South Africa	$n = 6235$	56% at least one BD	27%	27.9% Nurse 17.5% Doctor
Gu et al., 2023 [46]	Quantitative	China	$n = 1618$	78.4% at least one BD	41.8%	43.7% Physician 37% Nurse
Guarducci et al., 2023 [47]	Quantitative	Italy	$n = 1309$	96.5% one BD	NR	NR
Kolomba et al., 2024 [58]	Quantitative	Congo	$n = 514$	24.3% one BD	31.1%	23.1% Doctor
Krishna et al., 2023 [48]	Quantitative	India	$n = 535$	62.2% one BD	40%	NR
Lubad et al., 2023 [49]	Quantitative	Jordan	$n = 300$	NR	31.6%	NR

Table 1. *Cont.*

Author/Year (Ref.)	Study Type	Country	No of Participants	Vaccination History (%) Number of BDs Received	Vaccine Hesitancy (%)	Hesitancy Among HCPs by Specialty
Maraga et al., 2024 [22]	Quantitative	Palestine	$n = 919$	NR	66.5%	NR
Pandarathodiyil et al., 2024 [59]	Quantitative	Malaysa	$n = 392$	100% at least one BD	22%	NR
Paudel et al., 2023 [50]	Quantitative	Nepal	$n = 300$	29% one BD	12%	NR
Pristov al., 2024 [60]	Quantitative	Slovenia	$n = 560$	50.9% at least one BD	NR	NR
Ramot et al., 2023 [51]	Quantitative	Israel	$n = 124$	88.7% one BD 38.7% 2 BDs	61.3%	NR
Rathinakumar et al., 2024 [52]	Quantitative	South India	$n = 572$	12.6% one BD	19.7%	23.2% Paramedical workers 12.8% Doctor
Roberts et al. 2024 [61]	Quantitative	USA	$n = 182$	55% one BD	NR	NR
Russ et al., 2024 [62]	Quantitative	USA	$n = 3375$	85% one BD	NR	NR
Salah et al., 2023 [53]	Quantitative	Kingdom of Bahrain and Egypt	$n = 389$	NR	46.1%	46.1% Physicians 26% Nurses 34.6% Pharmacists
Sansone et al., 2024 [54]	Quantitative	Italy	$n = 521$	5.2% at least one BD	60.2%	NR
Viskupič et al., 2023 [55]	Quantitative	USA	$n = 1084$	63.2% one BD	NR	NR
Zoumpoulis et al., 2023 [56]	Quantitative	Greece	$n = 1224$	52.4% one BD 47.5% 2 BDs	27.4%	NR

BD: booster dose, HCP: healthcare professional, NR: not reported.

3.3. Measures

Sociodemographic characteristics were recorded in all of the studies included [22,40–62]. The majority of the studies assessed the participants' vaccination history, including the number of BDs received and the type of vaccine administered [22,40,46–48,52,53,57–62]. In addition, the studies included specific questions about willingness to take the COVID-19 vaccine BDs [22,40,48,49,51,52,54,57–59], vaccination trust [43,49,57], knowledge [50,53,54,57] and perceived benefit [22,46,47,49,53,56]. Questions related to attitudes about BDs [42,44–48,50–54,56,61], COVID-19 diagnosis and risk [44,46,60], barriers for BDs [46], health status factors [42,46,50,51,58,60] and psychological drivers for BDs [40] were also included and have been outlined in Table 1. Furthermore, specific assessment tools were used to evaluate vaccination hesitancy among HCPs, focusing on HCPs' knowledge, attitudes, and other factors associated with it. In particular, the specific tools used were the Belief Medicine Questionnaire Specific (BMQ) and the Belief Medicine Questionnaire General (BMQ), the Brief Illness Perception Questionnaire (BIPQ), the Oxford COVID-19 Vaccine Hesitancy Scale, and the Bespoke scale [41].

3.4. Vaccination History and Hesitancy

Regarding vaccination history (Table 1), the majority of HCPs had received at least one dose of the initial COVID-19 vaccine [22,40–62]. The percentages of HCPs receiving booster vaccinations have been found to vary widely in studies, with reported rates ranging from 4.9% to 100%. More specifically, the first BD has been administered to a considerable percentage of HCPs [40,42,43,45,47,48,50–52,55,57–62], while a smaller proportion have received the second BD [40,41,46,47,50,54,57,58,62]. The number of HCPs who have received the third BD is even lower [41,46,57]. There were substantial variations in HCPs' hesitancy towards BDs, ranging from 12% to 66.5% [22,40,42,44,45,49–54,56–59]. Hesitancy rates varied significantly across continents, with Asia ranging from 19.7% to 66.5%, Africa from 27% to 46.1%, and Europe from 14% to 60.2%. From the highest to the lowest rates of booster dose vaccination hesitancy, the countries were Palestine at 66.5% [22], Israel at 61.3% [51], Greece with rates ranging from 30.9 to 52.9% [44,56], Italy with rates ranging from 51.9% to 60.2%) [42,54], Egypt at 46.1% [53], Congo at 31.1% [58], Pakistan at 24.2% [40], South Africa at 20% [45], Malysia at 22% [59], South India at 19.7% [52], Jordan at 16% [49], Belgium at 14% [57], and Nepal at 12% [50]. Physicians displayed the most diverse hesitancy rates, ranging from 12.8% to 43.7%, whereas nurses and pharmacists exhibited rates between 26% and 37% and 26% to 34.6%, respectively.

3.5. Socio-Demographic Characteristics and COVID-19-Related Variables Associated with Vaccination Hesitancy

Socio-demographic characteristics related to vaccine booster dose hesitancy in HCPs were gender, age, type of HCPs included in studies, marital status, education level, co-morbidities, type of vaccine, and not being regularly vaccinated against influenza [22,40,42–47,49–60,62] (Table 2). When it comes to gender differences, females exhibited greater hesitancy towards receiving BDs than males [49,51,53,54,57,60]. Additionally, individuals without a chronic condition [33,45,58,60] and without medical training demonstrated a lower willingness compared to medical professionals to receive BDs [43,45,49,50,52,54,58]. Being in a younger age range [45,55–57,60,62], being single [40,52], and having a lower level of education [44,50,62] were also all factors that were positively associated with vaccine hesitancy. Family and friends were also identified as influential factors contributing to hesitancy [41,44,48,58]. On the other hand, individuals who had received mRNA-based vaccines in the past [40,46,47] and regularly received influenza vaccinations [22,44,45,55,56] were more inclined to be receptive to receiving a booster vaccine dose.

Table 2. Socio-demographic characteristics and COVID-19-related variables associated with vaccination hesitancy.

Factors	Associated with Hesitancy	Number of Studies
Age	Younger age [39,41,49–51,54,56].	7
Gender	Being male [34,39]. Being female [43,45,47,48,51,54].	8
Race	Black African [39]. Black [55]. Non-Hispanic Black [56]. Hispanic [56].	3
Education	Lower education [38,44,56].	3
Occupation	Non-prescribers [51]. Other than physicians [37–39,43,44,46,48,52]. Physicians [41,45,47]. Pharmacists [47]. Not in direct contact with patients [39]. Less job experience [39]. Working experience more than 5 years [52]. Wards of activity with lower risk of infection (Medical vs. Emergency/Critical/Infectious Disease wards) [48].	12
Political Leanings	Republican self-identification [49].	1
Marital Status	Single/not married [34,46]. Married [38].	3
Friends/family	Influence of friends/family [35,38,42,52].	4
Area of Residence	Rural [34,37]. Highly socially vulnerable census tract [56].	3
Low income	Low annual household income (<USD 50,000) [56].	1
Comorbidity/chronic illness	Absence of chronic conditions [38,39,52,54]. Permanent or temporary medical conditions [37]. History of allergy [40]. Obesity [47].	7
Health status	Good/very good self-perceived physical health [38]. Unhealthy dietary habits [54].	2
Time constraints	Lack of time [35]	1
Flu Vaccination	Lack of flu vaccination [17,38,39,49,50].	5
Hygiene measures	Increased compliance [38,41,52].	3
Relating to COVID-19	Previous COVID-19 infection [34,35,49]. No previous infection [38].	4
Relating to COVID-19 vaccination	No previous vaccination [34] Type of vaccine (non-mRNA COVID-19 vaccines) [34,53] Less previous vaccine doses [44,48,51,52] Uptake of the first booster dose [42] Previous side effects [34]	10

3.6. Vaccination Knowledge and Attitudes

In relation to vaccination attitudes, a notable percentage of HCPs (ranging from 6% to 77.1%) held the belief that the currently available BDs were not required, deemed unsafe, and lacked effectiveness [40,45–50,52,53,57,58] (Table 3). Furthermore, their belief was that vaccines do not provide adequate protection against severe cases of COVID-19 [40,42,51,52,57,59]. Consequently, there was a lack of trust in these vaccines, with percentages ranging from 20.9% to 26.8%. [43,44,49,57]. Fear of the side effects associated with COVID-19 booster vaccinations, [44–46,52,56], a belief in a low risk of COVID-19 infection [42,43,46,47,57], the non-compulsory nature of booster doses [41,43,44,52,56,57,59], and a history of COVID-19 infection [57] were also identified as contributing factors for vaccine hesitancy. Nevertheless, it seems that HCPs acknowledged receiving information about the efficacy of COVID-19 BDs [42], and expressed their willingness to receive additional information [42,51,54].

Table 3. Knowledge/attitudes associated with vaccine hesitancy.

Knowledge/Attitudes	Associated with Hesitancy	Number of Studies
Trust-related issues	Vaccine safety [34,35,38–43,45,47,52].	11
	Pregnancy safety [35].	
	Vaccine effectiveness [17,34,36,38–43,45–47,51–53,55].	16
	Vaccine necessity [35,36,38–40,45–47,52,55].	10
	Vaccine Side effects [17,36,37,46,50,52,55].	7
	Mistrust in government/scientists [37,42,43,50].	4
	Rapid development of the vaccines [37,42,50].	3
	Distrust due to racism and previous unethical treatment of minorities [37].	1
	Reliability of clinical trials (not including HCPs) [37].	1
	Low trust and satisfaction in COVID-19 vaccination [34,38,51].	3
	Wanting to wait more [37,42,43,45].	4
Information	Lack of information/misinformation [42,47,48].	3
Beliefs and attitudes about health and prevention	Low risk of COVID-19 infection [36,37,40,50,51].	5
	Immune system capable of fighting COVID-19 [43,51].	1
	Lower perception of the severity of COVID-19 [36,41,51,52].	4
	Against vaccines in general [50,52].	2
	Belief in greater efficacy of complementary alternative medicine [50].	1
Ethics	Mandatory Vaccination [39,41,48].	3
Other	Not being very likely to suggest the vaccine to patients [51].	1
	Tiredness due to the vaccination procedure [38].	1

4. Discussion

The objective of this scoping review was to evaluate the hesitancy of HCPs towards vaccination with COVID-19 BDs and identify associated factors. Our findings suggest that HCPs exhibit varying degrees of hesitancy across countries, indicating that HCPs still had concerns related to BDs. This hesitancy leads to a progressive decrease in the percentage of HCPs receiving the second and third booster doses. The prevalence of hesitancy towards BDs in HCPs was higher among females, younger and single individuals, those with lower education levels, and those who did not regularly receive flu vaccines. Notably, individuals with a history of COVID-19 infection, without chronic conditions, and non-physician HCPs also exhibited hesitancy. This review also identified the following key factors that prominently influenced BD hesitancy: uncertainties surrounding the vaccine's safety, efficacy, and necessity, a perception of low risk of contracting the infection, and that BDs were not mandatory.

In light of the evolving virus and the appearance of new variants, health authorities have endorsed the regular utilization of BDs to enhance and prolong vaccine-induced immunity [8–10]. However, our review indicates that a considerable portion of HCPs remain hesitant in receiving BDs of the COVID-19 vaccine. Literature research on vaccine hesitancy for COVID-19 in HCPs has produced varied results [63]. While HCPs generally exhibit lower vaccine hesitancy compared to non-healthcare workers [63], some studies have found no significant differences in vaccine hesitancy between these two groups [64,65]. Furthermore, the underlying factors contributing to vaccination hesitancy among HCPs appear to be similar to those documented within the general population [66]. This raises concerns since HCPs have traditionally been the primary and most trustworthy source of vaccine information [67]. It is to be expected that HCPs who have not been vaccinated are much less likely to suggest vaccinations to their patients [31]. However, even HCPs who have received their vaccinations need access to continually updated resources to effectively address vaccine hesitancy and discuss vaccines with their patients [31,68].

Another important finding of our review was the substantial variability in the hesitancy levels of HCPs across various countries. The COVID-19 vaccination hesitancy rates in Jordan at 16% [49], Belgium at 14% [57], and Nepal at 12% [50] were among the lowest worldwide, which could be attributed to significant efforts to build public trust in vaccines [69]. On the other hand, Palestine at 66.5% [22] and Israel at 61.3% [51] had the highest hesitancy rates. This variability aligns not only with other previous reviews conducted during the primary COVID-19 vaccination campaigns [12,70–72], but also with a subsequent review following the introduction of BDs [23]. Socioeconomic factors, such as race and income, are also significantly linked to geographic disparities in vaccine hesitancy [73]. A study analyzing COVID-19 vaccine hesitancy across 145 countries highlighted that hesitancy towards vaccination was a more prominent factor in determining uptake in low-income countries compared to high-income countries [74]. Lower availability or limited accessibility to COVID-19 vaccines [75,76], along with higher rates of COVID-19-related morbidity and mortality [70] in certain countries, may potentially explain the differences in hesitancy across countries regarding BD vaccinations. The widespread implementation of mandatory primary vaccinations for HCPs [77,78], and the resulting pressure to vaccinate, may also have contributed to hesitancy [77,79]. Nevertheless, and despite this considerable variation in hesitancy among HCPs worldwide, it is crucial to recognize the importance of implementing interventions that are tailored to each country's socioeconomical [80–82] and even religious conditions [83].

A major finding of the present study was that HCPs continue to express concerns about the vaccine's safety, necessity, and effectiveness, which are the same concerns that contributed to hesitancy towards the initial doses of the COVID-19 vaccine [12,70]. More specifically, HCPs have expressed concerns about negative effects of multiple boosters on the immune system [84,85], adverse events (AEs) and serious adverse events (SAEs) including myocarditis and pericarditis, particularly in younger males who have received mRNA vaccines [86,87]. There are also other rare but serious conditions, such as thrombosis with thrombocytopenia syndrome, that have contributed to unease among HCPs [88–90]. Although these AEs are statistically rare compared to the severe outcomes of COVID-19 infection (without a booster dose), they could have a significant impact on how HCPs perceive BDs [91–95]. To address these concerns and rebuild trust among HCPs, it is crucial to have transparent risk communication strategies and robust post-vaccine safety monitoring in place [96,97]. In support of this, evidence suggests that HCPs often express a desire for more convincing and comprehensive evidence, in terms of both quality and quantity, when deciding on vaccinations and whether to recommend them [42,98,99]. This emphasizes the necessity of ongoing training programs that focus on vaccine research, safety data, and effective communication strategies.

On the other hand, the belief that BDs of the COVID-19 vaccines are inadequate in providing protection against severe forms of COVID-19, as well as the lack of confidence in these vaccines, were also found to be significant factors contributing to vaccine hesitancy. Previous studies confirm these findings, since negative attitudes towards vaccines, lack of trust in government and institutions, and the belief that personal rights are being violated are all indicated as contributing factors to vaccine hesitancy [12,80]. Another important factor noted is the declining effectiveness of COVID-19 vaccines against infection as time goes on. Research has shown that vaccine-induced immunity, especially against new variants like Omicron, starts to decrease around five months following vaccination, after which "breakthrough" infections could occur [100]. Although breakthrough infections during this period are mostly mild, they have raised doubts about the long-term efficacy of BDs, especially for high-exposure groups like HCPs [100,101]. Behavioral science research indicates that deeper understanding has a stronger influence on decision making than statistical information, even among experts in the field [102]. This involves initiating a constructive dialogue, understanding the issues raised from the HCPs [103].

This review also found differences in vaccine hesitancy influenced by sociodemographic and medical history characteristics. More specifically, we found that characteristics such as female gender, lack of comorbidities, younger age, lower levels of education, being single, race/ethnicity (Blacks, Hispanics), and HCPs other than physician, have been identified as potential factors of vaccine hesitancy [25–30]. Consistent with prior research [40,45–47,50,51,53,54], female gender was identified as a key demographic factor contributing to hesitancy towards booster dose vaccination. In the past, women have shown more hesitancy towards receiving vaccinations for other diseases in comparison to men, and this tendency may also apply to the COVID-19 vaccine [104,105]. There are two main reasons for this. Firstly, the majority of reported side effects from the COVID-19 vaccine were observed in females, and secondly, women expressed concerns about the vaccine's potential impact on fertility [105–108]. Importantly, having underlying health conditions also appears to be a factor in determining vaccine acceptance. In addition, it seemed that younger HCPs, who tended to have lower levels of education and no flu vaccination in the previous season showed a greater tendency towards being hesitant about BDs. On the other hand, there is a scarcity of studies that have focused on the contribution of different types of healthcare personnel to the reception of COVID-19 BDs. The findings of this review indicate that HCPs displayed varying levels of hesitancy towards COVID-19 vaccination, with non-physicians exhibiting higher levels of hesitancy compared to physicians.

Finally, it is important to consider that given the unique characteristics of the COVID-19 virus, achieving herd immunity through widespread vaccination presents significant challenges [109,110]. This is because COVID-19 has the ability to infect various animal reservoirs, including minks, deer, and rodents [111–113]. From this point of view, it becomes clear that the health of humans is intimately tied to the health of domestic, wild, and farmed animals [111–113]. Therefore, addressing COVID-19 requires a more holistic and internationally coordinated strategy, involving collaboration among diverse disciplines like medicine and veterinary medicine. This effort should be guided by the "One Health" concept, recognizing the inherent interconnectedness between human and animal health, and the ecosystem [114].

Limitations

Our review makes a valuable contribution to the existing literature by thoroughly investigating the factors behind HCPs' hesitancy towards COVID-19 booster dose vaccination. Nevertheless, it is essential to recognize certain limitations as well. To begin with, we exclusively examined articles published in English, thereby narrowing down the selection of eligible studies. Moreover, the studies we selected were drawn from different contexts and populations, which posed challenges in terms of making comparisons and conducting further analysis. The majority of studies have also used self-reported surveys, increasing the likelihood of response bias. Differences in reported vaccine hesitancy across countries could also be partly explained by variations in measurement techniques, including the use of different survey questions or assessment tools. Furthermore, as real-world data emerge, we should anticipate potential changes in HCPs' views on COVID-19 vaccines. Longitudinal studies could offer valuable information about the evolving nature of attitudes in light of new developments and face-to-face interviews and focus groups could offer valuable insights into their beliefs and concerns that might not be captured by previous studies. Lastly, it should be noted that no evaluation was conducted on the articles' quality, and the conclusions were simply summarized without any supplementary analysis.

5. Conclusions

In summary, our review underscores the hesitancy among healthcare professionals (HCPs) towards receiving booster doses of the COVID-19 vaccine despite receiving the initial dose of the COVID-19 vaccine. This hesitancy is primarily influenced by sociodemographic factors and concerns surrounding vaccine safety, necessity, and effectiveness. Gaining insight into these factors underlying this hesitancy could guide future vaccination approaches. To better understand the nuances of vaccine knowledge, attitudes, and behaviors, future research should adopt a longitudinal qualitative approach to examine variations across time and regions with new developments.

Supplementary Materials: The following supporting information can be downloaded at: https://www.mdpi.com/article/10.3390/vaccines12121411/s1, Table S1: Preferred Reporting Items for Systematic reviews and Meta-Analyses extension for Scoping Reviews (PRISMA-ScR) Checklist.

Author Contributions: Conceptualization, A.C., I.B., A.A.-K., M.Z.-S. and I.T.; methodology, A.C., I.B., A.A.-K., M.Z.-S. and I.T.; formal analysis, A.C., I.B., A.A.-K., M.Z.-S. and I.T.; resources, A.C., I.B. and A.A.-K.; writing—original draft preparation, A.C., I.B. and A.A.-K.; writing—review and editing, A.C., I.B., A.A.-K., M.Z.-S. and I.T.; supervision, I.T. All authors have read and agreed to the published version of the manuscript.

Funding: This research received no external funding.

Conflicts of Interest: The authors declare no conflicts of interest.

References

1. Ashmore, P.; Sherwood, E. An overview of COVID-19 global epidemiology and discussion of potential drivers of variable global pandemic impacts. *J. Antimicrob. Chemother.* **2023**, *78*, ii2–ii11. [CrossRef] [PubMed]
2. Hodgson, S.H.; Mansatta, K.; Mallett, G.; Harris, V.; Emary, K.R.W.; Pollard, A.J. What defines an efficacious COVID-19 vaccine? A review of the challenges assessing the clinical efficacy of vaccines against SARS-CoV-2. *Lancet Infect. Dis.* **2021**, *21*, e26–e35. [CrossRef] [PubMed]
3. Adebisi, Y.A.; Alaran, A.J.; Bolarinwa, O.A.; Akande-Sholabi, W.; Lucero-Prisno, D.E. When it is available, will we take it? Social media users' perception of hypothetical COVID-19 vaccine in Nigeria. *Pan Afr. Med. J.* **2021**, *38*, 230. [CrossRef] [PubMed]
4. De Gier, B.; van Asten, L.; Boere, T.M.; van Roon, A.; van Roekel, C.; Pijpers, J.; van Werkhoven, C.H.H.; van den Ende, C.; Hahné, S.J.M.; de Melker, H.E.; et al. Effect of COVID-19 vaccination on mortality by COVID-19 and on mortality by other causes, the Netherlands, January 2021–January 2022. *Vaccine* **2023**, *41*, 4488–4496. [CrossRef]
5. Wouters, O.J.; Shadlen, K.C.; Salcher-Konrad, M.; Pollard, A.J.; Larson, H.J.; Teerawattananon, Y.; Jit, M. Challenges in ensuring global access to COVID-19 vaccines: Production, affordability, allocation, and deployment. *Lancet* **2021**, *397*, 1023–1034. [CrossRef]
6. Harder, T.; Koch, J.; Vygen-Bonnet, S.; Külper-Schiek, W.; Pilic, A.; Reda, S.; Scholz, S.; Wichmann, O. Efficacy and effectiveness of COVID-19 vaccines against SARS-CoV-2 infection: Interim results of a living systematic review, 1 January to 14 May 2021. *Eurosurveillance* **2021**, *26*, 2100563. [CrossRef]
7. Chakraborty, C.; Bhattacharya, M.; Dhama, K. SARS-CoV-2 vaccines, vaccine development technologies, and significant efforts in vaccine development during the pandemic: The lessons learned might help to fight against the next pandemic. *Vaccines* **2023**, *11*, 682. [CrossRef]
8. Wu, N.; Joyal-Desmarais, K.; Ribeiro, P.A.B.; Vieira, A.M.; Stojanovic, J.; Sanuade, C.; Yip, D.; Bacon, S.L. Long-term effectiveness of COVID-19 vaccines against infections, hospitalisations, and mortality in adults: Findings from a rapid living systematic evidence synthesis and meta-analysis up to December, 2022. *Lancet Respir. Med.* **2023**, *11*, 439–452. [CrossRef]
9. Naaber, P.; Tserel, L.; Kangro, K.; Sepp, E.; Jürjenson, V.; Adamson, A.; Haljasmägi, L.; Rumm, A.P.; Maruste, R.; Kärner, J.; et al. Dynamics of antibody response to BNT162b2 vaccine after six months: A longitudinal prospective study. *Lancet Reg. Health Eur.* **2021**, *10*, 100208. [CrossRef]
10. World Health Organization (WHO). Vaccine Efficacy, Effectiveness and Protection. Available online: https://www.who.int/news-room/feature-stories/detail/vaccine-efficacy-effectiveness-and-protection (accessed on 20 June 2024).
11. World Health Organization (WHO). WHO SAGE Roadmap on Uses of COVID-19 Vaccines in the Context of OMICRON and Substantial Population Immunity. Available online: https://iris.who.int/handle/10665/366671 (accessed on 14 April 2024).
12. Peterson, C.J.; Lee, B.; Nugent, K. COVID-19 Vaccination Hesitancy among Healthcare Workers—A Review. *Vaccines* **2022**, *10*, 948. [CrossRef]
13. Razai, M.S.; Oakeshott, P.; Esmail, A.; Wiysonge, C.S.; Viswanath, K.; Mills, M.C. COVID-19 vaccine hesitancy: The five Cs to tackle behavioural and sociodemographic factors. *J. R. Soc. Med.* **2021**, *114*, 295–298. [CrossRef] [PubMed]
14. Wang, L.; Wang, Y.; Cheng, X.; Li, X.; Yang, Y.; Li, J. Acceptance of coronavirus disease 2019 (COVID-19) vaccines among healthcare workers: A meta-analysis. *Front. Public Health* **2022**, *10*, 881903. [CrossRef] [PubMed]
15. Lin, C.; Mullen, J.; Smith, D.; Kotarba, M.; Kaplan, S.J.; Tu, P. Healthcare Providers' Vaccine Perceptions, Hesitancy, and Recommendation to Patients: A Systematic Review. *Vaccines* **2021**, *9*, 713. [CrossRef] [PubMed]
16. Ramonfaur, D.; Limaye, R.J.; Hinojosa-González, D.E.; Barrera, F.J.; Rodríguez-Gómez, G.P.; Castillo-Salgado, C. COVID-19 vaccine hesitancy prevalence in Mexico: A systematic review and metanalysis. *Vaccine X* **2024**, *18*, 100488. [CrossRef]

17. Rahbeni, T.A.; Satapathy, P.; Itumalla, R.; Marzo, R.R.; Mugheed, K.A.L.; Khatib, M.N.; Gaidhane, S.; Zahiruddin, Q.S.; Rabaan, A.A.; Alrasheed, H.A.; et al. COVID-19 Vaccine Hesitancy: Umbrella Review of Systematic Reviews and Meta-Analysis. *JMIR Public Health Surveill.* **2024**, *10*, e54769. [CrossRef]
18. Weinstein, N.; Schwarz, K.; Chan, I.; Kobau, R.; Alexander, R.; Kollar, L.; Rodriguez, L.; Mansergh, G.; Repetski, T.; Gandhi, P.; et al. COVID-19 Vaccine Hesitancy Among US Adults: Safety and Effectiveness Perceptions and Messaging to Increase Vaccine Confidence and Intent to Vaccinate. *Public Health Rep.* **2024**, *139*, 102–111. [CrossRef]
19. Bhattacharya, O.; Siddiquea, B.N.; Shetty, A.; Afroz, A.; Billah, B. COVID-19 vaccine hesitancy among pregnant women: A systematic review and meta-analysis. *BMJ Open* **2022**, *12*, e061477. [CrossRef]
20. Ma, Y.; Ren, J.; Zheng, Y.; Cai, D.; Li, S.; Li, Y. Chinese parents' willingness to vaccinate their children against COVID-19: A systematic review and meta-analysis. *Front. Public Health* **2022**, *10*, 1087295. [CrossRef]
21. Burrowes, S.A.B.; Casey, S.M.; Dobbins, S.; Hall, T.; Ma, M.; Bano, R.; Drainoni, M.L.; Schechter-Perkins, E.M.; Garofalo, C.; Perkins, R.B.; et al. Healthcare workers' perspectives on the COVID-19 vaccine and boosters for themselves, their patients, and their communities: A mixed methods study. *J. Public Health* **2024**, *32*, 123–136. [CrossRef]
22. Maraqa, B.; Nazzal, Z.; Baroud, H.; Douden, M.; El Hamshary, Y.; Jalamneh, T. Healthcare workers' attitudes toward and factors influencing their acceptance of an annual COVID-19 booster vaccine: A cross-sectional study in Palestine. *BMC Health Serv. Res.* **2024**, *24*, 624. [CrossRef]
23. Aldakhlan, H.A.; Khan, A.S.; Alabdulbaqi, D. Hesitancy Over the COVID-19 Vaccine Among Various Healthcare Workers: An International Narrative Review. *Cureus* **2024**, *16*, e53059. [CrossRef] [PubMed]
24. European Centre for Disease Prevention and Control (ECDC). Vaccine Hesitancy. Available online: https://www.ecdc.europa.eu/en/immunisation-vaccines/vaccine-hesitancy (accessed on 10 July 2024).
25. Oliver, K.; Raut, A.; Pierre, S.; Silvera, L.; Boulos, A.; Gale, A.; Baum, A.; Chory, A.; Davis, N.J.; D'Souza, D.; et al. Factors associated with COVID-19 vaccine receipt at two integrated healthcare systems in New York City: A cross-sectional study of healthcare workers. *BMJ Open* **2022**, *12*, e053641. [CrossRef] [PubMed]
26. Toth-Manikowski, S.M.; Swirsky, E.S.; Gandhi, R.; Piscitello, G. COVID-19 vaccination hesitancy among health care workers, communication, and policy-making. *Am. J. Infect. Control.* **2022**, *50*, 20–25. [CrossRef] [PubMed]
27. Wang, Q.; Yang, L.; Jin, H.; Lin, L. Vaccination against COVID-19: A systematic review and meta-analysis of acceptability and its predictors. *Prev. Med.* **2021**, *150*, 106694. [CrossRef] [PubMed]
28. Painter, E.M.; Ussery, E.N.; Patel, A.; Hughes, M.M.; Zell, E.R.; Moulia, D.L.; Scharf, L.G.; Lynch, M.; Ritchey, M.D.; Toblin, R.L.; et al. Demographic Characteristics of Persons Vaccinated During the First Month of the COVID-19 Vaccination Program—United States, December 14, 2020–January 14, 2021. *MMWR Morb. Mortal. Wkly. Rep.* **2021**, *70*, 174–177. [CrossRef]
29. Farah, W.; Breeher, L.; Shah, V.; Hainy, C.; Tommaso, C.P.; Swift, M.D. Disparities in COVID-19 vaccine uptake among health care workers. *Vaccine* **2022**, *40*, 2749–2754. [CrossRef]
30. Lee, J.T. Disparities in COVID-19 vaccination coverage among health care personnel working in long-term care facilities, by job category, National Healthcare Safety Network—United States, March 2021. *MMWR. Morb. Mortal. Wkly. Rep.* **2021**, *70*, 1036–1039. [CrossRef]
31. Wilpstra, C.D.; Morrell, S.; Mirza, N.A.; Ralph, J.L. Consequences of COVID-19 Vaccine Hesitancy Among Healthcare Providers During the First 10 Months of Vaccine Availability: Scoping Review. *Can. J. Nurs. Res.* **2024**, *56*, 204–224. [CrossRef]
32. Wróblewski, M.; Stankowska, J.; Kawiak-Jawor, E. 'We're at war.' Healthcare workers' experience with organisational change, uncertainty and vaccine hesitancy in 2021 and 2022 during the COVID-19 vaccination programe in Poland. *Int. J. Health Plan. Manag.* **2024**, *39*, 1298–1312. [CrossRef]
33. Zhang, L.; Wu, Y.; Jing, S.; Liu, X.; Ren, T.; Liu, X.; Dai, Z.; Fu, J.; Chen, X.; Xiao, W.; et al. The second dose of COVID-19 vaccine booster hesitancy among health care workers in China: A multicenter cross-sectional study. *Am. J. Infect. Control.* **2024**, *52*, 525–532. [CrossRef]
34. Thampy, P.; Sharma, S.; Joshi, P.; Raj, M.S.; Rupani, A.; Tyagi, S.; Joshi, A. COVID-19 Vaccine Hesitancy Among Healthcare Workers: A Phenomenological Study of Skepticism. *Cureus* **2024**, *16*, e58445. [CrossRef] [PubMed]
35. Thaivalappil, A.; Young, I.; MacKay, M.; Pearl, D.L.; Papadopoulos, A. A qualitative study exploring healthcare providers' and trainees' barriers to COVID-19 and influenza vaccine uptake. *Health Psychol. Behav. Med.* **2022**, *10*, 695–712. [CrossRef] [PubMed]
36. Bedston, S.; Lowthian, E.; Jarvis, C.I.; Akbari, A.; Beggs, J.; Bradley, D.; de Lusignan, S.; Griffiths, R.; Herbert, L.; Hobbs, R.; et al. COVID-19 booster vaccination uptake and infection breakthrough amongst health care workers in Wales: A national prospective cohort study. *Vaccine* **2023**, *41*, 1378–1389. [CrossRef]
37. Peters, M.D.; Godfrey, C.; McInerney, P.; Munn, Z.; Tricco, A.C.; Khalil, H. Chapter 11: Scoping reviews. *JBI Man. Evid. Synth.* **2020**, *169*, 467–473.
38. Tricco, A.C.; Lillie, E.; Zarin, W.; O'Brien, K.K.; Colquhoun, H.; Levac, D.; Moher, D.; Peters, M.D.J.; Horsley, T.; Weeks, L.; et al. PRISMA Extension for Scoping Reviews (PRISMA-ScR): Checklist and Explanation. *Ann. Intern. Med.* **2018**, *169*, 467–473. [CrossRef]
39. Mak, S.; Thomas, A. Steps for Conducting a Scoping Review. *J. Grad. Med. Educ.* **2022**, *14*, 565–567. [CrossRef]
40. Arshad, M.S.; Masood, I.; Imran, I.; Saeed, H.; Ahmad, I.; Ishaq, I.; Yaseen, H.; Akbar, M.; Chaudhry, M.O.; Rasool, M.F. COVID-19 Vaccine Booster Hesitancy (VBH) among Healthcare Professionals of Pakistan, a Nationwide Survey. *Vaccines* **2022**, *10*, 1736. [CrossRef]

41. Dale, C.; Seage, C.H.; Phillips, R.; James, D. The Role of Medication Beliefs in COVID-19 Vaccine and Booster Uptake in Healthcare Workers: An Exploratory Study. *Healthcare* **2023**, *11*, 1967. [CrossRef]
42. Della Polla, G.; Miraglia Del Giudice, G.; Folcarelli, L.; Napoli, A.; Angelillo, I.F. Willingness to accept a second COVID-19 vaccination booster dose among healthcare workers in Italy. *Front. Public Health* **2022**, *10*, 1051035. [CrossRef]
43. Dudley, M.Z.; Schuh, H.B.; Forr, A.; Shaw, J.; Salmon, D.A. Changes in vaccine attitudes and recommendations among US Healthcare Personnel during the COVID-19 pandemic. *NPJ Vaccines* **2024**, *9*, 49. [CrossRef]
44. Galanis, P.; Vraka, I.; Katsiroumpa, A.; Siskou, O.; Konstantakopoulou, O.; Katsoulas, T.; Mariolis-Sapsakos, T.; Kaitelidou, D. Predictors of second COVID-19 booster dose or new COVID-19 vaccine hesitancy among nurses: A cross-sectional study. *J. Clin. Nurs.* **2023**, *32*, 3943–3953. [CrossRef] [PubMed]
45. George, G.; Nota, P.; Strauss, M.; Lansdell, E.; Peters, R.P.H.; Brysiewicz, P.; Nadesan-Reddy, N.; Wassenaar, D. Examining the uptake of COVID-19 vaccine booster doses among healthcare workers in South Africa: A mixed-methods study. *PLoS Glob. Public Health* **2023**, *3*, e0002639. [CrossRef]
46. Gu, F.; Lin, H.; Chen, Z.; Ambler, G.; Chen, X.; Chen, X.; Xia, P.; Liu, N.; Du, H. Future COVID-19 Booster Vaccine Refusal in Healthcare Workers after a Massive Breakthrough Infection Wave, a Nationwide Survey-Based Study. *Vaccines* **2023**, *11*, 987. [CrossRef]
47. Guarducci, G.; Mereu, G.; Golinelli, D.; Galletti, G.; Gemmi, F.; Cartocci, A.; Holczer, N.; Bacci, L.; Sergi, A.; Messina, G.; et al. Factors Influencing the Healthcare Workers' Willingness to Receive the COVID-19 Booster Dose in Tuscany (Italy). *Vaccines* **2023**, *11*, 1751. [CrossRef]
48. Krishna, E.; Karthikeyan, V.; Ahmad, S.; Ranjan, A.; Hasan Km, A.; Pandey, S.; Kumar, P.; Singh, C.M. Acceptance of Annual Booster Doses of COVID-19 Vaccines Among Indian Healthcare Professionals: A Pan-India Cross-Sectional Survey. *Cureus* **2023**, *15*, e49363. [CrossRef]
49. Lubad, M.A.; Abu-Helalah, M.A.; Alahmad, I.F.; Al-Tamimi, M.M.; QawaQzeh, M.S.; Al-Kharabsheh, A.M.; Alzoubi, H.; Alnawafleh, A.H.; Kheirallah, K.A. Willingness of Healthcare Workers to Recommend or Receive a Third COVID-19 Vaccine Dose: A Cross-Sectional Study from Jordan. *Infect Dis. Rep.* **2023**, *15*, 210–221. [CrossRef]
50. Paudel, K.; Shah, S.; Bhusal, S.; Dahal, K.; Bhatta, N.; Pokhrel, S.; Dahal, S.; Gaihre, M.; Mudvari, A.; Gyanwali, P. Knowledge and attitude toward COVID-19 booster dose among health care professionals in Nepal: A cross-sectional study. *Ann. Med. Surg.* **2023**, *85*, 772–777. [CrossRef]
51. Ramot, S.; Tal, O. Attitudes of Healthcare Workers in Israel towards the Fourth Dose of COVID-19 Vaccine. *Vaccines* **2023**, *11*, 385. [CrossRef]
52. Rathinakumar, N.K.; Nishanthi, A.; Manickam, S. Perception and practices on COVID-19 vaccination and booster dose acceptability among health-care workers—A questionnaire-based study. *Perspect Clin. Res.* **2024**, *15*, 10–17. [CrossRef]
53. Salah, H.; Sinan, I.; Alsamani, O.; Abdelghani, L.S.; ElLithy, M.H.; Bukamal, N.; Jawad, H.; Hussein, R.R.S.; Elgendy, M.O.; Rabie, A.S.I.; et al. COVID-19 Booster Doses: A Multi-Center Study Reflecting Healthcare Providers' Perceptions. *Vaccines* **2023**, *11*, 1061. [CrossRef]
54. Sansone, V.; Miraglia Del Giudice, G.; Della Polla, G.; Angelillo, I.F. Impact of the COVID-19 pandemic on behavioral changes in healthcare workers in Italy. *Front. Public Health* **2024**, *12*, 1335953. [CrossRef] [PubMed]
55. Viskupič, F.; Wiltse, D.L. Drivers of COVID-19 booster uptake among nurses. *Am. J. Infect Control.* **2023**, *51*, 895–899. [CrossRef] [PubMed]
56. Zoumpoulis, G.; Deligiorgi, P.; Lamprinos, D.; Georgakopoulos, P.; Oikonomou, E.; Siasos, G.; Rachiotis, G.; Damaskos, C.; Papagiannis, D.; Papavassiliou, K.A.; et al. Attitudes and Practices Related to COVID-19 Vaccination with the Second Booster Dose among Members of Athens Medical Association: Results from a Cross-Sectional Study. *Vaccines* **2023**, *11*, 1480. [CrossRef]
57. Digregorio, M.; Van Ngoc, P.; Domen, J.; Bognar, Z.; Duysburgh, E.; Hendrickx, G.; Van Damme, P.; Coenen, S.; Scholtes, B. Primary Healthcare Providers' Views on Periodic COVID-19 Booster Vaccination for Themselves and Their Patients: A 2023 Nationwide Survey in Belgium. *Vaccines* **2024**, *12*, 740. [CrossRef]
58. Kolomba, B.M.; Kalenga Luhembwe, F.; Ndala, D.B.B.; Kanku Wa Ilunga, P.; Ciamala Mukendi, P.; Ngongo Kitenge, A.; Ngoy Lumbule, J.; Kilolo Ngoy, E.; Umba Ilunga, A.; Mbidi Miema, J.; et al. Healthcare workers' willingness to receive COVID-19 booster dose and associated factors in the Democratic Republic of the Congo. *Hum. Vaccin. Immunother.* **2024**, *20*, 2357214. [CrossRef]
59. Pandarathodiyil, A.K.; Veerabhadrappa, S.K.; Nabillah Ghani, W.M.; Termizi Bin Zamzuri, A. COVID-19 Booster Vaccination Adverse Effects and Willingness to Receive a Yearly Booster Dose among Members of Health Sciences Faculties: A Descriptive Cross-Sectional Study. *J. Pharm. Bioallied. Sci.* **2024**, *16*, S1776–S1783. [CrossRef]
60. Pristov, Z.; Lobe, B.; Sočan, M. Factors Influencing COVID-19 Vaccination among Primary Healthcare Nurses in the Pandemic and Post-Pandemic Period: Cross-Sectional Study. *Vaccines* **2024**, *12*, 602. [CrossRef]
61. Roberts, S.C.; Willebrand, K.; Fredrick, J.; Pischel, L.; Patel, K.; Murray, T.S.; Martinello, R.A. Characterizing healthcare personnel attitudes toward receipt of a voluntary bivalent COVID-19 booster vaccine during a COVID-19 outbreak at a behavioral health hospital in Connecticut. *Antimicrob. Steward. Healthc. Epidemiol.* **2024**, *4*, e87. [CrossRef]
62. Russ, S.; Myers, C.; Licherdell, E.; Bowden, A.; Chinchilli, E.; Dahhan, R.; Van Wijngaarden, E.; Plumb, I.D.; Dumyati, G. Sociodemographic and Occupational Characteristics Associated with Early and Continued COVID-19 Vaccine Uptake Among Healthcare Personnel: Monroe County, NY. *Vaccine* **2024**, *42*, 2585–2591. [CrossRef]

63. Baghani, M.; Fathalizade, F.; Loghman, A.H.; Samieefar, N.; Ghobadinezhad, F.; Rashedi, R.; Baghsheikhi, H.; Sodeifian, F.; Rahimzadegan, M.; Akhlaghdoust, M. COVID-19 vaccine hesitancy worldwide and its associated factors: A systematic review and meta-analysis. *Sci. One Health* **2023**, *2*, 100048. [CrossRef]
64. Dror, A.A.; Eisenbach, N.; Taiber, S.; Morozov, N.G.; Mizrachi, M.; Zigron, A.; Srouji, S.; Sela, E. Vaccine hesitancy: The next challenge in the fight against COVID-19. *Eur. J. Epidemiol.* **2020**, *35*, 775–779. [CrossRef] [PubMed]
65. Barello, S.; Nania, T.; Dellafiore, F.; Graffigna, G.; Caruso, R. 'Vaccine hesitancy' among university students in Italy during the COVID-19 pandemic. *Eur. J. Epidemiol.* **2020**, *35*, 781–783. [CrossRef] [PubMed]
66. Kaur, M.; Coppeta, L.; Olesen, O.F. Vaccine Hesitancy among Healthcare Workers in Europe: A Systematic Review. *Vaccines* **2023**, *11*, 1657. [CrossRef]
67. Dudley, M.Z.; Halsey, N.A.; Omer, S.B.; Orenstein, W.A.; T O'Leary, S.; Limaye, R.J.; Salmon, D.A. The state of vaccine safety science: Systematic reviews of the evidence. *Lancet Infect. Dis.* **2020**, *20*, e80–e89. [CrossRef]
68. Lip, A.; Pateman, M.; Fullerton, M.M.; Chen, H.M.; Bailey, L.; Houle, S.; Davidson, S.; Constantinescu, C. Vaccine hesitancy educational tools for healthcare providers and trainees: A scoping review. *Vaccine* **2023**, *41*, 23–35. [CrossRef]
69. Suliman, D.M.; Nawaz, F.A.; Mohanan, P.; Modber, M.; Musa, M.K.; Musa, M.B.; El Chbib, D.; Elhadi, Y.A.M.; Essar, M.Y.; Isa, M.A.; et al. UAE efforts in promoting COVID-19 vaccination and building vaccine confidence. *Vaccine* **2021**, *39*, 6341–6345. [CrossRef]
70. Bianchi, F.P.; Stefanizzi, P.; Brescia, N.; Lattanzio, S.; Martinelli, A.; Tafuri, S. COVID-19 vaccination hesitancy in Italian healthcare workers: A systematic review and meta-analysis. *Expert Rev. Vaccines* **2022**, *21*, 1289–1300. [CrossRef]
71. Hall, C.M.; Northam, H.; Webster, A.; Strickland, K. Determinants of seasonal influenza vaccination hesitancy among healthcare personnel: An integrative review. *J. Clin. Nurs.* **2022**, *31*, 2112–2124. [CrossRef]
72. Alalawi, M.; Alsalloum, M.A.; Garwan, Y.M.; Abuzeid, M.; Alalawi, H.; Eljaaly, K.; Thabit, A.K.; Jose, J. COVID-19 vaccine hesitancy among healthcare workers in Arab Countries: A systematic review and meta-analysis. *PLoS ONE* **2024**, *19*, e0296432. [CrossRef]
73. Mollalo, A.; Tatar, M. Spatial Modeling of COVID-19 Vaccine Hesitancy in the United States. *Int. J. Environ. Res. Public Health* **2021**, *18*, 9488. [CrossRef] [PubMed]
74. Moradpour, J.; Shajarizadeh, A.; Carter, J.; Chit, A.; Grootendorst, P. The impact of national income and vaccine hesitancy on country-level COVID-19 vaccine uptake. *PLoS ONE* **2023**, *18*, e0293184. [CrossRef] [PubMed]
75. Schaefer, G.O.; Leland, R.; Emanuel, E.J. Making vaccines available to other countries before offering domestic booster vaccinations. *JAMA* **2021**, *326*, 903–904. [CrossRef]
76. Diseases, T.L.I. COVID-19 vaccine equity and booster doses. *Lancet. Infect. Dis.* **2021**, *21*, 1193. [CrossRef]
77. Tselebis, A.; Sikaras, C.; Milionis, C.; Sideri, E.P.; Fytsilis, K.; Papageorgiou, S.M.; Ilias, I.; Pachi, A. A Moderated Mediation Model of the Influence of Cynical Distrust, Medical Mistrust, and Anger on Vaccination Hesitancy in Nursing Staff. *Eur. J. Investig. Health Psychol. Educ.* **2023**, *13*, 2373–2387. [CrossRef]
78. Galanis, P.; Moisoglou, I.; Vraka, I.; Siskou, O.; Konstantakopoulou, O.; Katsiroumpa, A.; Kaitelidou, D. Predictors of COVID-19 vaccine uptake in healthcare workers: A cross-sectional study in Greece. *J. Occup. Environ. Med.* **2022**, *64*, e191–e196. [CrossRef]
79. Bell, S.; Clarke, R.M.; Ismail, S.A.; Ojo-Aromokudu, O.; Naqvi, H.; Coghill, Y.; Donovan, H.; Letley, L.; Paterson, P.; Mounier-Jack, S. COVID-19 vaccination beliefs, attitudes, and behaviours among health and social care workers in the UK: A mixed-methods study. *PLoS ONE* **2022**, *17*, e0260949. [CrossRef]
80. Kigongo, E.; Kabunga, A.; Tumwesigye, R.; Musinguzi, M.; Izaruku, R.; Acup, W. Prevalence and predictors of COVID-19 vaccination hesitancy among healthcare workers in Sub-Saharan Africa: A systematic review and meta-analysis. *PLoS ONE* **2023**, *18*, e0289295. [CrossRef]
81. Wang, Y.; Liu, Y. Multilevel determinants of COVID-19 vaccination hesitancy in the United States: A rapid systematic review. *Prev. Med. Rep.* **2022**, *25*, 101673. [CrossRef]
82. Bianchi, F.P.; Stefanizzi, P.; Cuscianna, E.; Riformato, G.; Di Lorenzo, A.; Giordano, P.; Germinario, C.A.; Tafuri, S. COVID-19 vaccination hesitancy among Italian parents: A systematic review and meta-analysis. *Hum. Vaccin. Immunother.* **2023**, *19*, 2171185. [CrossRef]
83. Issaris, V.; Kalogerakos, G.; Milas, G.P. Vaccination Hesitancy Among Greek Orthodox Christians: Is There a Conflict Between Religion and Science? *J. Relig. Health* **2023**, *62*, 1373–1378. [CrossRef]
84. Irrgang, P.; Gerling, J.; Kocher, K.; Lapuente, D.; Steininger, P.; Habenicht, K.; Wytopil, M.; Beileke, S.; Schäfer, S.; Zhong, J.; et al. Class switch toward noninflammatory, spike-specific IgG4 antibodies after repeated SARS-CoV-2 mRNA vaccination. *Sci. Immunol.* **2023**, *8*, eade2798. [CrossRef]
85. Uversky, V.N.; Redwan, E.M.; Makis, W.; Rubio-Casillas, A. IgG4 Antibodies Induced by Repeated Vaccination May Generate Immune Tolerance to the SARS-CoV-2 Spike Protein. *Vaccines* **2023**, *11*, 991. [CrossRef]
86. Stowe, J.; Miller, E.; Andrews, N.; Whitaker, H.J. Risk of myocarditis and pericarditis after a COVID-19 mRNA vaccine booster and after COVID-19 in those with and without prior SARS-CoV-2 infection: A self-controlled case series analysis in England. *PLoS Med.* **2023**, *20*, e1004245. [CrossRef]
87. Abraham, N.; Spruin, S.; Rossi, T.; Fireman, B.; Zafack, J.; Blaser, C.; Shaw, A.; Hutchings, K.; Ogunnaike-Cooke, S. Myocarditis and/or pericarditis risk after mRNA COVID-19 vaccination: A Canadian head to head comparison of BNT162b2 and mRNA-1273 vaccines. *Vaccine* **2022**, *40*, 4663–4671. [CrossRef]

88. Jain, N.; Chaudhary, P.; Shrivastava, A.; Kaur, T.; Kaur, S.; Brar, H.S.; Jindal, R. Thrombosis with Thrombocytopenia Syndrome (TTS) After ChAdOx1 nCoV-19 Immunization: An Investigative Case Report. *Am. J. Case Rep.* **2023**, *24*, e938878. [CrossRef]
89. Islam, A.; Bashir, M.S.; Joyce, K.; Rashid, H.; Laher, I.; Elshazly, S. An Update on COVID-19 Vaccine Induced Thrombotic Thrombocytopenia Syndrome and Some Management Recommendations. *Molecules* **2021**, *26*, 5004. [CrossRef]
90. Tran, H.A.; Deng, L.; Wood, N.; Choi, P.; Singleton, S.; Clarke, L.; Khanlari, S.; Maitland-Scott, I.; Bird, R.; Brown, S.; et al. The clinicopathological features of thrombosis with thrombocytopenia syndrome following ChAdOx1-S (AZD1222) vaccination and case outcomes in Australia: A population-based study. *Lancet Reg. Health West. Pac.* **2023**, *40*, 100894. [CrossRef]
91. Lang, A.L.; Hohmuth, N.; Višković, V.; Konigorski, S.; Scholz, S.; Balzer, F.; Remschmidt, C.; Leistner, R. COVID-19 Vaccine Effectiveness and Digital Pandemic Surveillance in Germany (eCOV Study): Web Application-Based Prospective Observational Cohort Study. *J. Med. Internet. Res.* **2024**, *26*, e47070. [CrossRef]
92. Gram, M.A.; Emborg, H.D.; Schelde, A.B.; Friis, N.U.; Nielsen, K.F.; Moustsen-Helms, I.R.; Legarth, R.; Lam, J.U.H.; Chaine, M.; Malik, A.Z.; et al. Vaccine effectiveness against SARS-CoV-2 infection or COVID-19 hospitalization with the Alpha, Delta, or Omicron SARS-CoV-2 variant: A nationwide Danish cohort study. *PLoS Med.* **2022**, *19*, e1003992. [CrossRef] [PubMed]
93. Garrett, M.E.; Galloway, J.G.; Wolf, C.; Logue, J.K.; Franko, N.; Chu, H.Y.; Matsen, F.A.t.; Overbaugh, J.M. Comprehensive characterization of the antibody responses to SARS-CoV-2 Spike protein finds additional vaccine-induced epitopes beyond those for mild infection. *Elife* **2022**, *11*, e73490. [CrossRef] [PubMed]
94. Katz, M.A.; Rojas Castro, M.Y.; Chakhunashvili, G.; Chitadze, N.; Ward, C.L.; McKnight, C.J.; Lucaccioni, H.; Finci, I.; Zardiashvili, T.; Pebody, R.; et al. Primary series COVID-19 vaccine effectiveness among health care workers in the country of Georgia, March–December 2021. *PLoS ONE* **2024**, *19*, e0307805. [CrossRef]
95. Haas, E.J.; Angulo, F.J.; McLaughlin, J.M.; Anis, E.; Singer, S.R.; Khan, F.; Brooks, N.; Smaja, M.; Mircus, G.; Pan, K.; et al. Impact and effectiveness of mRNA BNT162b2 vaccine against SARS-CoV-2 infections and COVID-19 cases, hospitalisations, and deaths following a nationwide vaccination campaign in Israel: An observational study using national surveillance data. *Lancet* **2021**, *397*, 1819–1829. [CrossRef]
96. Haque, A.; Pant, A.B. Mitigating Covid-19 in the face of emerging virus variants, breakthrough infections and vaccine hesitancy. *J. Autoimmun.* **2022**, *127*, 102792. [CrossRef]
97. Graña, C.; Ghosn, L.; Evrenoglou, T.; Jarde, A.; Minozzi, S.; Bergman, H.; Buckley, B.S.; Probyn, K.; Villanueva, G.; Henschke, N.; et al. Efficacy and safety of COVID-19 vaccines. *Cochrane Database Syst. Rev.* **2022**, *12*, Cd015477. [CrossRef]
98. De Waele, A.; Hendrickx, G.; Valckx, S.; Domínguez, À.; Toledo, D.; Castilla, J.; Tuells, J.; Van Damme, P. The Vaccine Training Barometer: Assessing healthcare providers' confidence to answer vaccine-related questions and their training needs. *Vaccine* **2024**, *42*, 2421–2428. [CrossRef]
99. Paterson, P.; Meurice, F.; Stanberry, L.R.; Glismann, S.; Rosenthal, S.L.; Larson, H.J. Vaccine hesitancy and healthcare providers. *Vaccine* **2016**, *34*, 6700–6706. [CrossRef]
100. Moghnieh, R.; Haddad, W.; Jbeily, N.; El-Hassan, S.; Eid, S.; Baba, H.; Sily, M.; Saber, Y.; Abdallah, D.; Bizri, A.R.; et al. Immunogenicity and real-world effectiveness of COVID-19 vaccines in Lebanon: Insights from primary and booster schemes, variants, infections, and hospitalization. *PLoS ONE* **2024**, *19*, e0306457. [CrossRef]
101. Barosa, M.; Ioannidis, J.P.A.; Prasad, V. Evidence base for yearly respiratory virus vaccines: Current status and proposed improved strategies. *Eur. J. Clin. Investig.* **2024**, *54*, e14286. [CrossRef] [PubMed]
102. Nusbaum, N.J. The COVID Vaccination Hesitancy Epidemic. *J. Community Health* **2024**, *49*, 377–378. [CrossRef]
103. Diekema, D.S. Responding to parental refusals of immunization of children. *Pediatrics* **2005**, *115*, 1428–1431. [CrossRef]
104. Alya, W.A.; Maraqa, B.; Nazzal, Z.; Odeh, M.; Makhalfa, R.; Nassif, A.; Aabed, M. COVID-19 vaccine uptake and its associated factors among Palestinian healthcare workers: Expectations beaten by reality. *Vaccine* **2022**, *40*, 3713–3719. [CrossRef]
105. Zintel, S.; Flock, C.; Arbogast, A.L.; Forster, A.; von Wagner, C.; Sieverding, M. Gender differences in the intention to get vaccinated against COVID-19: A systematic review and meta-analysis. *J. Public Health* **2023**, *31*, 1303–1327. [CrossRef]
106. Nachtigall, I.; Bonsignore, M.; Hohenstein, S.; Bollmann, A.; Günther, R.; Kodde, C.; Englisch, M.; Ahmad-Nejad, P.; Schröder, A.; Glenz, C.; et al. Effect of gender, age and vaccine on reactogenicity and incapacity to work after COVID-19 vaccination: A survey among health care workers. *BMC Infect. Dis.* **2022**, *22*, 291. [CrossRef]
107. Di Resta, C.; Ferrari, D.; Viganò, M.; Moro, M.; Sabetta, E.; Minerva, M.; Ambrosio, A.; Locatelli, M.; Tomaiuolo, R. The Gender Impact Assessment among Healthcare Workers in the SARS-CoV-2 Vaccination—An Analysis of Serological Response and Side Effects. *Vaccines* **2021**, *9*, 522. [CrossRef] [PubMed]
108. Sallam, M.; Dababseh, D.; Eid, H.; Al-Mahzoum, K.; Al-Haidar, A.; Taim, D.; Yaseen, A.; Ababneh, N.A.; Bakri, F.G.; Mahafzah, A. High rates of COVID-19 vaccine hesitancy and its association with conspiracy beliefs: A study in Jordan and Kuwait among other Arab countries. *Vaccines* **2021**, *9*, 42. [CrossRef]
109. She, J.; Hou, D.; Chen, C.; Bi, J.; Song, Y. Challenges of vaccination and herd immunity in COVID-19 and management strategies. *Clin. Respir. J.* **2022**, *16*, 708–716. [CrossRef]
110. Dassarma, B.; Tripathy, S.; Chabalala, M.; Matsabisa, M.G. Challenges in Establishing Vaccine Induced Herd Immunity through Age Specific Community Vaccinations. *Aging Dis.* **2022**, *13*, 29–36. [CrossRef]
111. Goldberg, A.R.; Langwig, K.E.; Brown, K.L.; Marano, J.M.; Rai, P.; King, K.M.; Sharp, A.K.; Ceci, A.; Kailing, C.D.; Kailing, M.J.; et al. Widespread exposure to SARS-CoV-2 in wildlife communities. *Nat. Commun.* **2024**, *15*, 6210. [CrossRef]

112. Delahay, R.J.; de la Fuente, J.; Smith, G.C.; Sharun, K.; Snary, E.L.; Flores Girón, L.; Nziza, J.; Fooks, A.R.; Brookes, S.M.; Lean, F.Z.X.; et al. Assessing the risks of SARS-CoV-2 in wildlife. *One Health Outlook* **2021**, *3*, 7. [CrossRef]
113. Valencak, T.G.; Csiszar, A.; Szalai, G.; Podlutsky, A.; Tarantini, S.; Fazekas-Pongor, V.; Papp, M.; Ungvari, Z. Animal reservoirs of SARS-CoV-2: Calculable COVID-19 risk for older adults from animal to human transmission. *Geroscience* **2021**, *43*, 2305–2320. [CrossRef]
114. Shaheen, M.N.F. The concept of one health applied to the problem of zoonotic diseases. *Rev. Med. Virol.* **2022**, *32*, e2326. [CrossRef]

vaccines

Article

Acceptance of the COVID-19 Vaccine by Prisoners and Staff in Spanish Prisons

Nancy Vicente-Alcalde [1,*], Sorina Madalina Sferle [2], Carlos Franco-Paredes [3] and José Tuells [4]

1 Penitentiary Center Alicante II, Carretera N-330, Km. 66, 03400 Villena, Spain
2 Instituto Universitario de Matemática Multidisciplinar, Universitat Politècnica de València, Camino de Vera, s/n, 46022 Valencia, Spain; smsferle@doctor.upv.es
3 Department of Microbiology, Immunology and Pathology, Children's Hospital of Mexico Federico Gomez, Dr. Márquez 162, Ciudad de Mexico 06720, Mexico; carlos.franco.paredes@gmail.com
4 Department of Community Nursing, Preventive Medicine and Public Health and History of Science, University of Alicante, San Vicente del Raspeig, 03690 Alicante, Spain; tuells@ua.es
* Correspondence: nanvical@gmail.com

Abstract: The COVID-19 vaccination of prisoners and prison staff represents a public health intervention to reduce the impact of the pandemic in conglomerate settings. In Spanish prisons, the road map of the Ministry of Health was followed to protect the population at risk. We conducted a cross-sectional study to assess the acceptance of COVID-19 vaccination by prisoners and prison staff in a prison in Alicante, Spain. We analyzed data obtained through a standardized, self-administered, and anonymous questionnaire; 1016 prisoners and 288 prison staff responded to the survey. The majority of inmates and staff reported no history of symptomatic COVID-19, 90.15% and 91.66%, respectively. Respondents reported that 88.72% agreed to be vaccinated and 89.64% would recommend the vaccine to others. Approximately 89% believe that the benefit of getting vaccinated against COVID-19 is greater than the risk, and 70.55% reported that vaccination should be mandatory for inmates and staff to participate in some activities. The acceptance of COVID-19 vaccination among prisoners and prison staff is high in a Provincial Prison in Spain. Elevated acceptance of COVID-19 vaccination in prisons is a major factor in public health intervention and vaccine equity.

Keywords: COVID-19; vaccine; acceptance; prisons; public health

1. Introduction

Prisons are dynamic ecological environments in which prisoners, staff, officers, and visitors transit daily between the prison and the larger community [1]. Incarcerated individuals live in confined spaces, often with poor ventilation and overcrowding. These factors are conducive to the spread and amplification of infectious diseases inside and outside prisons, making carceral settings more vulnerable to outbreaks of coronavirus disease (COVID-19) [2,3]. The Ministry of Health in Spain paid close attention to the COVID-19 pandemic by establishing guidelines to address the vulnerability of prisoners and prison staff [4–6]. As a result, the COVID-19 vaccination of prisoners and prison staff was considered a crucial public health intervention [6–9].

Vaccination coverage against COVID-19 in prisons (incarcerated individuals and staff) in certain countries reached levels similar to that of the general population even during periods of limited vaccine supply [10–12]. However, globally, there is evidence that vaccination against COVID-19 among inmates and prison staff was not considered a public health priority [10–12].

Vaccination in Spanish prisons began in April 2021 [13], responding to the national strategy to deploy the COVID-19 vaccination to high-risk populations [14] and following the World Health Organization (WHO) vaccination against COVID-19 guidelines [15]. COVID-19 vaccination in Spain was offered on a voluntary basis [16]. During the initial deployment of the COVID-19 vaccination, the prison population in Spain amounted to more than 51,000 people and the number of workers laboring inside penitentiary institutions was 28,460, corresponding to a ratio of 1.9 prisoner/worker, which places Spain above the European average for this proportion [17,18].

The availability and wide deployment of a newly introduced vaccine to protect against a life-threatening infection does not imply an immediate acceptance of vaccination by the general population. According to the 5Cs model, vaccine acceptability is contingent upon trust, risk perception, information-seeking behavior, and the willingness to protect others [19]. The effect described as "Pandemic Public Health Paradox" associates the acceptance of a vaccine with the influence of the media rather than with the epidemiological dynamics of the disease [20]. Indeed, there are different factors that can pose an obstacle to vaccine acceptance, including ease of access to reach vaccination sites, geographical location, accessibility, availability, health system factors, and the affordability of vaccines, as well as cultural, psychological, emotional, cognitive, social, and political factors [21].

The objective of this study was to ascertain the level of acceptance of vaccination against COVID-19 in Spanish prisoners and prison workers.

2. Materials and Methods

2.1. Design and Participants

We conducted a cross-sectional study to assess the degree of COVID-19 vaccine acceptance in prisoners of the Alicante II-Villena Penitentiary Center and Spanish prison workers. The exclusion criteria were refusal to participate in the study or answering the survey inappropriately or with information not requested for the study.

2.2. Tools

We used a self-administered, anonymous, and standardized questionnaire to evaluate the acceptance of the COVID-19 vaccine in prisoners and prison staff. The questionnaire, designed "Ad hoc" for this project, consisted of a total of 36 questions, including sociodemographic variables, some of them posed with multiple answers and others on a nominal scale. Its structure was divided into three sections: (i) baseline socio-demographic questionnaire (sex, age, origin, marital status, number of children) and personal health variables (items 1 to 5: suffering from chronic disease, smoking, alcohol, psychotropic drugs); (ii) COVID-19 variables (items 6 to 16: suffering from COVID-19 disease, contagion in a prison environment, need for quarantine, death of a family member or friend due to COVID-19, PCR performance, PCR results); (iii) acceptance of the COVID-19 vaccine (items 17 to 36: vaccination, previous influenza vaccination, adverse effects of vaccination, confidence in the recommendations of the health authorities, reasons for acceptance or rejection of the vaccine). We developed the questions in this survey based on a review of the medical literature and approval by consensus from all researchers.

2.3. Study

At the time of the study, the Alicante II Penitentiary Center had 1037 prisoners and 312 workers. We included 1304 participants (1016 (98%) prisoners and 288 (92.3%) workers) who responded to a voluntarily self-administered survey during the months of April to June 2021. To use an appropriate sampling frame, it was decided to recruit participants through the prison health team, providing them with information about the project, requests to participate by obtaining an informed consent, and the actual survey.

All prisoners and prison staff who showed a willingness to participate and who met the inclusion criteria were included. Sample selection was carried out in a "non-probabilistic" manner, using convenience sampling.

2.4. Statistical Analysis

We conducted a descriptive univariate analysis on all the variables. For categorical variables we calculated frequencies and percentages, and continuous variables, such as age, were categorized by age group. We also carried out a descriptive bivariate analysis. For pairs of categorical variables, we generated contingency tables and calculated the corresponding column percentages. In such cases, we employed the Chi-squared test to assess the association between these variables. To assess factors influencing the response to questions related to COVID-19 vaccine acceptance, logistic regression analysis was performed for cases in which the response variable had two categories and multinomial logistic regression analysis for those with more than two categories. To determine whether each predictor variable has a statistically significant effect on the response variable, we obtained *p*-values using the Wald test. We exponentiated the coefficients to better interpret the results obtained, thus providing odds ratios (OR) for the logistic model and relative risk ratios (RRR) for the multinomial model, with their respective 95% confidence intervals (CI95%). Before performing these analyses, we determined whether there was an association or dependence between the categorical variables using the chi-squared test or Fisher's exact test, when the sample size of the resulting contingency tables was small. We set the significance level at $\alpha = 0.05$. All analyses were performed using RStudio, specifically version 4.0.2 of the open-source software.

2.5. Ethical Considerations

The study was approved by the General Secretary of Penitentiary Institutions, Subdirectorate General of Institutional Relations and Territorial Coordination (number 395714). Participation in the survey was conducted anonymously and voluntarily, and the analysis of the questionnaire was completely confidential, ensuring the privacy of the data of all respondents. For this study, we followed the ethical principles for medical research involving human subjects set out in the Declaration of Helsinki and EU Regulation 134 2016/679 (GDPR) regarding the processing of personal data.

3. Results

3.1. Population Description

We analyzed data obtained from 1304 surveys, of which 1016 were from incarcerated individuals. Of these, most were Spanish citizens (92.61%), and most were men (89.96%), married (59.84%), had children (70.37%), and were between 40 and 60 years of age (45.67%). Approximately 98% of prisoners in the Alicante Penitentiary participated in the survey. Just over half of the prisoners said they were not suffering from any chronic medical disease (65.45%), most were smokers (75%), and most did not consume alcohol (78.24%) (Table 1). However, 33.27% reported the active use of psychotropic drugs. Almost all prison staff who responded to the survey were Spanish citizens (99.31%), 51.04% were men, 44% were married, 61.8% had children, and the ages ranged from 40 to 60 years old (71.88%). From the *p*-values obtained using the chi-squared test, we can conclude that there was a relationship between each of the categorical variables (those shown in the first column) and the response variable composed of the prisoners and prison staff categories. In other words, the test indicates that demographic characteristics are associated with differences in professionalism among participants.

3.2. Variables Related to COVID-19 Disease

At the time of conducting the study, a high percentage of participants had not suffered from symptomatic COVID-19 infection (90.15% of prisoners and 91.66% of workers) (Table 2). However, 69.68% of prisoners had been placed in quarantine due to close contact with a confirmed case and 18.89% reported the death of a family member or friend due to COVID-19. Approximately 67.42% had to undergo PCR testing or antigen testing to detect SARS-CoV-2. Results were negative in 85.40% of tests performed. Just 32.48% of prisoners reported limiting their contacts or social relationships with others during the pandemic.

Table 1. Demographic characteristics (n = 1304).

	Prisoners *n* (%)	**Prison Staff** *n* (%)	***p*-Value**	**Total** *n* (%)
	1016 (77.91)	288 (22.08)		1304 (100)
Sex			<0.001	
Male	914 (89.96)	147 (51.04)		1061 (81.36)
Female	102 (10.03)	141 (48.95)		243 (18.63)
Nationality			<0.001	
Spanish	941 (92.61)	286 (99.31)		1227 (94.10)
Non-Spanish	75 (7.38)	2 (0.69)		77 (5.9)
Cohabitation			<0.001	
Only	408 (40.15)	69 (23.95)		477 (36.57)
As a couple	608 (59.84)	219 (44.4)		827 (63.42)
Age (years)			<0.001	
18–<40	455 (44.78)	76 (26.38)		531 (40.72)
40–<60	464 (45.67)	207 (71.88)		671 (51.46)
>60	97 (9.55)	5 (1.74)		102 (7.82)
Children			0.007126	
No	301 (29.62)	110 (38.19)		411 (31.52)
Yes	715 (70.37)	178 (61.8)		893 (68.48)
Chronic disease			<0.001	
No	665 (65.45)	233 (80.90)		898 (68.86)
Yes	351 (34.54)	55 (19.09)		406 (31.13)
Tobacco use			<0.001	
No	254 (25.0)	272 (94.44)		526 (40.34)
Yes	762 (75.0)	16 (5.55)		778 (59.66)
Alcohol use			<0.001	
No	795 (78.24)	282 (97.91)		1077 (82.59)
Yes	221 (21.75)	6 (2.1)		227 (17.41)
Use of psychotropic drugs			<0.001	
No	678 (66.73)	285 (98.96)		963 (73.85)
Yes	338 (33.27)	3 (1.04)		341 (26.15)

Among prison staff, 24.30% had been placed in quarantine due to contact with a confirmed case and 18.40% reported the death of a family member or friend due to COVID-19. Over half of the survey respondents (52.08%) underwent PCR testing or antigen testing to detect SARS-CoV-2. Results were negative in 92% of tests performed. Almost all prison staff (98.95%) reported limiting their social interactions during the pandemic.

With respect to the *p*-values, we observed that having or not having COVID-19 disease (0.5113), and whether or not an acquaintance had died from this infectious disease (0.9169), was not related to the response variable. In practical terms, this means that there is no statistically significant association between having had COVID-19 or having an acquaintance who died and professionalism among inmates and prison staff. However, the variables related to having undergone quarantine (<0.001), having taken a diagnostic test (<0.001) and having reduced social interactions (<0.001) were related to the response variable. Therefore, these do depend on whether one is a prisoner or prison staff; for example, with respect to the last variable there is a clear difference in that prisoners are negligent in continuing to have social contact.

Table 2. COVID-19 disease in prisoners and workers surveyed (n = 1304).

	Prisoners n (%)	Prison Staff n (%)	p-Value	Total n (%)
	1016 (77.91)	288 (22.08)		1304 (100)
Have you had COVID-19 disease?				
Yes	100 (9.84)	24 (8.33)	0.5113	124 (9.5)
No	916 (90.15)	264 (91.66)		1180 (90.5)
Have you had to quarantine for contact with a COVID-19 case?				
Yes	708 (69.68)	70 (24.30)	<0.001	778 (59.66)
No	308 (30.31)	218 (75.69)		526 (40.33)
Has a family member or friend died from COVID-19?				
Yes	192 (18.89)	53 (18.40)	0.9169	245 (18.78)
No	824 (81.10)	235 (81.59)		1059 (81.21)
Have you had any diagnostic tests, antigen tests or PCRs to detect SARS-CoV-2 at any time during this pandemic?				
Yes	685 (67.42)	150 (52.08)	<0.001	835 (64.03)
No	331 (32.57)	138 (47.91)		469 (35.96)
What were the results of the antigen test or PCR test to detect SARS-CoV-2?				
Positive	100 (14.59)	12 (8)	0.04384	112 (13.41)
Negative	585 (85.40)	138 (92)		723 (86.58)
Have you reduced your social interactions (visits, contacts with other groups, etc.) during the pandemic?				
Yes	330 (32.48)	285 (98.95)	<0.001	615 (47.16)
No	686 (67.51)	3 (1.05)		689 (52.84)

3.3. *Variables Related to COVID-19 Vaccine Acceptance and Attitude towards Vaccination*

As depicted in Table 3, 88.72% of the prisoners and prison staff who responded to the survey reported that they would accept COVID-19 vaccination, and 89.64% would recommend the vaccine to others. However, recommending the vaccine to children was reported only by 67.71% of study participants. Approximately 89% believe that the benefit of undergoing COVID-19 vaccination is greater than the risk, and 70.55% reported that vaccination should be mandatory for prisoners and staff to participate in some activities. It is important to note that vaccine acceptance for the seasonal influenza vaccine during the 2019–2020 season was low, resulting in 86.71 prisoners and 44.44% prison staff not receiving the influenza vaccination.

Most prisoners who were vaccinated (97.24%) received Jcovden® and prison staff who were vaccinated (88.89%) received mostly Vaxzervria®.

We can see that all questions were associated with the response variable, since the p-values were below the significance level (p-values < 0.05). All of these significant values collectively point to the fact that there are pronounced differences between inmates and prison staff in their attitudes and behaviors related to COVID-19 vaccines.

3.4. *Relative Risk Ratios from the Multinomial Logistic Regression Model and Odds Ratios from the Logistic Regression Model by Age, Sex and Comorbidity*

Important factors to evaluate for our study are sex, gender and comorbidity. We can see that in most cases all three are related to the questions based on COVID-19 vaccine acceptance. For a more comprehensive interpretation of these relationships, we focused on the RRRs and ORs of those statistically significant cases, i.e., when the p-values were less than 0.05 (Table 4).

Table 3. COVID-19 vaccine acceptance and attitude toward vaccination (n = 1304).

	Prisoners *n* (%)	Prison Staff *n* (%)	*p*-Value	Total *n* (%)
	1016 (77.91)	288 (22.08)		1304 (100)
If the COVID-19 vaccine were available to you, would you get vaccinated?				
Yes	885 (87.10)	272 (94.44)	<0.001	1157 (88.72)
No	117 (11.51)	4 (1.38)		121 (9.2)
I would wait a few more months	6 (0.59)	7 (2.43)		13 (0.99)
I would wait for others to try it before	8 (0.78)	5 (1.73)		13 (0.99)
Would you vaccinate your children when the COVID-19 vaccine is available for them?				
Yes	659 (64.86)	224 (77.77)	<0.001	883 (67.71)
No	106 (10.43)	23 (7.98)		129 (9.89)
I would wait a few more months	92 (9.05)	25 (8.68)		117 (8.97)
I would wait for others to try it before	159 (15.65)	16 (5.55)		175 (13.42)
Would you recommend the COVID-19 vaccine?				
Yes	891 (87.70)	278 (96.53)	<0.001	1169 (89.64)
No	125 (12.30)	10 (3.47)		135 (10.35)
Do you think the benefit of getting vaccinated outweighs that of not getting vaccinated?				
Yes	879 (86.52)	278 (96.53)	<0.001	1157 (88.73)
No	137 (13.48)	10 (3.47)		147 (11.27)
Would it seem appropriate to be required to be vaccinated for certain activities?				
Yes	711 (69.98)	209 (72.57)	0.4368	920 (70.55)
No	305 (30.02)	79 (27.43)		384 (29.45)
Did you get the flu vaccine during the 2019–2020 vaccination campaign?				
Yes	135 (13.29)	160 (55.56)	<0.001	295 (22.62)
No	881 (86.71)	128 (44.44)		1009 (77.38)
Have you received the COVID-19 vaccine?				
Yes	988 (97.24)	256 (88.89)	<0.001	1244 (95.39)
No	28 (2.76)	32 (11.11)		60 (4.61)
If you have received it, what vaccine did you receive?				
Pfizer/BioNTech Comirnaty®	91 (9.21)	66 (25.78)	<0.001	157 (12.62)
Spikevax® by Moderna	12 (1.21)	38 (14.84)		50 (4.01)
Vaxzevria® by AstraZeneca	86 (8.70)	151 (58.98)		237 (19.05)
Jcovden® Janssen	799 (80.87)	1 (0.39)		800 (64.30)

Males were 67% less likely to choose "yes" (getting vaccinated) compared to females. The p-value (p = 0.0015) indicates that the difference is statistically significant, so there is strong evidence that being male is associated with a lower probability of choosing to be vaccinated.

The extreme values associated with the ">60" category of the age variable were due to the presence of zero cell counts, since all participants in this category responded affirmatively, which caused calculation problems.

Being in the "40–<60" age group did not significantly affect the likelihood of choosing to be vaccinated or waiting a few more months; however, individuals aged over 60 were more likely to choose "yes" compared to those in the "18–<40" age group.

Individuals with a chronic disease were 1.86 times more likely to be willing to be vaccinated than those without a chronic disease, where the p-value = 0.008 indicates that the association between having a chronic disease and being willing to be vaccinated is statistically significant. Having chronic diseases appears to be associated with an increased likelihood of answering "yes" to all questions related to COVID-19 vaccine acceptance, except in the case of agreeing that it would seem appropriate to be required to be vaccinated for certain activities, where the difference may not be statistically significant (p-value = 0.06).

Table 4. Relative risk ratios from the multinomial logistic regression model and odds ratios from the logistic regression model.

Questions Related to COVID-19 Vaccine Acceptance									***p*-Value**
If the COVID-19 Vaccine Were Available to You, Would You Get Vaccinated?									
		No	**Yes**		**I would wait a few more months**		**I would wait for others to try it before**		
			RRR (CI95%)	***p*-value**	**RRR (CI95%)**	***p*-value**	**RRR (CI95%)**	***p*-value**	
Sex	Female	Ref.	Ref.		Ref.		Ref.		0.0031
	Male	Ref.	0.33 (0.16–0.65)	0.0015	0.27 (0.06–1.15)	0.077	0.44 (0.08–2.31)	0.333	
Age	18–<40	Ref.	Ref.		Ref.		Ref.		<0.001
	40–<60	Ref.	1.31 (0.89–1.89)	0.17	0.44 (0.18–1.49)	0.19	0.61 (0.19–1.98)	0.41	
	>60	Ref.	8.73×10^{13}	0.00	7.2×10^{-5}	NaN	7.2×10^{-5}	0.00	
Chronic disease	No	Ref.	Ref.		Ref.		Ref.		0.0015
	Yes	Ref.	1.86 (1.18–2.94)	0.008	4.2×10^{-13}	0.00	1.15 (0.29–4.51)	0.84	
Would you vaccinate your children when the COVID-19 vaccine is available for them?									
		No	**Yes**		**I would wait a few more months**		**I would wait for others to try it before**		
			RRR (CI95%)	***p*-value**	**RRR (CI95%)**	***p*-value**	**RRR (CI95%)**	***p*-value**	
Sex	Female	Ref.	Ref.		Ref.		Ref.		<0.001
	Male	Ref.	0.83 (0.49–1.39)	0.48	0.21 (0.11–0.38)	<0.001	1.42 (0.72–2.8)	0.32	
Age	18–<40	Ref.	Ref.		Ref.		Ref.		<0.001
	40–<60	Ref.	1.28 (0.88–1.88)	0.19	0.29 (0.17–0.5)	<0.001	0.48 (0.3–0.7)	0.002	
	>60	Ref.	7928.78 (6.1×10^{-14}–1.1×10^{21})	0.66	0.28 (2.3×10^{-32}–3.41×10^{30})	0.97	0.38 (1.9×10^{-27}–7.5×10^{25})	0.97	
Chronic disease	No	Ref.	Ref.		Ref.		Ref.		<0.001
	Yes	Ref.	2.89 (1.77–4.71)	<0.001	1.19 (0.61–2.3)	0.6	1.78 (0.99–3.17)	0.05	

Table 4. *Cont.*

Questions Related to COVID-19 Vaccine Acceptance					***p*-Value**
Would you recommend the COVID-19 vaccine?					
		No	**Yes**		
			OR (CI95%)	***p*-value**	
Sex	Female	Ref.	Ref.		0.0014
	Male	Ref.	0.36 (0.18–0.65)	0.0015	
Age	18–<40	Ref.	Ref.		<0.001
	40–<60	Ref.	1.42 (0.98–2.03)	0.06	
	>60	Ref.	6.5×10^6	0.97	
Chronic disease	No	Ref.	Ref.		0.0043
	Yes	Ref.	1.92 (1.26–3.03)	0.0036	
Do you think the benefit of getting vaccinated outweighs that of not getting vaccinated?					
		No	**Yes**		
			OR (CI95%)	***p*-value**	
Sex	Female	Ref.	Ref.		<0.001
	Male	Ref.	0.36 (0.18–0.63)	<0.001	
Age	18–<40	Ref.	Ref.		<0.001
	40–<60	Ref.	1.76 (1.24–2.5)	0.0015	
	>60	Ref.	7.88×10^6	0.97	
Chronic disease	No	Ref.	Ref.		<0.001
	Yes	Ref.	2.16 (1.42–3.41)	<0.001	
Would it seem appropriate to be required to be vaccinated for certain activities?					
		No	**Yes**		
			OR (CI95%)	***p*-value**	
Sex	Female	Ref.	Ref.		0.042
	Male	Ref.	0.71 (0.51–0.97)	0.035	
Age	18–<40	Ref.	Ref.		<0.001
	40–<60	Ref.	0.82 (0.64–1.04)	0.1	
	>60	Ref.	6.54 (3.04–17.02)	<0.001	

Table 4. *Cont.*

Questions Related to COVID-19 Vaccine Acceptance					***p*-Value**
Chronic disease	No	Ref.	Ref.		0.06
	Yes	Ref.	1.3 (0.99–1.68)	0.06	
Did you get the flu vaccine during the 2019–2020 vaccination campaign?					
		No	**Yes**		
			OR (CI95%)	***p*-value**	
Sex	Female	Ref.	Ref.		<0.001
	Male	Ref.	0.42 (0.31–0.56)	<0.001	
Age	18–<40	Ref.	Ref.		<0.001
	40–<60	Ref.	2.8 (2.04–3.88)	<0.001	
	>60	Ref.	12.4 (7.71–20.21)	<0.001	
Chronic disease	No	Ref.	Ref.		<0.001
	Yes	Ref.	3.04 (2.33–3.98)	<0.001	

There was no statistical difference in the willingness to vaccinate their children between males and females; however, there were statistically significant differences in preferences for waiting periods, since males were significantly less likely (0.21 times and p-value < 0.001) to prefer waiting a few more months compared to females.

Age appeared to be significantly associated with preferences regarding waiting times for vaccination among children. Individuals aged "40–<60" were significantly less likely to prefer waiting a few more months (0.29 times and p-value < 0.001) or waiting for others to try the vaccine (0.48 times and p-values = 0.002) before vaccinating their children compared to those aged "18–<40". However, the age group ">60" showed no significant differences in these preferences compared to the "18–<40" group.

The OR = 0.36 with p-value = 0.0015 suggests that gender had a significant influence on the recommendation of the COVID-19 vaccine, with females being more likely to recommend it than males.

The analysis suggests that gender is strongly associated (p-value < 0.001) with the perception of the benefit of COVID-19 vaccination. Females were more likely to believe that being vaccinated is beneficial. The OR = 0.71 (p-value = 0.035) indicates that gender appears to have a significant effect on the perception of whether vaccination should be required for certain activities, with males being less likely to agree with such a requirement compared to females.

Individuals in the "40–<60" age group were more likely, compared to those in the "18–< 40" age group, to hold the belief that the benefits of vaccination outweigh those of not vaccinating, as indicated by the OR of 1.76 (p-value = 0.0015). The odds of agreeing that it would seem appropriate to be required to be vaccinated for certain activities were 6.54 times the odds for the "18–<40" age group. However, the difference in the "40–<60" age group may not be statistically significant.

Finally, being female, being in the "40–<60" or ">60" age groups, and having a chronic disease were associated with higher odds of having received the flu vaccine during the 2019–2020 vaccination campaign. These associations were statistically significant.

3.5. Reasons for COVID-19 Vaccines Acceptance or Refusal

The reasons for the acceptance or rejection of the COVID-19 vaccine are shown in Figure 1. The main reasons for accepting a COVID-19 vaccine were associated with individual protection against the disease. Likewise, the reasons for acceptance referred to by most prisoners and workers were: (1) Protection of oneself. (2) The benefits of vaccines. (3) Return to normal. (4) For work reasons or protection towards the family. Regarding prisoners, self-protection and a return to normality predominated over the benefits of the vaccine and work or family protection reasons. On the other hand, in the case of prison staff, the majority reported accepting COVID-19 vaccination for all four stated reasons and benefits.

3.6. Beliefs and Occurrence of Adverse Effects after the Administration of the COVID-19 Vaccine

Table 5 shows that both prisoners (83.17%) and prison staff (66.67%) reported that COVID-19 vaccination is not associated with more adverse effects than other vaccines, but on the contrary, they believed that there were unknown adverse effects (71.06% prisoners and 57.99% prison staff). Approximately 61.11% reported that the accelerated pace of vaccine production had no effect in reducing its safety and 81.82% reported to trust recommendations made by public health authorities. Regarding the adverse effects suffered by the administration of the vaccine, 56.11% reported having suffered them, with prison staff reporting a higher frequency than prisoners; 69.92% and 52.53%, respectively. The most frequent adverse effects reported were pain at the injection site (69.91%), generalized muscle aches (59.45%) and chills (57.59%). In addition, the column associated with the p-values suggests that there was a statistically significant association between each variable (questions) and the response variable. This result implies that the groups (prisoners and prison staff) do not have the same views about adverse effects following the COVID-19 vaccination.

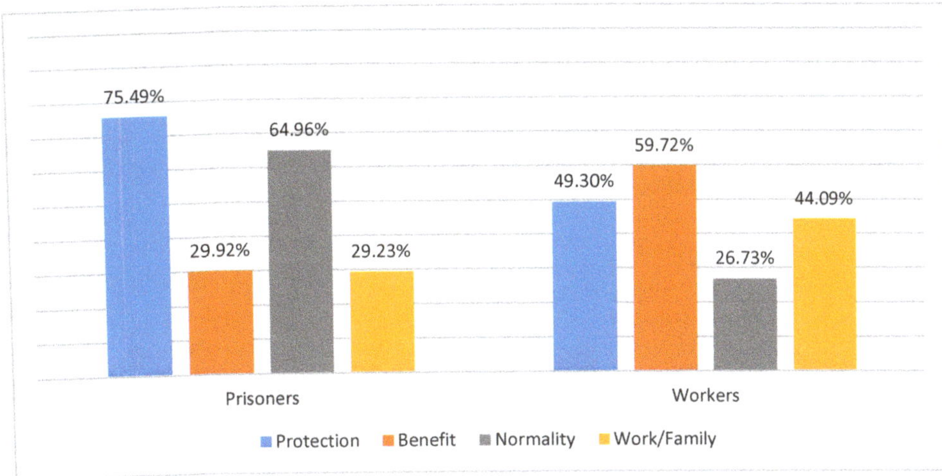

Figure 1. Acceptance of COVID-19 vaccines in prisoners and prison staff of the Alicante II Penitentiary Center.

Table 5. Beliefs and occurrence of adverse effects following COVID-19 vaccine.

	Prisoners *n* (%)	Prison Staff *n* (%)	*p*-Value	Total *n* (%)
	1016 (77.91)	288 (22.08)		1304 (100)
Do they produce more adverse effects than other vaccines?				
Yes	171 (16.83)	96 (33.33)	<0.001	267 (20.47)
No	845 (83.17)	192 (66.67)		1037 (79.52)
Are there any unknown adverse effects from the COVID-19 vaccine?				
Yes	722 (71.06)	167 (57.99)	<0.001	889 (68.17)
No	294 (28.94)	121 (42.01)		415 (31.82)
Does the accelerated pace of vaccine production reduce its safety?				
Yes	376 (37.01)	131 (45.49)	0.01119	507 (38.88)
No	640 (62.99)	157 (54.51)		797 (61.11)
Do you trust the recommendations of the health authorities?				
Yes	817 (80.41)	250 (86.81)	0.01656	1067 (81.82)
No	199 (19.59)	38 (13.19)		237 (18.17)
After vaccination, have you experienced adverse effects? (*n* = 1244)				
Yes	519 (52.53)	179 (69.92)	<0.001	698 (56.11)
No	469 (47.47)	77 (30.08)		546 (43.89)
Which side effects have you experienced? (*n* = 698)				
Pain site of administration	350 (67.43)	138 (77.09)	<0.001	488 (69.91)
Fatigue	270 (52.02)	119 (66.48)		389 (55.73)
Fever	165 (31.79)	97 (54.10)		262 (37.53)
Generalized muscle aches	304 (58.57)	111 (62.01)		415 (59.45)
Headache	279 (53.75)	88 (49.16)		367 (52.57)
Chills	303 (58.38)	99 (55.30)		402 (57.59)
Inflammation	11 (2.11)	13 (7.26)		24 (3.43)
Vomiting	17 (3.2)	6 (3.35)		23 (3.29)

4. Discussion

The COVID-19 pandemic substantially impacted congregate facilities such as jails and prisons. Correctional facilities concentrate large populations of incarcerated individuals, and many of them have underlying chronic medical conditions that predispose them to negative clinical outcomes during outbreaks of highly transmissible infectious pathogens. As such, it is crucial to implement interventions to reduce the impact of infectious outbreaks among prison staff and incarcerated individuals from a medical and public health perspective. In this regard, vaccination against COVID-19 offers the possibility to reduce medical complications associated with SARS-CoV-2 infections for incarcerated individuals and staff working in correctional facilities.

To our knowledge, this study is the first conducted on the acceptance of the COVID-19 vaccine among incarcerated individuals and prison staff in Spanish prisons. Most reports are from the United States, the country with the highest number of incarcerated individuals worldwide. Our results are similar to those reported in other carceral settings [5,11,12,22–24]. According to studies conducted in carceral settings in the U.S. the incidence of COVID-19 infections in prisons was identified in some jails and prisons to be 5.5 times higher than in the community [4,25,26]. Prior to the start of the COVID-19 vaccination campaign in prisons, the pandemic forced the adoption of a series of restrictive measures to prevent infections in prisons [27]. However, there is evidence to suggest that, in the prison settings, with the implementation of COVID-19 vaccinations, the number of cases and fatalities due to COVID-19 were reduced substantially, demonstrating the effectiveness of COVID-19 vaccination in incarcerated individuals and prison staff [22,27].

Ismail, N et al. in their review study concluded that conducting more empirical research on the acceptability of COVID-19 vaccination would help to reduce the impact of COVID-19 on the prison population, prevent community transmission, improve vaccine acceptance in prisons, encourage political accountability and inform future decision-making [10].

Our study highlights the high acceptance of COVID-19 vaccination by Spanish prisoners and prison staff, which almost reached the levels of vaccination coverage in the general population, as it has been reported in the United Kingdom and Wales [28]. Among prisons in Catalonia, full vaccination against COVID-19 was achieved in 72.9% of their prison populations, in contrast to that achieved in Alicante, of 95.39%. There was a variability of COVID-19 vaccination acceptance, leading to highly susceptible populations being unprotected in other settings. For example, studies carried out in jails and prisons in the United States show lower vaccine acceptance, similar to the overall low vaccination acceptance in the larger community [11,12,22,24,29].

Our study shows that at the time of administration of the COVID-19 vaccine, acceptance was higher than that reported by prisoners initially. Other studies have shown that among prisoners who initially declined the first dose of the vaccine, a significant fraction accepted it when it was reoffered, so vaccine hesitancy is not permanent [11,22,24]. According to our study, one of the main reasons for accepting the COVID-19 vaccine among Spanish prisoners was the desire to return to normality after the institution of social distancing and restrictive measures, which highlights the trust of this population in recommendations made by health authorities. This last point turned out to be a determining factor in the acceptance or not of the vaccine against COVID-19, as can be seen in other, similar studies, in which a lack of trust in health personnel was a key factor in accepting or refusing vaccination [12,30,31].

On the other hand, we observed that vaccination among Spanish prison staff was slightly lower than that of prisoners. This fact was also reflected in studies carried out in the U.S. [11,22,32]. Among our findings, nearly half of prison staff believe that the accelerated pace of vaccine production reduced their safety; this belief was also reported as the main reason for COVID-19 vaccination refusal among prison staff in Massachusetts [29].

Currently, in Spanish prisons, high vaccination coverage against COVID-19, along with immunity generated from natural infections, allows us to consider that the majority of the prison population is currently protected against COVID-19 [33,34].

5. Conclusions

The SARS-CoV-2 pandemic has highlighted the vulnerability of incarcerated individuals and prison staff. The high levels of acceptance and vaccination against COVID-19 in Spanish prisons are a measure of responses to public health needs of incarcerated individuals and prison staff. The results of this study demonstrate that vaccine acceptability was high in a prison system during a public health emergency such during a pandemic. While we cannot extrapolate these results to other settings, to prevent relegating these vulnerable populations to not receiving vaccination based on assumptions that vaccination acceptability would be low, the results of this study are promising, encouraging the implementation of vaccination not only during public health emergencies, but also as part of routine immunization catch-up programs in prisons. Improving vaccination coverage in adults residing in prisons reduces health inequities among marginalized populations.

Author Contributions: Conceptualization, J.T. and N.V-A.; methodology, N.V-A. and J.T.; investigation, N.V.-A.; data curation, analysis and software S.M.S.; writing—original draft preparation J.T., C.F.-P. and N.V-A.; writing—review and editing, J.T., C.F.-P. and N.V-A. All authors have read and agreed to the published version of the manuscript.

Funding: This research received no external funding.

Institutional Review Board Statement: The study was approved by the General Secretary of Penitentiary Institutions, Sub-directorate General of Institutional Relations and Territorial Coordination (number 395714). Participation in the survey was conducted anonymously and voluntarily, and the analysis of the questionnaire was completely confidential, ensuring the privacy of the data of all respondents. For this study, we followed the ethical principles for medical research involving human subjects set out in the Declaration of Helsinki and EU Regulation 134 2016/679 (GDPR) regarding the processing of personal data.

Informed Consent Statement: Informed consent was obtained from all subjects involved in the study.

Data Availability Statement: Data is unavailable due to privacy or ethical restrictions.

Conflicts of Interest: The authors declare no conflict of interest.

References

1. Crowley, D.; Cullen, W.; O'Donnell, P.; Van Hout, M.C. Prison and opportunities for the management of COVID-19. *BJGP Open. R. Coll. Gen. Pract.* 2020. [CrossRef]
2. World Health Organization. Frequently Asked Questions about Prevention and Control of COVID-19 in Prisons and Other Places of Detention. 2020. Available online: http://www.euro.who.int/en/health-topics/healthdeterminants/prisons-and-health (accessed on 5 March 2022).
3. Marco, A.; Guerrero, R.; Turu, E. El control de la infección por SARS-CoV-2 en prisiones [Control of SARS-CoV-2 in prisons]. *Semergen* **2021**, *47*, 47–55. [CrossRef] [PubMed]
4. Ministry of the Interior. Secretariat of Penitentiary Institutions. Adaptation of the Measures of the Strategy for Early Detection, Surveillance and Control of COVID-19 after the Acute Phase of the Pandemic for Prisons Dependent on the General Secretariat of Penitentiary Institutions. Available online: https://www.sanidad.gob.es/profesionales/saludPublica/ccayes/alertasActual/nCov/documentos/COVID-19_Adaptacion_Estrategia_Vigilancia_Centros_Penitenciarios.pdf (accessed on 20 August 2022).
5. Macmadu, A.; Berk, J.; Kaplowitz, E.; Mercedes, M.; Rich, J.D.; Brinkley-Rubinstein, L. COVID-19 and mass incarceration: A call for urgent action. *Lancet Public Health* **2020**, *5*, e571–e572. [CrossRef] [PubMed]
6. Byrne, J.; Rapisarda, S.S.; Hummer, D.; Kras, K.R. An Imperfect Storm: Identifying the Root Causes of COVID-19 Outbreaks in the World's Largest Corrections Systems. *Vict. Offenders.* **2020**, *15*, 862–909. [CrossRef]
7. Wang, E.A.; Zenilman, J.; Brinkley-Rubinstein, L. Ethical Considerations for COVID-19 Vaccine Trials in Correctional Facilities. *JAMA* **2020**, *324*, 1031–1032. [CrossRef]
8. Simpson, P.L.; Levy, M.; Butler, T. Incarcerated people should be prioritized for COVID-19 vaccination. *BMJ* **2021**, *373*, n859. [CrossRef]

9. Berk, J.; Rich, J.D.; Brinkley-Rubinstein, L. Why we vaccinate incarcerated people first. *EClinicalMedicine* **2021**, *35*, 100864. [CrossRef]
10. Ismail, N.; Tavoschi, L.; Moazen, B.; Roselló, A.; Plugge, E. COVID-19 vaccine for people who live and work in prisons worldwide: A scoping review. *PLoS ONE* **2022**, *17*, e0267070. [CrossRef]
11. Vicente-Alcalde, N.; Ruescas-Escolano, E.; Harboe, Z.B.; Tuells, J. Vaccination Coverage among Prisoners: A Systematic Review. *Int. J. Environ. Res. Public Health.* **2020**, *17*, 7589. [CrossRef]
12. Hagan, L.M.; Dusseau, C.; Crockett, M.; Rodriguez, T.; Long, M.J. COVID-19 vaccination in the Federal Bureau of Prisons, December 2020-April 2021. *Vaccine* **2021**, *39*, 5883–5890. [CrossRef]
13. Stern, M.F.; Piasecki, A.M.; Strick, L.B.; Rajeshwar, P.; Tyagi, E.; Dolovich, S.; Patel, P.R.; Fukunaga, R.; Furukawa, N.W. Willingness to Receive a COVID-19 Vaccination Among Incarcerated or Detained Persons in Correctional and Detention Facilities—Four States, September-December 2020. *MMWR* **2021**, *70*, 473–477. [CrossRef] [PubMed]
14. National Health System. Interterritorial Council. Vaccination Strategy against COVID-19 in Spain. Update 6. Available online: https://www.sanidad.gob.es/en/profesionales/saludPublica/prevPromocion/vacunaciones/covid19/Actualizaciones_Estrategia_Vacunacion/docs/COVID19_Actualizacion6_EstrategiaVacunacion.pdf (accessed on 20 August 2022).
15. National Health System. Interterritorial Council. Vaccination Strategy against COVID-19 in Spain. Update 7. Available online: https://www.sanidad.gob.es/profesionales/saludPublica/prevPromocion/vacunaciones/covid19/Actualizaciones_Estrategia7_Vacunacion/docs/COVID-19_EstrategiaVacunacion.pdf (accessed on 21 October 2022).
16. World Health Organization. WHO SAGE Values Framework for the Allocation and Prioritization of COVID-19 Vaccination. 2020. Available online: https://apps.who.int/iris/bitstream/handle/10665/334299/WHO-2019-nCoV-SAGE_Framework-Allocation_and_prioritization-2020.1-eng.pdf (accessed on 12 December 2022).
17. National Health System. Interterritorial Council. Vaccination Strategy against COVID-19 in Spain. Update 1. Available online: https://www.sanidad.gob.es/profesionales/saludPublica/prevPromocion/vacunaciones/covid19/Actualizaciones_Estrategia_Vacunacion/docs/COVID-19_Actualizacion1_EstrategiaVacunacion.pdf (accessed on 15 July 2022).
18. Ministry of the Interior. Secretariat of Penitentiary Institutions. Statistics of the Prison Population. [Internet]. 2021. Available online: https://www.poderjudicial.es/cgpj/es/Temas/Estadistica-Judicial/Estadistica-por-temas/Datos-penales{-}{-}civiles-y-laborales/Cumplimiento-de-penas/Estadistica-de-la-Poblacion-Reclusa/ (accessed on 20 August 2022).
19. Aebi, M.F.; Cocco, E.; Molnar, L.; Tiago, M.M. *Prisons and Prisoners in Europe 2022: Key Findings of the SPACE I Report*; Series UNILCRIM 2023/2; Council of Europe and University of Lausanne: Lausanne, Switzerland, 2022.
20. Betsch, C.; Schmid, P.; Heinemeier, D.; Korn, L.; Holtmann, C.; Böhm, R. Beyond confidence: Development of a measure assessing the 5C psychological antecedents of vaccination. *PLoS ONE* **2018**, *13*, e0208601. [CrossRef] [PubMed]
21. Reintjes, R.; Das, E.; Klemm, C.; Richardus, J.H.; Keßler, V.; Ahmad, A. "Pandemic Public Health Paradox": Time Series Analysis of the 2009/10 Influenza A/H1N1 Epidemiology, Media Attention, Risk Perception and Public Reactions in 5 European Countries. *PLoS ONE* **2016**, *11*, e0151258. [CrossRef]
22. Thomson, A.; Vallée-Tourangeau, G.; Suggs, L.S. Strategies to increase vaccine acceptance and uptake: From behavioral insights to context-specific, culturally-appropriate, evidence-based communications and interventions. *Vaccine* **2018**, *36*, 6457–6458. [CrossRef] [PubMed]
23. Berk, J.; Murphy, M.; Kane, K.; Chan, P.; Rich, J.; Brinkley-Rubinstein, L. Initial SARS-CoV-2 Vaccination Uptake in a Correctional Setting: Cross-sectional Study. *JMIRx Med.* **2021**, *2*, e30176. [CrossRef]
24. Ortiz-Paredes, D.; Varsaneux, O.; Worthington, J.; Park, H.; MacDonald, S.E.; Basta, N.E.; Lebouché, B.; Cox, J.; Ismail, S.J.; Kronfli, N. Reasons for COVID-19 vaccine refusal among people incarcerated in Canadian federal prisons. *PLoS ONE* **2022**, *17*, e0264145. [CrossRef]
25. Chin, E.T.; Ryckman, T.; Prince, L.; Leidner, D.; Alarid-Escudero, F.; Andrews, J.R.; Salomon, J.A.; Studdert, D.M.; Goldhaber-Fiebert, J.D. COVID-19 in the California State Prison System: An Observational Study of Decarceration, Ongoing Risks, and Risk Factors. *J. Gen. Intern. Med.* **2021**, *36*, 3096–3102. [CrossRef]
26. Saloner, B.; Parish, K.; Ward, J.A.; DiLaura, G.; Dolovich, S. COVID-19 Cases and Deaths in Federal and State Prisons. *JAMA* **2020**, *324*, 602–603. [CrossRef]
27. Vicente-Alcalde, N.; Ruescas-Escolano, E.; Franco-Paredes, C.; Tuells, J. Control of a COVID-19 Outbreak in a Spanish Prison: Lessons Learned in Outbreak Control. *Front. Med.* **2022**, *9*, 806438. [CrossRef]
28. Brinkley-Rubinstein, L.; Peterson, M.; Martin, R.; Chan, P.; Berk, J. Breakthrough SARS-CoV-2 Infections in Prison after Vaccination. *N. Engl. J. Med.* **2021**, *385*, 1051–1052. [CrossRef]
29. Braithwaite, I.; Edge, C.; Lewer, D.; Hard, J. High COVID-19 death rates in prisons in England and Wales, and the need for early vaccination. *Lancet Respir Med.* **2021**, *9*, 569–570. [CrossRef]
30. Augustynowicz, A.; Bachurska, B.; Wójcik, M.; Borowska, M.; Czerw, A.; Opolski, J.; Słabicka, K.; Pinkas, J. COVID-19-Infections and Immunization of Inmates in Penitentiary Institutions in Poland in 2021. *Int. J. Environ. Res. Public Health.* **2022**, *19*, 13725. [CrossRef]
31. Khorasani, S.B.; Koutoujian, P.J.; Zubiago, J.; Guardado, R.; Siddiqi, K.; Wurcel, A.G. COVID-19 Vaccine Interest among Corrections Officers and People Who Are Incarcerated at Middlesex County Jail, Massachusetts. *J. Urban Health.* **2021**, *98*, 459–463. [CrossRef] [PubMed]

32. Lessard, D.; Ortiz-Paredes, D.; Park, H.; Varsaneux, O.; Worthington, J.; Basta, N.E.; MacDonald, S.E.; Lebouché, B.; Cox, J.; Ismail, S.J.; et al. Barriers and facilitators to COVID-19 vaccine acceptability among people incarcerated in Canadian federal prisons: A qualitative study. *Vaccine X.* **2022**, *10*, 100150. [CrossRef] [PubMed]
33. Prince, L.; Long, E.; Studdert, D.M.; Leidner, D.; Chin, E.T.; Andrews, J.R.; Salomon, J.A.; Goldhaber-Fiebert, J.D. Uptake of COVID-19 Vaccination Among Frontline Workers in California State Prisons. *JAMA Health Forum.* **2022**, *3*, e220099. [CrossRef] [PubMed]
34. Iglesias, S. Transmission and prevention of SARS-CoV-2 (COVID-19) in prisons. *Rev. Esp. Sanid. Penit.* **2020**, *22*, 87–90. [CrossRef]

vaccines

MDPI

Review

Living with HIV and Getting Vaccinated: A Narrative Review

Andrea De Vito [1,*,†], Agnese Colpani [1,†], Mattia Trunfio [2], Vito Fiore [1], Giulia Moi [1], Marco Fois [1], Nicola Leoni [1], Stefano Ruiu [1], Sergio Babudieri [1], Andrea Calcagno [2] and Giordano Madeddu [1]

1 Unit of Infectious Diseases, Department of Medicine, Surgery, and Pharmacy, University of Sassari, 07100 Sassari, Italy; colpani.agnese@gmail.com (A.C.); giordano@uniss.it (Giordano Madeddu)
2 Unit of Infectious Diseases, Department of Medical Sciences, University of Turin, 10149 Torino, Italy
* Correspondence: andreadevitoaho@gmail.com; Tel.: +39-3404704834
† These authors contributed equally to this work.

Abstract: After 40 years of its appearance, human immunodeficiency virus (HIV) infection remains a leading public health challenge worldwide. Since the introduction of antiretroviral treatment (ART), HIV infection has become a chronic condition, and people living with HIV could have life expectancies close to those of the general population. People with HIV often have an increased risk of infection or experience more severe morbidity following exposure to vaccine-preventable diseases. Nowadays, several vaccines are available against bacteria and viruses. However, national and international vaccination guidelines for people with HIV are heterogeneous, and not every vaccine is included. For these reasons, we aimed to perform a narrative review about the vaccinations available for adults living with HIV, reporting the most updated studies performed for each vaccine among this population. We performed a comprehensive literature search through electronic databases (Pubmed—MEDLINE and Embase) and search engines (Google Scholar). We included English peer-reviewed publications (articles and reviews) on HIV and vaccination. Despite widespread use and guideline recommendations, few vaccine trials have been conducted in people with HIV. In addition, not all vaccines are recommended for people with HIV, especially for those with low CD4 cells count. Clinicians should carefully collect the history of vaccinations and patients' acceptance and preferences and regularly check the presence of antibodies for vaccine-preventable pathogens.

Keywords: HIV; vaccination; preventable diseases; HBV; HPV; HAV; SARS-CoV-2; MPox

1. Introduction

After 40 years of its appearance, human immunodeficiency virus (HIV) infection remains a leading public health challenge worldwide. Since the introduction of antiretroviral treatment (ART), HIV infection has become a chronic condition, and people living with HIV (PWH) could have life expectancies close to those of the general population [1,2]. This implies that PWH are becoming older, with an increase in the comorbidity burden that HIV specialists have to manage [3–12]. However, despite ART, many people do not have a complete CD4 recovery [13–16], and PWH with low CD4 cell count have an estimated life expectancy of 30 years lower than the general population [1].

People with HIV often have an increased risk of infection or experience more severe morbidity following exposure to vaccine-preventable diseases. Therefore, it is fundamental to prevent non-communicable and infective diseases [17,18]. Nowadays, several vaccines are available against bacteria and viruses. Different vaccinal technologies have been developed over the years (e.g., live-attenuated, whole inactivate vaccine, virus-like particles, polysaccharide, mRNA), with varying routes of administration (e.g., oral, subcutaneous, nasal) [19,20]. However, not all vaccines could be administered in PWH, particularly in those people with a low CD4 cells count. For example, the use of a trivalent live-attenuated vaccine against measles, mumps, and rubella is contraindicated in PWH with a CD4 cell count <200 cell/mm^3 for the high risk of developing the disease [21–23]. Therefore, it is clear that focusing on the vaccination of PWH is mandatory, balancing the pros and cons of each available vaccine.

National and international vaccination guidelines in PWH are heterogeneous, and not every vaccine is included [22–27] (Tables 1, 2, 5–7 and 9). For these reasons, we aimed to perform a narrative review about the vaccinations available for adults living with HIV, reporting the most updated studies performed for each vaccine among this population.

2. Vaccines

2.1. Hepatitis A Virus

Hepatitis A is an acute infectious disease transmitted through contaminated food or water by fecal–oral route. Hepatitis A virus (HAV) has an icosahedral structure, and human beings are the only reservoir in its biological cycle. Therefore, it is a cosmopolitan infection. However, its circulation is influenced by hygiene and socioeconomic condition; thus, it is an endemic disease in developing countries commonly acquired during childhood. In non-endemic countries such as Europe, HAV infection is acquired in adulthood. Risk factors include travel to an endemic country, intravenous drug use, or homelessness and being men who have sex with men (MSM) [28].

No specific disease manifestations in immunocompromised hosts or PWH have been described. However, Lin et al. showed that people with HIV are more infectious and for a more extended period than people without HIV [29]. Therefore, the normalization of transaminase levels may also be prolonged in these patients [30]. However, some cases of fibrosing cholestatic hepatitis in PWH with severe immunodeficiency have been described, with severe jaundice, coagulation deficit, and encephalopathy with rapid evolution until death [31].

Specific treatment for HAV is not available. Hospitalization is mandatory only in fulminant hepatic failure, requiring a liver transplant. Predictors of disease evolution are age (<10 or >40 years old), creatinine $\geq$2–3 mg/dl, and prothrombin time $\geq$50 s. Otherwise, supportive care and symptomatic treatment are sufficient [32].

Prevention measures for HAV infection include vaccination, immunoglobulin administration, and careful personal hygiene. Vaccination of high-risk adults such as travellers in super-endemic countries, MSM, patients with chronic liver disease, and individuals with one year or more of HIV infection is recommended. The HAV vaccine contains purified and inactivated viruses boosted by an aluminium salt as an adjuvant. Two doses are required in a range of six to eight months [33]. The vaccine is safe and immunogenic in 97–99% of the cases two weeks after the second dose. However, the efficacy is inferior in HIV co-infected patients, and the seroconversion rates range from 52% to 94% [34]. Recommendations of the different guidelines are summarized in Table 1.

Patients with CD4 cells count <200 cells/mm^3 and those with detectable HIV-RNA have a higher risk of poor response to the vaccine. For these reasons, some authors suggest an additional dose of the HAV vaccine to improve the durability of seroprotection in PWH with low CD4 cells count [29]. Chen et al. found that PWH who have lost their anti-HAV antibodies after primary vaccination had a faster and better serological response to a single dose of HAV revaccination than PWH who received the first dose [35]. Regarding the durability of HAV response, Jablonowska and Kuydowicz evaluated 234 PWH, of which about 30% had anti-HAV antibodies [36]. Of the 83 PWH who received a complete vaccination, 79.5 had a good response (anti-HAV-T >20 IU/L after one month since the booster dose). In addition, they confirmed that having less than 200 CD4/mm^3 and HIV/HCV coinfection were associated with a worse response [36].

The most common adverse events are fever, injection site reaction, rash, and headache [37]. In addition, severe events, such as Guillain-Barrè syndrome, have been reported, although their relationship with vaccination is uncertain. No difference regarding safety has been seen in PWH [34]. Finally, Crisinel et al. reported a 100% seroconversion rate after two doses of HAV vaccination in children living with HIV without severe symptoms or immunosuppression. Despite a high seroconversion rate, children with CD4 counts of <750/mm^3

have lower anti-HAV antibodies, which could reflect less lasting protection. For this reason, serological monitoring and additional boosting doses should be considered for these children [38].

Table 1. Comparison of five HIV guideline recommendations for the HAV vaccine administration.

	BHIVA [22,25]	EACS [24]	NIH [23]	SIMIT [27]	WHO [26]
Who to vaccine?	According to risk profile (travel, close contact with children, MSM, IVDU, active hepatitis B or C infection, chronic liver disease), and with a negative anti-HAV IgG antibodies	According to risk profile (travel, close contact with children, MSM, IVDU, active hepatitis B or C infection, chronic liver disease), and with a negative anti-HAV IgG antibodies	Any person without evidence of immunity to HAV	According to risk profile (travel, close contact with children, MSM, IVDU, active hepatitis B or C infection, chronic liver disease), and with a negative anti-HAV IgG antibodies	No specific recommendation
Difference for people with low CD4/mm^3	>350 CD4/mm^3: two vaccines doses at 0 and 6 months <350 CD4/mm^3: three vaccines doses at 0, 1, and 6 months	No	<200 CD4 with risk factors: do vaccination and check antibodies response after 1–2 months. If negative, revaccinate when CD4 are >200. <200 CD4/mm^3 without risk factors: waiting for CD4 > 200/mm^3	No	No specific recommendation
Boosting?	Every 10 years	NP	NP	The cited BHIVA's recommendation of performing a booster every 10 years in high-risk people	NP

NP: not present.

Although vaccination against HAV is essential for HIV-infected patients, the uptake of HAV vaccine is reported to be very low [39]. For this reason, further efforts are needed to improve HAV vaccine offer and acceptance.

2.2. Hepatitis B Virus

Hepatitis B virus (HBV) is one of the principal causes of chronic viral liver disease worldwide. As for HIV, no definitive cure is currently known.

Hepatitis B virus could be transmitted by blood, semen and other bodily fluids, or through vertical transmission [40–43]. People with HIV are less likely to develop a clinical recovery after acute infection, given the lower HBV surface antibody (HBsAb) production rates. For this reason, these patients are more likely to develop a chronic infection, with liver cirrhosis, end-stage liver disease, and hepatocellular carcinoma (HCC) than the general population [44–49].

HBV surface antibody production is less commonly observed with low CD4+ cell counts, high HIV viral loads, HCV co-infection, and other comorbidities [50].

Even in the ART era, there is evidence of higher mortality among PWH with HBV infection [51]. For this reason, achieving long-term immunity protection is still challenging, and vaccination remains one of the most important weapons for HBV prevention [52].

Consequently, targeted interventions for assessing immunity and primary prevention with vaccines should be prioritized, especially for those people who need to switch to a dual-regimen treatment without an active drug against HBV.

Regarding vaccination, there available different effective formulations. They consist of recombinant, combined, or mammalian cell-derived vaccines.

(i) Recombinant HBV vaccines include Recombivax HB® [containing 10 mcg HBV surface antigen (HBsAg)/mL], Engerix-B® (containing 20 mcg HBsAg/mL), and Heplisav-B® (HepB-CpG; containing 20 mcg HBsAg/0.5 mL). Recombivax HB® has been available since 1983 and is widely available [53]. It typically requires three doses. Engerix-B® has been available since 1989 and usually requires three doses. Finally, HepB-CpG (an adjuvanted vaccine) was approved in 2017, only in adults. It is administrated in two separate doses at one month of distance [54–56].

(ii) Combined vaccines: The combined vaccine (Twinrix®) contains 720 enzyme-linked immunosorbent assay units of inactivated hepatitis A virus and 20 mcg of recombinant HBsAg [57].

The different recommendations are summarized in Table 2.

Table 2. Comparison of five HIV guideline recommendations for the HBV vaccine administration.

	BHIVA [22,25]	EACS [24]	NIH [23]	SIMIT [27]	WHO [26]
Who to vaccinate?	All if seronegative	All if seronegative	All if seronegative	All if seronegative	All if seronegative
Type of vaccine and doses	Yeast-based: 40 µg Adjuvanted: 20 µg Four doses: 0, 1, 2, 6 months	According to national guidelines	Yeast-based: 40µg Adjuvanted: 20 µg Three doses	Yeast-based: 40 µg Adjuvanted (preferred): 20 µg Three doses	Suggest using double doses
Target IgG	>100 UI/L 8 weeks after the last doses	>100 UI/L	≥10 mIU/mL 8 weeks after the last doses	>100 UI/L	>100 UI/L
Occult HBV*	One dose; check HBsAb two weeks later; if HBsAg < 10 IU/L, offer full vaccination	NP	NP	One dose; check HBsAb two weeks later; if HBsAg < 10 IU/L, offer full vaccination	NP
Differences for people with low CD4/mm^3	No differences in doses; repeat HBsAb screening more frequently if CD4 cell/mm^3 < 350	For people with "particularly low CD4", consider a double dose (40 µg) or use a more immunogenetic vaccine	No difference in doses. For non-responder people with CD4/mm^3 < 200: delay re-vaccination until CD4 > 200/mm^3	No difference in doses. For non-responder people with CD4/mm^3 < 500: delay re-vaccination until CD4 > 500/mm^3	NP
Boosting	People with HBsAg < 10 UI/L: three more doses People with HBsAg < 100 UI/L but >10 UI/L: one dose	People with HBsAg < 10 UI/L: three more doses People with HBsAg < 100 UI/L but >10 UI/L: one dose	Non-responder: revaccinate with 3–4 doses For people whose HBsAg level fall below 10 UI/L: one dose if not receiving tenofovir-based regimen	People with HBsAg < 10 UI/L: three more doses People with HBsAg < 100 UI/L but >10 UI/L: one dose	People with HBsAg < 10 UI/L: three more doses People with HBsAg < 100 UI/L but >10 UI/L: one dose

* HBsAg negative, HBcAb positive, and HBsAb negative. NP: not present.

According to all national and international guidelines, PWH should be assessed for HBV infection before choosing vaccination. In particular, every patient should be screened for HBsAg, HBsAb, and HBV core antigen–antibody (HBcAb) [23–26,58]. Depending on the results of this test, we could face different situations:

People with HIV who never received HBV vaccine and who have never encountered the virus (anti-HBs, HBsAg, anti-HBc negative)

In this case, HBV vaccination is recommended for all PWH regardless of HIV viral load (VL) and CD4+ cells count, given their HBV susceptibility.

Four randomized controlled trials (RCTs) on PWH were conducted from 2005 to 2013, analyzing various schedules [59–62]. In almost all cases, there was an advantage to a higher dose of vaccine in this population. Interestingly, Cornejo-Juárez et al. showed no relevant differences when comparing a 10 μg to a 40 μg schedule [60]. Furthermore, an RCT conducted by Chaiklang et al. in 2013 highlighted no statistical differences between the study groups; they also observed a higher response rate in classic schedules than in every previous study [63]. However, results showed a response ranging from 16% to 18.2% lower at 12 months in the group receiving the standard dose (Table 3). Even if not statistically significant, this result could be considered clinically relevant when coming to practice. Finally, in 2013, a meta-analysis carried out by Ni et al. confirmed the advantage of higher doses to increase response rates (pooled OR for increased dose = 1.96 (95% CI 1.47–2.61)) [64].

Table 3. Randomized controlled trials on HBV vaccination among PWH who never received vaccine.

Study	Year	Included Patients	Schedule	Rates of Response	*p*-Value
Fonseca et al. [61]	2005	210	20 μg vs. 40 μg Month 0–1–6	34% vs. 47%	0.07
Cornejo-Suarez et al. [60]	2006	79	10 μg vs. 40 μg Month 0–1–6	60% vs. 61.5%	-
Launay et al. [62]	2011	437	20 μg Month 0–1–6 40 μg Month 0–1–2–6 4 mg ID Month 0–1–2–6	65% 82% 77%	- <0.01 0.02
Chaiklang et al. [64]	2013	132	20 μg Month 0–1–6 40 μg Month 0–1–2–6 4 mg ID Month 0–1–2–6	70.4% 86.4% 88.6%	- 0.119 0.062

People with HIV who did not respond to a vaccine cycle (anti-HBs, HBsAg, anti-HBc negative with a known history of vaccination)

People with HIV who did not respond to a vaccine cycle are considered susceptible to HBV. For this reason, a new vaccine cycle should be considered for this population to obtain an acceptable serological response. However, there are no univocal indications regarding revaccination or the schedule to use. For example, in the United States and in France, a second series is recommended [23,65]. Instead, British recommendations consider three vaccines with high doses [25].

Over the years, several non-randomized studies have been conducted, but only a few RCTs.

In 2010, Psevdos et al. analyzed the response differences between supplementary double or standard doses among 101 PWH non-responders to the first HBV vaccine schedule [66]. They found a difference of ~30% in response rates in favor of double dose ($p = 0.006$).

In 2015, Rey et al. conducted a study on 178 PWH assessing the efficacy of a double vs. standard dose vaccine among non-responders to a 20 μg booster after the first vaccine cycle [67]. As a result, they found a significant difference at week 72 of follow-up (54% vs. 31%, respectively; $p = 0.01$).

Recently, Vargas et al. compared the efficacy of a high-dose vs. standard-dose HBV revaccination schedule in an RCT including 107 PWH. From December 2013 to March 2018, they enrolled patients with HBs-Ab titers <10 IU/L after the first HBV vaccination regimen [68]. The high-dose group received three doses of 40μg recombinant HBV vaccine; the other one received 20 μg at 0, 1, and 2 months. At one year of follow-up, they demonstrated 40% higher response rates among people receiving a 40 μg dose (80% vs. 39.1%; $p = 0.01$) (Table 4).

All this considered, a double-dose revaccination seems to be the best practice among PWH who did not respond to the first vaccine cycle.

Table 4. Randomized controlled trials on HBV vaccination among PWH who did not respond to vaccine.

Study	Year	Included Patients	Revaccination Schedule	Rates of Response	*p*-Value
Psevdos et al. [67]	2010	101	40 μg (3 doses) vs. 20 μg (3 to 8 doses) after classic schedule	85% vs. 59%	0.006
Rey et al. [68]	2015	178	Double vs. standard schedule	54% vs. 31%	0.001
Vargas et al. [69]	2021	107	20 μg vs. 40 μg Month 0-1-2	80% vs. 39.1%	0.01

People with HIV with positive HBcAb

Literature data showed how up to 20% of PWH tested positive for HBcAb [69–73] However, there is no international consensus about vaccination in this case. For example, the European AIDS Clinical Society (EACS) guidelines report that "vaccination is not recommended in this population" [21], while the National Institute of Health (NIH) suggest performing one standard dose of HepB (Table 2).

Unfortunately, few studies about this population are present. In 2003, Gahndi et al. found that among 42 PWH positive only for HBcAb, one had a positive HBV-DNA, supporting the idea that occult hepatitis B viremia may occur even after apparent clearance of infection [74]. In 2016, Piroth et al. conducted a clinical trial in this population, enrolling 54 PWH with isolated HBcAg positivity. All people received one dose (20 μg) of the recombinant HBV vaccine. At 4 weeks, only 25 (46%) patients were responders, and only 14/24 (58%) maintained an anti-Hbs level >10 mIU/mL at 28 weeks (one LTFU). Those who at 4 weeks were non-responders (anti-HBs level of <10 mIU/mL) received three additional double doses. Among them, 24/27 (89%) and 81% (21 of 26) had an anti-HBs level of ≥10 mIU/mL at week 28 and month 18, respectively. The authors concluded, "All of the patients with an isolated anti-HBc profile who did not have an anti-HBs titer of >100 mIU/mL 4 weeks after a single recall dose of HBV vaccine should be further vaccinated with a reinforced triple double-dose scheme" [75]. Finally, from 2005 to 2016, some prospective studies aimed to evaluate response rates with different schedules, and vaccine success was reported in up to 89%. For this reason, we agree with NIH guidelines since the HBV vaccine represents an added value among these patients, reducing the risk of new infections [74–77].

HBV surface antigen positive

In this case, vaccination is not recommended, and patients should be treated with a triple-drug regimen containing two Nucleoside Reverse Transcriptase Inhibitors (NRTI), as suggested by guidelines [23–25].

In conclusion, the management of HBV vaccination is still debated in the literature, and further studies with longer follow-ups are needed. In the meantime, the suggestion is to monitor the HBsAg title yearly and use a tiple-drug treatment containing tenofovir in the non-responder subjects.

2.3. Human Papillomavirus

Human papillomavirus (HPV) is the most common sexually transmitted disease worldwide. Among the >200 identified genotypes so far, most can cause anogenital warts and respiratory papillomatosis, whereas about 40 genotypes have been associated with premalignant and malignant lesions of the cervix, anus, vulva, vagina, penis, and oropharynx [78]. Worldwide, genotypes 16 and 18 cause about 70% of cervical cancers (the fourth most common cancer in women), while HPV-6 and 11 are the most frequent causes of benign lesions [78,79].

People with HIV, even on effective ART, have increased risk and rate of HPV acquisition, persistence, and re-infection after clearance, higher carriage of multiple HPV genotypes, and a more rapid progression to HPV-associated malignancies [80–82]. Furthermore, HIV-positive MSM have the highest HPV-related anal warts and cancer risk. At the same time, women with HIV show a six-fold greater incidence of cervical cancer than HIV-negative women [83]. The worse epidemiology of HPV infection in PWH is due to behavioral habits and immunological reasons related to HIV-induced NK, B, and T-cell dysfunction, chronic inflammation, and persistent mucosal/epithelial alterations [84]. Furthermore, HPV infection can increase by two-fold the likelihood of HIV acquisition [85]. HPV vaccination may have a relevant impact in settings featured by low HIV prevention coverage, where mathematical models showed that the cumulative number of HIV infections that could be averted by HPV vaccination over 50 years could reach up to 27,812 cases in women and 14,693 cases in men [86].

Four types of prophylactic recombinant vaccines based on virus-like particles are currently available: two bivalent (Cervarix®, Glaxosmith-Kline, UK, and Cecolin®, Xiamen Innovax Biotech, China), the quadrivalent, and the nonavalent (Gardasil® and Gardasil-9®, Merck, Rahway, NJ, USA). The two bivalent vaccines protect against HPV-16 and 18, while Gardasil® and Gardasil-9® protect against HPV-6, 11, 16, and 18, and against HPV-6, 11, 16, 18, 31, 33, 45, 52, and 58, respectively.

In the general population, HPV vaccines showed outstanding safety and effectiveness against vaccine-included genotypes, anogenital warts, and high-grade intraepithelial neoplasia up to 14 years after vaccination [87]. As a result, vaccination regimes for young girls and boys (9–14 years) have moved from the original licensed 3 doses to 2 doses. In addition, there is growing interest in evaluating whether one shot is insufficient for long-lasting protection [88].

Despite HPV vaccination being also recommended for immunocompromised subjects, including PWH, robust consolidated evidence on its efficacy and safety is missing in PWH. Several studies suggest these vaccines are safe and immunogenic. Still, there has been no formal assessment of the influence of vaccine type, number of doses, baseline HPV serostatus, nor of the age and timing of vaccination along the course of HIV infection stages. Guideline recommendations are summarized in Table 5.

A 2022 meta-analysis of 18 longitudinal studies, including about 3900 participants, evaluated HPV vaccines immunogenicity, safety, and efficacy in PWH according to baseline HPV status [89]. Overall, their findings support that PWH develop a valid immune response following HPV vaccination and that all the vaccines are as well tolerated and safe as for HIV-negative populations. Nevertheless, the pooled follow-up was 1–2 years, no study assessed the effects of one or two doses only, and only one reported on Gardasil-9® and none on Cecolin®, recently licensed [89]. Furthermore, most of the participants included in the meta-analysis were relatively healthy but also more representative of old HIV-positive cohorts compared to PWH attending clinics nowadays: they presented an average long duration of infection off ART and old ART regimens.

As for immunogenicity, among PWH who were seronegative for HPV-16 and -18 prior to vaccination, seroconversion rates were high (>94%) at 7 months from the first dose across all vaccines [89]. Seropositivity after the third dose remained high despite some decline over time, which was more pronounced in PWH as compared to HIV-negative participants and greater for HPV-18 and with the quadrivalent vaccine; consequently, increases in seropositivity after a fourth dose was more pronounced for this genotype and with Gardasil® [89]. Due to heterogeneity and limited statistical power, there was only modest evidence suggesting that antibody titers and seroconversion rates were lower in PWH with lower CD4+ counts or detectable plasma viremia. Therefore, no conclusion was drawn for the potential contributions of ART [89]. Previously, lower antibody titers and seroconversion rates after HPV vaccination in PWH with CD4+ count $\leq$200 cells/mm^3, positive correlations between CD4+ count and antibody titers, no difference in antibody titers by CD4 nadir, and higher antibody titers in PWH on ART (vs. off ART) and in those virally suppressed (vs. non-suppressed) were reported [90–94]. Interestingly, genotype- and timing-specific differences in seropositivity between HIV-negative and PWH after three doses could also occur [89].

Table 5. Comparison of five HIV guideline recommendations for HPV vaccine administration.

	BHIVA [22,25]	EACS [24]	NIH [23]	SIMIT [27]	WHO [26]
Who to vaccinate?	All aged $\leq$ 26 yo; MSM and women aged < 40; Defer if CD4 < 200/mm^3	All people aged between 9 and 45	All aged $\leq$ 26 For people between 27 and 45 years old, depending on risk factors	All aged $\leq$ 26 For people with more than 26 years evaluate risk/benefit	Girls aged between 9 and 14; females aged $\geq$ 15 years or males are recommended only if this is feasible, affordable, cost-effective, and does not divert resources from vaccination of the primary target population
Type of vaccine and doses	If available, prefer the 9-valent vaccine; otherwise, use the 4-valent vaccine For both, perform three doses: 0, 1–2, and 6 months	Prefer the 9-valent vaccine	If available, prefer the 9-valent vaccine; otherwise, use the 4-valent vaccine For both, perform three doses: 0, 1–2, and 6 months	If available, prefer the 9-valent vaccine; otherwise, use the 4-valent vaccine For both, perform three doses	Depending on which is available Performing three doses
Differences for people with low CD4/mm^3	Naïve people with CD4 < 200/mm^3: deferred until the ART starts	NP	NP	NP	NP
People with HPV disease	Perform vaccine despite age to reduce risk of recurrences	Perform vaccine despite age to reduce risk of recurrences	NP	NP	NP

NP: not present.

To date, no reliable estimate of any biological effect of HPV vaccination in PWH has been carried out; thereby, most evidence relies on immunological responses with no robust and unbiased data about the clinical counterpart of such responses, such as post-vaccination cytology results or rates of HPV infection and anogenital warts and cancers [89]. For instance, and partially differing from the results in adult PWH, among perinatally infected youths receiving Gardasil®, viro-immunological parameters were marginally associated with abnormal cytology but not with antibody titers or vaccine doses [95]. Eventually, the 2022 meta-analysis concluded that PWH who have not been vaccinated prior to acquiring HIV can still benefit from receiving the vaccine. However, the higher likelihood of HPV-positivity in PWH may hinder the net benefit of vaccination independently from other determinants, such as immune competence [89].

More data are also required to confirm the alleged superior immunogenicity of Cervarix® compared to the other HPV vaccines in PWH [81,88,96]; this observation could be potentially explained by the fact that among the licensed vaccines, only Cervarix® contains AS04. This peculiar adjuvant is a detoxified form of lipopolysaccharide that acts as a Toll-like receptor 4 (TLR) agonist. Previous evidence about anti-HBV vaccination suggested that TLR agonist adjuvant-based vaccines can improve PWH immunogenicity by overcoming T follicular helper dysfunctions [81,97]. However, considering the greater prevalence of infections by concurrent multiple HPV genotypes in PWH, the cross-protection towards a wider spectrum of genotypes induced by Cervarix® may be lower compared to quadri- and nonavalent vaccines. Therefore, mixed vaccination regimens may be regarded with interest in PWH. However, the general population still has limited data supporting this approach [98].

In conclusion, further research is warranted to detail the influence of prior HPV exposure, the role of immune suppression, HIV infection stages, the timing of ART initiation and its duration, and the age of vaccination, as all could potentially affect the efficacy and duration of protection in PWH.

2.4. *Influenza Virus*

Human Influenza A and B viruses cause annual outbreaks of Influenza in temperate climates during winter. Influenza C virus is less common and causes milder diseases, while Influenza D virus does not affect humans. Seasonal Influenza symptoms include dry cough, fever, myalgia, arthralgia, headache, and malaise [99]. Most people recover without medical attention; however, high-risk individuals can develop severe illnesses and death. Mortality is estimated to be between 290,000 and 560,000 deaths per year. People at greater risk of disease progression are pregnant women, children under 59 months of age, people with chronic morbidities, elderly people, and people affected by immunosuppressive conditions, including PWH. Transmission easily occurs through droplets and can be prevented with face masks and frequent hand hygiene [100].

A safe and constantly updated inactivated vaccine is available, and its administration is recommended to all people aged >6 years, with high priority among at-risk individuals. A trivalent vaccine containing two strains of virus A and one of virus B was first introduced; in 2013–2014, a fourth component targeting B strain was added. The vaccine is not always consistent with the circulating virus due to the high variability of Influenza virus. However, it is updated twice yearly. Even if not perfectly matching, it can still confer protection against severe illness and hospitalization [101].

People with HIV have always been at higher risk of disease progression, even if hospitalization due to Influenza has decreased since the introduction of ART. Still, PWH are considered at higher risk of disease complications and severe illness; thus, annual vaccination with a tetravalent vaccine is recommended [102–104].

A systematic review by Remschmidt et al. conducted in 2014 aimed to assess Influenza vaccine safety and efficacy among PWH. Overall, they collected two randomized clinical trials, three cohort studies including adults with HIV, and one trial including children. All data collected refer to the trivalent vaccine, the only one available at the research time. Authors highlighted that the vaccine prevents Influenza in adults, but no evidence regarding pneumonia, hospitalization, and mortality was reported. No difference according to CD4+ cells count and HIV viral load was encountered.

On the contrary, effectiveness among children under six years old was not demonstrated. This group reported an inferior antibody response compared to its healthy counterparts. However, few data are available among children with and without HIV [105].

A cohort study conducted during seasonal Influenza 2013–2014, 2014–2015, and 2015–2016 involving PWH and HIV-negative subjects grouped by age showed a lower prevalence of vaccine responders among PWH. No clinical outcome was evaluated [106]. An analysis from the same cohort shows that dysfunctional peripheral antigen-specific T helper cells are associated with this impaired response and may be affected by ageing and HIV infection [107].

Regarding the tetravalent inactivated vaccine, no data regarding PWH are available. However, encouraging data from the trivalent vaccine among PWH and data regarding the tetravalent vaccine among the general population support safety and efficacy of the tetravalent vaccine among PWH [108,109].

Regarding safety, no differences have been seen in the adverse events in PWH and the general population. On the impact of vaccination on HIV viral load and CD4 cell count, controversial results have been published. Some authors showed HIV viral load rebound and a decrease in CD4 cell count after vaccination for Influenza. The HIV rebound has been attributed to the activation of quiescent HIV-infected CD4 cells. However, most of these studies were conducted between 1995 and 2010, when Integrasis inhibitors were unavailable [110].

The available literature pushes towards promoting vaccination among PWH. However, further studies are needed to assess the safety and efficacy of the quadrivalent inactivated Influenza vaccine among children and adults living with HIV.

2.5. *Measles Morbillivirus*

Measles is a severe disease caused by a Morbillivirus. It is highly contagious and particularly threatening for immunocompromised individuals [111–114]. Its incidence has been decreasing since the introduction of an effective vaccine; however, the reluctance to vaccine uptake is undermining the achievement of herd immunity in many countries [115,116]. Measle vaccination is part of the routinely administered vaccines during childhood. Its immunogenicity and safety among children living with HIV and exposed uninfected children have been studied in past years.

A systematic review published in 2019, including only randomized control trials and cohort studies with HIV-negative children matching cohort, reported good immunogenicity with greater waning in children with HIV [117]. This is consistent with what was reported for other vaccines given before immune recovery. Immunologic recovery, intended as the recovery in the CD4 cell count, in children, is achieved through naïve cells; thus, immunity acquired with vaccines administered before immunologic recovery cannot be re-established (differently from what we can see in adults PWH). These findings support the administration of a booster vaccine after immunologic recovery.

Interesting data emerged from another review from the same period, including cross-sectional studies, case reports, and case series. The Authors reported pooled data suggesting a better response to the vaccine from children on ART and with rapid ART initiation. In comparison, a poorer response was recorded when ART was differed or not prescribed. Despite the small sample size and the numerous confounders, these data reinforce the need to start treatment promptly in children living with HIV [118]. In addition, confirmation came from a recently published prospective study; during a two-year follow-up, Bruzzese et al. reported an 87% coverage among children with HIV on stable ART, with better response among children who received the vaccine after starting ART [119]. Regarding safety, no serious adverse events were reported in the two reviews. However, long follow-up data on immunogenicity and long-term efficacy are missing [117,118].

Regarding adults and adolescents, Loevinsohn et al. published a systematic review in 2019, including 9607 PWH. Immunogenicity was highly variable across the studies, significantly improving after ART introduction. However, despite complete ART coverage, the waning of immunity reaching 50% was also reported. Nevertheless, no severe adverse events were reported [120]. In this regard, only a case of vaccine-strain severe pneumonia in an HIV-infected young adult is well known; in this case, the CD4+ cell count was "too few to enumerate" when receiving the vaccine [121].

Studies reported are widely variable, and the characteristics of people included are heterogeneous; thus, more rigorous investigations regarding immunogenicity, efficacy, and safety of the measles vaccine among adults PWH are advocated. Despite the lack of punctual data on long-term immunogenicity and efficacy, based on severe outcomes of Morbillivirus infection and safety and immunogenicity data from cohort studies and randomized trials, the measles vaccine is recommended by HIV guidelines in PWH with CD4+ count >200 cells/mm^3 and on stable ART [102,104]. Given the low rate of Morbillivirus antibodies among the population [122–124], far from reaching herd immunity, the pros and cons of recommending vaccination should be considered when evaluating a new patient.

2.6. Mpox Virus

Mpox virus (MPV) is a zoonotic orthopoxvirus that is in the same genus as variola virus (causative agent of smallpox), vaccinia, ectromelia, camelpox, and cowpox viruses. In particular, MPV is considered the most important orthopoxvirus infecting human beings since the eradication of smallpox, confirmed by WHO in 1980 [125].

MPV was identified in 1958; however, the first documented human infection was described in 1970 in a 9-year-old child from the Democratic Republic of Congo [126].

Since 1970, monkeypox has continued spreading in central and western Africa, which is now endemic. The first outbreak in Western countries was in the United States in 2003. Since then, sporadic outbreaks have been reported in several countries [127]. The most recent outbreak dates to May 2022 and is still ongoing; in this case, however, the person-to-person transmission would seem to be the main route of contagion, unlike the previous outbreaks [128].

The disease caused by MPV infection is usually characterized by a febrile prodrome with lymphadenopathy, headache, and fatigue (typically 0 to 5 days) followed, after 1 to 3 days, by a vescicopapular rash with lesions that generally start on the face and then spread to the whole body (including palms and soles). In addition, many atypical cases have been reported during the current outbreak, with skin lesions mainly localized at oral and anogenital levels, probably due to the sexual transmission route [129].

In most cases, the infection progresses benign, with complete healing after 2–4 weeks. However, cases of severe disease and complications have been described. The risk of developing a more serious disease also correlates with the patient's immune status.

From preliminary data regarding the current outbreak, it seems to be a connection between MPV infection and HIV. Thornhill et al. reported that of 528 people infected between April and June 2022, 41% had HIV infection [130].

Even before 2022, data from Africa had shown that in people with uncontrolled HIV, especially when they presented with AIDS features, the course of monkeypox was more severe (e.g., more extensive lesions, more significant complications, and increased mortality) [131]. On the contrary, this discrepancy has not been highlighted for PWH on ART [132].

Currently, there are two types of vaccines against smallpox and MPV: a replication-deficient modified vaccinia Ankara (MVA) vaccine and a replication-competent smallpox vaccine (ACAM2000).

The MVA vaccine is a second-generation smallpox vaccine. It represents the first choice due to its excellent safety profile, even in immunocompromised people. It is administered subcutaneously in two doses, 28 to 35 days apart. However, intradermal administration might be considered in outbreak situations if supplies are limited, as it requires a lower dose [133].

Greenberg et al. evaluated the safety and immunogenicity of MVA as a smallpox vaccine with a phase I/II clinical study comparing the safety and immunogenicity of MVA in 91 vaccinia-naive HIV-infected subjects (CD4+ T-cell counts, >350/mm^3) and 60 uninfected subjects [134]. To measure the potential efficacy of MVA, the ability to boost the memory response in people previously vaccinated against smallpox was evaluated by enrolling vaccinia-experienced HIV-infected and HIV-uninfected subjects in two additional groups [134]. They found that MVA was well tolerated and immunogenic in all subjects, with an antibody response comparable between people without HIV (PWoH) and PWH. In 2020, Overton et al. conducted a phase II trial on PWH, enrolling 87 participants [135].

They were divided into three groups: (i) people who received two standard doses on weeks 0 and 4; (ii) people who received two standard double doses on the same schedule in the double dose; (iii) people who received standard doses on weeks 0 and 4 weeks, plus a standard boosted dose at week 12. No differences in safety and immune response have been reported in the three groups. Therefore, the authors concluded that a booster dose does not appear necessary.

On the contrary, Pugliese et al. propose to perform the third dose for people with a CD4 cells count below 200 cells/mm^3 or 15% [136].

Agunbiade et al. recently conducted a cohort study of 10,068 (including also PWH) high-risk people who received MVA-BN vaccination [137]. They registered only 15 cases of Mpox, and 3 were HIV-positive. To note, the median time between vaccination and Mpox occurrence was 4 days (IQR 3–9).

The ACAM2000 vaccine, approved in 2007 to replace the original Dryvax vaccine used to eradicate smallpox, is a replication-competent vaccine with high immunogenic power. However, it can only be used in specific cases due to the frequent occurrence of severe adverse events secondary to the injection (acute vaccinia syndrome, postvaccinal encephalitis, progressive vaccinia, eczema vaccinatum, generalized vaccinia, and cardiac complications). The risk of developing these adverse events is particularly high in people with immunodeficiency and chronic skin diseases; therefore, these vaccines are contraindicated in PWH and diagnosed with atopic dermatitis [138].

Adverse events occurring after vaccination with replication-competent vaccines seem to be closely related to the immune status of the subject. In a study by Tasker et al. of 10 individuals with undiagnosed HIV-1 infection and CD4 counts >200 cells/mm^3 at the time of smallpox vaccination, none developed adverse events [139]. On the other hand, in a case report by Redfield et al., the patient who developed disseminated vaccinia had a CD4 cells count below 25 cells/mm^3 and active cryptococcal meningitis [140]. Therefore, in the interim Guidance for Prevention and Treatment of Monkeypox in Persons with HIV Infection, O'Shea et al. do not recommend using ACAM2000 in PWH for the risk of severe adverse effects [141].

In conclusion, the development of third-generation vaccines such as MVA has made it possible to expand the subjects to whom smallpox and MPX vaccines should be administered, including PWH.

2.7. *Severe Acute Respiratory Syndrome Coronavirus 2 (SARS-CoV-2)*

Severe acute respiratory syndrome coronavirus 2 (SARS-CoV-2) belongs to the coronavirus family and shares 79% sequence with SARS-CoV [142]. The main symptoms of Coronavirus Disease 19 (COVID-19) are fever, cough, and dyspnoea; a low proportion complains of gastrointestinal symptoms, anosmia, dysgeusia, headache, and skin lesions [143–149]. Most people develop asymptomatic or paucisymptomatic forms of infection [150,151]. However, the disease can evolve into a life-threatening systemic inflammation, respiratory failure, and multiorgan dysfunction [152–155]. Several studies have been conducted to evaluate if having an HIV infection represents a risk factor for developing severe disease. People with HIV with low CD4 cells count or detectable HIV-RNA seem to have an increased risk of severe COVID-19, while people with an undetectable HIV-RNA and a CD4 count higher than 200 cells/mm^3 appear to have the same risk as people without HIV [156–158]. For these reasons, having HIV was considered among the conditions prioritized for receiving a vaccination and eligible for early antiviral treatment against SARS-CoV-2 [159,160].

In addition, some studies showed that HIV treatments could act against SARS-CoV-2 [161,162]; in particular, treatment with tenofovir disoproxil fumarate (TDF)/emtricitabine (FTC) seems associated with a lower risk of infection and disease progression [163,164].

At the end of 2020, the first vaccine against SARS-CoV-2 was already available. Currently, nine vaccines have been approved by the WHO and administered worldwide [165–174], with many others approved only in one country (e.g., EpiVacCorona fully approved in Turkmenistan) or whose trials are still ongoing [175].

Several studies have evaluated the vaccine acceptance, efficacy, and safety in PWH.

Efficacy

Only one trial to investigate the efficacy of SARS-CoV-2 vaccination in PWH has been conducted, particularly on the AZD1222/ChAdOx1 vaccine. In the interim analysis, they presented data about 103 PWH (52 received vaccine, 51 received placebo) and 58 PWoH (29 received the vaccine, 29 received placebo). All PWH had an undetectable HIV-RNA and a CD4 cells count above 350 cells/mm^3. In the interim analysis, the authors compared 54 PWH with 50 PWoH who received two vaccine doses. They found that PWH showed cross-reactive binding antibodies to the beta variant and wild-type Asp614Gly. High responders retained neutralization against beta [176]. In the final analysis, they compared 54 PWH who received two doses with 50 PWoH. They have not found a correlation between the magnitude of anti-spike IgG and CD4 cell count, and there is no difference between the two cohorts [177].

More studies have been conducted on mRNA vaccines BNT162b2 and mRNA-1273. Schmidt et al. found a significantly lower level of SARS-CoV-2-specific IgA in PWH than in PWoH, indicating a moderately lower functionality of the humoral vaccine response [178,179]. Likewise, Hefdtal et al. and Xu et al. showed that PWH had a lower level of IgG than PWoH [179,180]. Several studies confirmed these data [178,181].

Other studies found a significant difference in neutralizing antibody responses between PWH with a CD4:CD8 ratio < 0.5 or less than 200/250 CD4 cells/mm^3 [182–186]. On the contrary, Portillo et al. found no evidence of poorer viral neutralization in PWH compared to PWoH [187].

Many of these studies, and we agree with them, concluded that PWH might become a target population for prioritization to receive booster vaccinations.

Regarding Ad26.COV2.S, Khan et al. enrolled 73 PWoH and 26 PWH, and as a comparison group, they included unvaccinated participants (28 PWoH and 34 PWH) with prior documented SARS-CoV-2 infection. They found a similar neutralization response in both groups [188].

About the inactivated vaccine, Coronavac and BBiBP CorV, Netto et al. conducted a cohort study including 215 PWH and 296 PWoH. They found that people with less than 500 CD4/mm^3 had a lower antibody level than people with more than 500 CD4/mm^3 [189]. In addition, they found lower S-RBD-IgG antibody seropositivity rates and levels in PWH than in PWoH. Similar results were found by Zeng et al. and Liu et al. [190,191]; however, they found a lower antibody level in people with less than 350 CD4 cells/mm^3.

Regarding the other inactivated vaccine, WIBP-CorV, Zou et al. found a delayed and low immunogenicity peak in PWH compared to PWoH; however, no significant difference was found in six-month immunogenicity between the two groups [192].

Finally, Gushchin et al. reported data about the Sputnik vaccine, including 24,423 PWH. Of them, 2543 (10.4%) were fully vaccinated, 17,592 (72.0%) were unvaccinated, and 4288 (17.5%) received only one dose. They found a general vaccination efficiency of 76.3%, while in PWH with more than 350 CD4 cells/mm^3, it was 79.4%. In addition, vaccination avoided hospitalization in 90.1% of cases and gave protection from moderate or severe disease in 97.1%. For the delta variant, they observed a reduction in action (efficiency 65.3%, avoided hospitalization 75.7%, and protection from moderate/severe disease 93.1%) [193].

Safety

Most of the studies present in the literature have not reported notable adverse events. In the AZD1222 trial, the authors have not reported any serious adverse events. At the same time, local and systemic reactions occurred during the first seven days after vaccination. The most common were pain at the injection site (49%), fatigue (47%), headache (47%), and malaise (34%) [176]. However, some studies reported a detectable HIV-RNA in a part of the vaccinated subject in the following months [187]. In the Gianserra et al. study, one patient vaccinated with BNT162b2 developed a reversible sensorineural hearing loss 24 h after boosting [185]. Finally, Chaabouni et al. reported a case of herpetic meningoencephalitis after having received one dose of inactivated vaccine [194]. Atiyat et al. reported a case of a 36-year-old man with HIV that had a Varicella-Zoster Virus (VZV) reactivation two days after he received the second dose of BNT162b2 vaccine. To note, he had a low CD4 cell count (158 cells/mm^3), and he was not on ART (HIV-RNA 20600 copies/mL) [195].

In conclusion, many studies have been published on SARS-CoV-2 vaccination in PWH. The majority agree that the neutralizing antibodies level was lower in PWH than in PWoH, especially when a low CD4 cell count was present. However, the sample size in many studies is small; for this reason, we believe that other studies are needed, with larger sample sizes, to better understand the different vaccines' efficacy. Until then, PWH represents a high-risk population, and they should have priority in receiving the boosting doses.

2.8. *Varicella-Zoster Virus*

Varicella-Zoster Virus is one of the known herpes viruses which infect humans. The infection confers life-long immunity; however, the virus remains latent in the ganglia and can reactivate. It can provoke two different clinical diseases. The first infection (Varicella or chickenpox) leads to a vesicular rash that usually spreads to the whole body, particularly affecting the face and trunk. While it is usually a self-limited disease, complications such as soft tissue infection, pneumonia, hepatitis, and encephalitis may affect at-risk individuals (e.g., immunocompromised and pregnant women). Herpes Zoster (HZ) reactivation (shingles) usually involves one or two contiguous dermatomes with a painful vesicular rash; among its complications, postherpetic neuralgia is common in older and immunocompromised patients; eyes, visceral, and neurological involvement are also possible. In pregnant women, HZ may cause foetus injuries [196].

Herpes Zoster has always been common among PWH before the introduction of ART. Ever since, its incidence has been declining [197]; however, PWH are still at higher risk of HZ and its complications compared to the general population [198]. Moreover, in people with VZV or HZ, the treatment must be promptly started to be effective. However, even in the best conditions, it is unlikely to protect from post-herpetic neuralgia and other complications alone [199]. Thus, prevention remains the best chance to reduce the burden of the disease, especially on immunocompromised patients.

Regarding chickenpox prevention, two vaccines are available in Europe: Varivax and Varilrix, both live-attenuated vaccines. After reconstitution, one dose (0.5 mL) of Varivax contains no less than 1350 UFP VZV live-attenuated Oka/Merck strain. After reconstitution, one dose (0.5 mL) of Varilrix contains no less than $10^{3.3}$ PFU VZV live-attenuated Oka/Merck strain. Guideline recommendations are summarized in Table 6.

Several data regarding the safety and efficacy of these vaccines among the general population are available. On the contrary, few data about using live-attenuated VZV vaccines among PWH can be found in the literature. A systematic review including all published literature up to 2013 conducted by the World Health Organization (WHO) confirmed their efficacy in preventing disease of any severity in immunocompetent individuals. The same review reported a possible benefit for HIV-infected children; nonetheless, more evidence was warranted to clarify its role in this population [200]. While further studies were later published regarding safety and efficacy among children living with HIV [201], there are almost no data on adult PWH. One study conducted to assess the role of attenuated VZV vaccine as a booster to prevent HZ among adult PWH suggests its safety and good tolerability among this population [202]. Nonetheless, given the high risk of a possible fulminant or complicated chickenpox course and relying on safety and efficacy data among children, vaccination is recommended in seronegative individuals with $\geq$200 CD4+ cells/mm^3 [102,104].

Regarding HZ reactivation, live-attenuated VZV vaccines have been used as boosters in children and adults living with HIV [201,203]. Weinberg et al. enrolled 82 subjects with positive serology for VZV; the first group included PWH on stable ART and with >400 CD4+ cells/mm^3, and the second included PWH with CD4 cells count between

201 cells/mm^3 and 400 cells/mm^3 at study entry, and one cohort of HIV-negative subjects. In each cohort, subjects were randomized to Varivax or placebo: the study reported excellent tolerability and moderate immunogenicity in PWH enrolled.

Table 6. Comparison of five HIV guideline recommendations for the Varicella-Zoster vaccine administration.

	BHIVA [22,25]	EACS [24]	NIH [23]	SIMIT [27]	WHO [26]
VZV					
Who to vaccinate?	All with a negative or uncertain history of chickenpox or shingles	All with a negative serology	All with a negative serology	All with a negative serology	All if seronegative
IgG testing	Yes, to determine susceptibility to primary infection and reactivation	Yes	Only HIV without a history of prior varicella or varicella vaccination	NP	NP
Differences for people with low CD4/mm^3	Only in people with CD4 > 200/mm^3	Contraindicated if CD4 count <200 cells/μL (14%) and/or AIDS	Only in people with CD4 > 200/mm^3	Only in people with CD4 > 200/mm^3	NP
Zoster prevention					
Who to vaccinate?	VZV IgG seropositive with more than 60 years	NP	VZV IgG seropositive with more than 18 years	NA	NP
Differences for people with low CD4/mm^3	Only in people with CD4 > 200/mm^3	NP	No data identify the optimal vaccination timing for persons with a CD4 < 200/mm^3. Some experts would administer the RZV vaccination series after CD4 count recovery	NA	NP

NA: not available at the moment of guidelines publication. NP: not present.

In 2006, the first vaccine against HZ was licensed (Zostavax)—a live-attenuated vaccine. After reconstitution, one dose (0.65 mL) contains no less than 19,400 PFU VZV live-attenuated Oka/Merck strain. Due to its characteristic, few studies are available among immunocompromised patients, including PWH. Therefore, a randomized, double-blind, placebo-controlled, multicenter study has been conducted to assess the efficacy and safety of the heat-attenuated formulation among PWH with less than 200 CD4+ cells/mm^3 within 90 days before the first dose administration; four doses were administered approximately 30 days apart. Although the vaccine was safe and well-tolerated, results were unsatisfactory regarding immunogenicity, with a weak immunogenic response unlikely to be protective against VZV reactivation [204]. More encouraging results were reported from PWH with a better immunologic profile. A randomized, double-blind, placebo-controlled trial in virally suppressed PWH, and with at least 200 CD4+ cells/mm^{3,} demonstrated the safety and immunogenicity of HZ live-attenuated vaccine even though the 24-weeks follow-up could not guarantee the durability of this effect [205]. However, being a live-attenuated vaccine, some concerns exist about its use in an immunocompromised population.

The recently approved recombinant, adjuvanted HZ vaccine (Shingrix) may be a more suitable alternative. The adjuvanted VZV glycoprotein E subunit vaccine was recently authorized for immunocompromised adults [102,104]. Results from older adults demonstrated efficacy and tolerability [206–208]. A phase 1/2a, randomized, observer-masked, placebo-controlled, multicenter trial conducted among PWH confirmed Shingrix's effectiveness in soliciting an immune response. A two-doses course was associated with a significant increase in cellular and humoral immunity compared with a single dose, while a third dose was reported as not significantly beneficial [209]. The same study reported excellent tolerability, with pain at the injection site and fatigue as the most reported symptoms; no vaccine-related severe adverse event leading to withdrawal was reported [209].

Safety and tolerability among immunocompromised individuals were confirmed by a review of six trials addressing this wide population. Data from oncologic, transplanted, and seropositive patients were reported, confirming the clinically acceptable profile of the vaccine [210]. In addition, real-life data from the Medicare population (n = 15.589.546) confirmed the beneficial impact of Shingrix among immunocompromised individuals. Izurieta et al. reported significantly higher immunogenicity following the second dose, despite lower effectiveness than reported among the general population (64.1% vs. 70.9%) [211]. However, the authors did not provide which were the underlying conditions of the subjects involved. In addition, the study was published only two years after licensure; thus, further surveillance data should follow to confirm preliminary results.

In conclusion, we have different strategies to address Varicella and Zoster reactivation among a fragile population such as PWH. The newest vaccine (Shingrix) seems promising, effective, and well-tolerated. However, long-term, real-life data are needed to better inform vaccination campaigns.

2.9. *Neisseria Meningitidis*

Neisseria meningitidis is a gram-negative, facultatively anaerobic diplococcus that exclusively infects humans. It was first isolated in 1887 from observing the cerebral spinal fluid of patients with meningitis [212].

It is the etiologic agent of severe meningitis and systemic infections that primarily affect children and young adults, named invasive meningococcal disease (IMD). Five main serogroups cause IMD: A, B, C, W, and Y. According to the last ECDC report, updated in 2018, the notification rate remained relatively stable in the last three years. Serogroup B is confirmed to be responsible for most cases (51%), followed by serogroups W and C; Serogroup A is more common in Africa, Asia, South America, and ex-Soviet Republics; Serogroup Y accounts for about one-third of cases in the United States [213].

Fever, myalgias, nausea, vomiting, and headache characterize the initial symptomatology of IMD. Subsequently, loss of consciousness, confusion, meningism, and hemorrhagic rash may onset. Treatment should not be delayed more than one hour to reduce the mortality risk; thus, a prompt diagnosis is crucial [214,215].

People with HIV are at increased risk of developing invasive *N. meningitidis* disease, regardless of sexual habits [216]. Some factors appear to be associated with an increased risk of IMD in PWH. Among these, the higher risk of bacteremia compared to patients without HIV infection is relevant [217]. The mortality rate seems directly proportional to the CD4 cell count, suggesting that the elevated risk for IMD among PWH is at least partially a result of HIV-related immune suppression [216]. In addition, atypical infections due to N. meningitidis, such as septic arthritis, have been described in PWH [217,218].

Three types of vaccine are available: the tetravalent MenACWY, against the serogroups A, C, W, and Y; the monovalent vaccine against B serogroup (MenB); the monovalent glycoconjugate-vaccine against meningococcal C vaccine (Menjugate) [219].

The tetravalent vaccines are as follows: (i) MenACWY-D (Menactra), that it is a conjugate vaccine with polysaccharide diphtheria [220]; (ii) MenACWY-CRM (Menveo), a conjugate vaccine with the oligosaccharide diphtheria CRM_{197} [221]; (iii) MenACWY-TT (MenQuadfi), a conjugate vaccine with polysaccharide tetanus toxoid [222].

The available vaccines against serogroup B are as follows: (i) MenB-FHbp (Trumenba) consists of two purified recombinant lipidated FHbp antigens, one from each FHbp subfamily (A and B) [223]; (ii) MenB-4C consists of three recombinant proteins (neisserial adhesin A [NadA], factor H binding protein [FHbp] fusion protein from subfamily B, and neisserial heparin-binding antigen [NhbA] fusion protein), and outer membrane vesicles (OMVs) containing outer membrane protein porin A (PorA) serosubtype P1.4 [224].

All guidelines suggest vaccination for *N. meningitidis* in PWH; however, each guideline suggests a different approach. For example, EACS suggests performing the quadrivalent vaccination every five years according to the risk factors and does not recommend the MenB vaccine [24]. NIH suggests vaccinating all PWH over 18 years old with the quadrivalent vaccine, while MenB is not routinely indicated [23] (Table 7).

Table 7. Comparison of five HIV guideline recommendations for the Neisseria meningitidis vaccine administration.

	BHIVA [22,25]	EACS [24]	NIH [23]	SIMIT [27]	WHO [26]
Who to vaccinate?	All aged < 25 if not already vaccinated or if they received the last MenC doses below the age of 10 years; Presence of specific risk factors: asplenia or persistent complement component deficiency; Risk of exposure through travel	According to the risk profile: - Travel - MSM - Contact with Children	All aged > 18 years if not already vaccinated	All people	Recommended for children in some high-risk populations
Type of vaccine	MenC, MenACWY, Men B in people < 25 years MenC, MenB, and/or MenACWY for high-risk people; MenACWY: exposed to travel	MenACWY; MenB according to national guidelines	MenACWY; MenB not indicated	MenACWY; MenB	NP
Interval doses	Two doses with 2 months interval	Two doses with 2 months interval	Two doses with 2 months interval	MenACWY: two doses with 2–3 months interval MenB: two doses with at least one-month interval	NP
Booster	MenACWY every five years if ongoing risk through travel or due to underlying condition	NP	Repeat vaccination every 5 years throughout life	Considerer repeat vaccination with MenACWY every 5 years to keep high immunity	NP

NP: not present.

However, few studies have been conducted among PWH to assess the immunogenicity in this specific population. Siberry et al. conducted a Phase I/II trial among children and youth with HIV (11–24 years old). One dose of quadrivalent Polysaccharide Diphtheria Toxoid Conjugate Vaccine was administered to all participants (317). Then, all people with CD4 cells < 15% received a second dose at 24 weeks; the other participants were randomized to receive or not a second dose. They found that immunogenicity was weaker than in the general population, especially for people with low CD4 cells count and detectable viral load [225]. These data were confirmed by Lujan-Zilbermann et al. [226]. Frota et al., in their study among children and young PWH, found that one dose of the quadrivalent vaccine was insufficient and suggested performing the second dose [227,228]. These studies also showed the excellent safety of the vaccines with a very low incidence of adverse events [225–228].

Regarding the MenB, no studies have been conducted on PWH to assess immunogenicity and safety. Of interest, in a recent study, Raccagni et al. evaluated the incidence of *Neisseria gonorrhoea* in MSM living with HIV with a recent history of sexually transmitted infections [229]. They observed how, during the follow-up (median 3.8 years), people who received two doses of MenB vaccination had a 44% reduced risk of gonorrhoea, confirming what was described by Paynter et al. and Petousis-Harris in the general population [230,231].

Further studies are needed to assess these vaccines' efficacy in adult PWH. However, due to its high efficacy, vaccination should be recommended for all PWH, especially those with an increased risk of infection [232,233]. A recent review conducted in the United States shows a relatively low vaccination rate, even in newly diagnosed patients [234]. In this regard, we believe that informing people about the cross-efficacy of the vaccine for gonorrhoea could be an incentive for vaccination and an opportunity for counselling about meningitis and sexually transmitted infections [235].

2.10. Pertussis, Diphtheria, and Tetanus

Pertussis (Whooping cough) is a highly contagious bacterial infection caused by *Bordetella pertussis* and mainly affects the high respiratory tract [236]. It is effectively preventable by inactivated vaccine, although it does not confer life-long immunity. Whooping cough is considered a childhood disease; however, its prevalence among adults may be underreported. Studies among adult PWH are anecdotal, but a cross-sectional seroprevalence study conducted in the United States showed a 1000-fold higher prevalence among PWH than the general population [237]. In addition, case reports show a severe course of the diseases among people with AIDS [238,239].

Diphtheria is caused by *Corynebacterium diphtheriae* and *Corynebacterium ulcerans*; it affects the high respiratory tract and skin [240]. It is preventable thanks to the toxoid vaccine. Data regarding disease prevalence and severity among PWH are lacking, as are vaccine safety and efficacy among this population; however, it seems that PWH, especially with low CD4 cell count, develop a lower antibody titre than the general population [241,242].

Tetanus is caused by neurotoxins released by *Clostridium tetani*. It causes general rigidity and spasms, leading to respiratory and cardiac failure and death [243]. It is preventable through a toxoid vaccine, with a long, although not lifelong, lasting immunity; reinforcing doses are recommended every 10 years. It is not known if the clinical course and mortality rate differ in PWH compared to the general population; however, data regarding immunogenicity suggest a poorer immunological response in PWH. A trial published in 2019 reported a lower memory response in children with HIV not on ART, while a similar kinetic was reported in children with HIV on ART and children unexposed to HIV [244]. In addition, there was a greater waning in immunity; thus, earlier booster doses should be considered in children with HIV [245]. A study conducted in Senegal confirmed a lower immunogenic response in PWH than in the general population [246]. Dauby et al. estimated the durability of tetanus toxoid-specific seroprotection, finding a half-life of 9.9 years. In addition, in their analysis, people born outside Europe had a shorter half-life (4.4 years), probably due to their low CD4 cell count at the time of immunization and the low CD4 nadir. They concluded that longer intervals of booster vaccination, as recommended in the general population, might not be appropriate in this subgroup of PWH [247]. Regarding safety, no data regarding increased adverse events are reported.

Pertussis, diphtheria, and tetanus vaccines are often administered together in a pediatric (DTPa) or adult ($\geq$7 years old) formulation with a reduced component of diphtheria and pertussis (dTpa). They can also be found combined with the polio vaccine in a tetravalent formulation (dTpaIPV).

In conclusion, all guidelines reported that the indication for these three pathogens is no different in people with HIV and suggested following standard recommendations.

2.11. Streptococcus Pneumoniae

Streptococcus pneumoniae is a Gram-positive bacteria with alfa- and beta-hemolytic features in aerobiotic and anaerobiotic conditions. It causes a broad spectrum of infections, such as pneumonia, meningitis, otitis, bronchitis, conjunctivitis, sepsis, osteomyelitis, and others [248,249].

HIV-related immunological deficiency exposes PWH to an increased risk of pneumococcal infections and severe manifestations [250,251]. The risk of pneumococcal infection is from 10- to 100-fold higher in PWH receiving and not receiving ART; the risk increases with a lower CD4 cell count (<350 cells/mm^3) [250,252].

To date, four different vaccines are available: 23-valent unconjugated purified polysaccharide vaccine (PPSV23), 13-valent vaccine conjugate vaccine (PCV-13), 15-valent pneumococcal conjugate vaccine (PCV15), and the 20-valent pneumococcal conjugate vaccine (PCV20). The first conjugate vaccine, PCV-7, is no more used (Table 8).

Several studies about the pneumococcal vaccine in PWH have been conducted with variable results.

Table 8. Comparison between the four available vaccines for *Streptococcus pneumoniae*.

	PPSV-23	PCV-13	PCV-15	PCV-20
Year of introduction	1983	2010	2021	2021
Serotypes included	1,2, 3, 4, 5, 6B, 7F, 8, 9N, 9V, 10A, 11A, 12F, 14, 15B, 17F, 18C, 19F, 19A, 20, 22F, 23F, 33F	1, 3, 4, 5, 6A, 6B, 7F, 9V, 14, 18C, 19F, 19A, 23F	1, 3, 4, 5, 6A, 6B, 7F, 9V, 14, 18C, 19A, 19F, 22F, 23F, 33F	1, 3, 4, 5, 6A, 6B, 7F, 8, 9V, 10A, 11A, 12F, 14, 15B, 18C, 19F, 19A, 22F, 23F, 33F
Advantages	Low Cost; High number of serotypes; Trial conducted in PWH	Longer lasting immunity; Trial conducted in PWH	Longer lasting immunity; High number of serotypes; Trial conducted in PWH only for immunogenicity	High number of serotypes
Disadvantages	Need of re-vaccinations every 3–5 years	Few serotypes covered	No clinical data on the efficacy	No clinical data about efficacy; Lack of immunogenicity in immunocompromised hosts

The recommendation for the general population is to utilize either PCV20 alone or PCV15 in association with the PPSV23 [253]. However, HIV guidelines have different suggestions due to the lack of data in PWH. For example, EACS suggest administering one dose of any PCV vaccine [13,15,20] to all PWH according to national guidelines, even if they already received PPSV-23 [24]. In addition, they recommend one dose of PPSV-23 in those who received PCV-13 or PCV-15. NIH, on the contrary, suggests PPSV-23 in all people with more than 200 CD4/mm^3. In those who received PCV-13, NIH suggests administering one dose of PPSV-23 [23] (Table 9).

It was suggested that PPSV-23 might not be the appropriate vaccination strategy for PWH because of some characteristics of this vaccine. Specifically, it contains purified polysaccharide antigens of the pneumococcal capsule and produces immunity through activating B-cells without T-cells involvement. Because of this, no immune memory is produced, and adjunctive doses do not elicit an additional immune response [254]. On the other hand, conjugated vaccines like PCV stimulate B- and T-cell activation, providing a sustained immune memory.

Lesprit et al. enrolled 213 adults infected with HIV and randomized them to receive either one dose of PCV-7 followed by one dose of PPSV-23 after four weeks or one dose of PPSV-23 at week four. The two-dose group showed higher immune responses than those receiving only one PPV dose at weeks 8 and 24 [255]. Similar results were obtained by Feikin et al. in a randomized trial where they found a better immune response in those who received two doses of PCV-7 or one of PCV-7 and one of PPSV-23 versus a third group that received one dose of placebo and one of PPSV-23 [256]. In addition, Bhorat et al. conducted a trial on PWH by administering three doses of PCV-13 followed by one dose of PPSV-23 at 1-month intervals with good tolerability and showing that PWH achieved a significant immune response after the first dose of PCV-13, with only modest increases in antibody titres following the other doses.

Table 9. Comparison of five HIV guideline recommendations for the *Streptococcus pneumoniae* vaccine administration.

	BHIVA [22,25]	EACS [24]	NIH [23]	SIMIT [27]	WHO [26]
PCV-13	All once (PVC-13)	If PCV-15 is not available	Non more recommended	All once	NP
PPV-23	At-risk individuals, according to national plan	At-risk individuals, according to national plan: one dose of PPSV-23 after PCV-13 or 15	Only in people previously vaccinated with PCV-13; Booster dose after five years in those previously vaccinated with PCV-13 or PPV-23; If the second PPV-23 dose is performed before 65 years, a third dose with 5 years interval should be offered	One dose in those previously vaccinated with PCV-13 with 2 months interval; Two doses in those never vaccinated with one-year intervals, and a third dose after five years	NP
PCV-15	NA	All once	All once (except those vaccinated with PCV-20), including those already vaccinated with one PPV-23 dose	NA	NP
PCV-20	NA	All once if not vaccinated before	All once (except those vaccinated with PCV-15), including those already vaccinated with one PPV-23 dose	NA	NP

NA: not available at the moment of guidelines publication. NP: not present.

The only clinical efficacy study was performed by French et al. from 2003 to 2007, involving both people with CD4 cell count lower and higher than 200 cells/mm^3; among the 439 PWH enrolled in the study, only 13% were receiving ART. Nevertheless, they found that in the group vaccinated with PCV-7, the one-year efficacy was 85% [257]. A meta-analysis by Garrido et al. conducted in 2020 concluded that the combination of PCV-13 and PPSV-23 has good immunogenicity; however, the durability of this vaccination remains unknown. In addition, data suggested delaying the PCV administration until the CD4 cells count is above 200 cells/mm^3.

In 2022, Mohapi et al. published a randomized, double-blinded clinical trial to compare the immunogenicity and safety of PCV-15 and PCV-13; they included 302 PWH. PCV-15 was generally well tolerated; immune responses were elicited for all 15 pneumococcal serotypes. However, no clinical data about this vaccine are available.

In conclusion, there is scarce clinical evidence about the efficacy of PCV in PWH. Further studies are needed both for clinical efficacy and to assess the immunogenicity of the new PCV vaccine in this specific population. However, considering the severity of pneumococcal pneumonia among immunocompromised individuals, physicians should recommend the combination of PCV-PPSV, according to international guidelines. Special attention should be given to PWH with <200 CD4 cells/mm^3.

2.12. *Vaccines for Travel*

The immunization of international travelers is mandatory to prevent the spread of infections between countries and reduce the risk of severe disease and death [258]. However, these vaccines' acceptance is low [259–262]. Below, we briefly report the suggested vaccination for travelers and the available information and recommendation for PWH.

- **Cholera**: it could be present in the area without a clean water supply or modern sewage system or in case of environmental changes due to natural disasters (such as tsunamis) or human-driven events (such as wars or massive migrations). People with HIV have a higher risk of contracting the infection and suffering severe consequences [263]. Many vaccines are available for cholera. CVD103-HgR (replicating—live-attenuated) has been proven safe and immunogenetic in PWH;

however, it is not currently available worldwide [264]. According to the NIH, it could be administered in at-risk PWH with more than 200 CD4 cells/mm^3. If CVD103-HgR is unavailable, according to BHIVA guidelines, WC/rBS vaccine (inactivated) could be administered. It is essential to know that PWH with less than 100 CD4/mm^3 may be expected to respond poorly to it [265].

- **Flu Vaccine**: see paragraph "Influenza".
- **HAV**: see paragraph "HAV".
- **HBV**: see paragraph "HBV".
- **Japanese encephalitis (JEV)**: it is caused by a *Flavivirus* transmitted by mosquito bites. This virus is present only in Asia. In most people, it is asymptomatic; however, it is symptomatic in approximately 1 patient out of 250 infections. The severity of infection ranges from flu-like to encephalitis, which could be life-threatening in 20–30% of cases. Many vaccines for JEV are available worldwide (inactivated, live-attenuated, and live-recombinant) [266]. For PWH, the inactivated vaccine (IXARO®) is suggested. However, no study in adult PWH have been conducted, and only BHIVA guidelines provide recommendations regarding this vaccine [25].
- ***N. meningitidis***: see paragraph "*Neisseria meningitidis*".
- **Rabies**: it is transmitted by infected animals (present worldwide), generally with a bite or a scratch. It causes acute encephalomyelitis, sometimes associated with ascending flaccid paralysis. If not rapidly treated with immunoglobulins, patient death is very likely, with only a few reported survivors [240]. The vaccine against rabies is inactivated and administered in three doses. The vaccine induces satisfactory antibody production in more than 95% of vaccinated subjects. However, in PWH, the immunogenicity is influenced by CD4 count and viral load; in particular, low or absent antibody responses were reported in some patients with CD4 cell counts <250 CD4/mm^3 [267,268].
- **Polioviruses**: three serotypes of polioviruses could infect humans. They spread through the fecal–oral and respiratory routes. They usually cause gastrointestinal symptoms, but in some cases, they could give severe neurological manifestations, including meningitis, encephalitis, and poliomyelitis syndrome with acute onset of flaccid paralysis. Two vaccines against polioviruses are available [269]; however, the live-attenuated oral poliovirus vaccine is not used anymore in many countries due to its side effects since it could cause vaccine-associated paralytic polio, especially in immunocompromised people, including PWH [270]. The trivalent inactivated poliovirus vaccine is the most used, combined with tetanus and the diphtheria toxoid (Td/IPV). People with HIV should receive three doses if they are not vaccinated or have an uncertain vaccination history, followed by two booster doses after 5 and 10 years. Then, a booster every 10 years is suggested.
- **Tuberculosis:** it is present worldwide, with a higher incidence in Asia, Africa, and South America. In most people, it remains latent; however, latent TB could reactivate in 5–15% of immunocompetent adults [271,272]. In PWH, the risk of activation is higher, especially in those people with a low CD4 cells count. The Bacille Calmette-Guerin (BCF) vaccine is a live-attenuated vaccine from *Mycobacterium bovis* strains. Its efficacy is controversial since the protection rate varies widely among different trials [273]. According to HIV guidelines, the BCG vaccine is contraindicated in PWH regardless of CD4 cells count, ART, viral load, and clinical status since some studies described a higher risk of local and systemic complications among this population, including disseminated BCG [21,25].
- **Typhoid Fever**: it is a cosmopolitan infection; however, higher-risk areas are characterized by poor sanitation and hygiene (Africa, India, South-East Asia, and South America). Three vaccines are available: (i) Vi (polysaccharide vaccine—one intramuscular dose); (ii) Ty21a (live-attenuated—tablets); (iii) Combined with HAV (polysaccharide vaccine—intramuscular). Ty21a is not recommended in PWH, especially in those with less than 200 CD4 cells/mm^3, since it contains live samples of *Salmonella typhi*. On

the contrary, VI vaccination is recommended in all PWH and should be performed at least one week before exposure [274].

- **Yellow fever:** it is caused by a virus transmitted through the bite of an infected *Aedes aegypti* mosquito. It is present in tropical and subtropical regions of Africa and South America. The infection is often symptomatic [275]; however, it sometimes causes severe hepatitis, jaundice, and bleeding, with high mortality rates. It is not known if PWH have an increased risk of severe forms. The vaccine contains a replicating live-attenuated virus. A single dose protects around 90% after 10 days and 99% after 30 days [276]. In 2014 a systematic review investigated the immunogenicity and safety of the yellow fever vaccine in PWH. They found that PWH (compared with PWoH) developed significantly lower concentrations of neutralizing antibodies in the first year post-immunization; however, the decay patterns were similar for recipients regardless of HIV infection. Furthermore, no study patient with HIV infection suffered serious adverse events due to vaccination [277]. However, since it contains a replicating live-attenuated virus, this vaccine is suggested only in PWH with more than 200 CD4/mm^3 and aged <60 years old.

In conclusion, many vaccines are not recommended in PWH with low CD4 counts. A thorough analysis of the pros and cons is needed for these patients. In addition, we recommend postponing travels, when possible, until immunological recovery.

3. Conclusions

Vaccinations represent a powerful tool to avoid vaccine-preventable infectious diseases also in PWH. Therefore, clinicians should carefully collect the history of vaccinations in all new patients and regularly check the presence of antibodies for each vaccine-preventable pathogen, especially in people with low CD4 numbers, who have a higher antibody-waning rate. Although vaccinations for PWH are strongly recommended, data on immunogenicity, tolerability, and clinical efficacy are limited for this specific population. For this reason, further studies are needed to assess these features and harmonize different guidelines. In addition, the acceptance rate can and must be improved.

Author Contributions: Conceptualization: A.D.V., A.C. (Agnese Colpani), A.C. (Andrea Calcagno) and G.M. (Giordano Madeddu). Resources: all authors; Writing—original draft preparation: all authors; writing—review and editing: all authors; supervision: A.C. (Andrea Calcagno) and G.M. (Giordano Madeddu). All authors have read and agreed to the published version of the manuscript.

Funding: This research received no external funding.

Institutional Review Board Statement: Not applicable.

Informed Consent Statement: Not applicable.

Data Availability Statement: Not applicable.

Conflicts of Interest: The authors declare no conflict of interest.

References

1. Trickey, A.; Zhang, L.; Sabin, C.A.; Sterne, J.A.C. Life expectancy of people with HIV on long-term antiretroviral therapy in Europe and North America: A cohort study. *Lancet Healthy Longev.* **2022**, *3*, S2. [CrossRef]
2. Deeks, S.G.; Lewin, S.R.; Havlir, D.V. The end of AIDS: HIV infection as a chronic disease. *Lancet* **2013**, *382*, 1525–1533. [CrossRef]
3. Deeks, S.G.; Phillips, A.N. HIV infection, antiretroviral treatment, ageing, and non-AIDS related morbidity. *BMJ* **2009**, *338*, a3172. [CrossRef] [PubMed]
4. Guaraldi, G.; Rockwood, K. Geriatric-HIV Medicine Is Born. *Clin. Infect. Dis.* **2017**, *65*, 507–509. [CrossRef]
5. Guaraldi, G.; Milic, J.; Mussini, C. Aging with HIV. *Curr. HIV/AIDS Rep.* **2019**, *16*, 475–481. [CrossRef] [PubMed]
6. Trunfio, M.; Vai, D.; Montrucchio, C.; Alcantarini, C.; Livelli, A.; Tettoni, M.; Orofino, G.; Audagnotto, S.; Imperiale, D.; Bonora, S.; et al. Diagnostic accuracy of new and old cognitive screening tools for HIV-associated neurocognitive disorders. *HIV Med.* **2018**, *19*, 455–464. [CrossRef]
7. Calcagno, A.; Celani, L.; Trunfio, M.; Orofino, G.; Imperiale, D.; Atzori, C.; Arena, V.; Ettorre, G.D.; Guaraldi, G.; Gisslen, M.; et al. Alzheimer Dementia in People Living with HIV. *Neurol. Clin. Pract.* **2021**, *11*, e627–e633. [CrossRef]

8. Mazzitelli, M.; Isabel, P.B.; Muramatsu, T.; Chirwa, M.; Mandalia, S.; Moyle, G.; Marta, B.; Milinkovic, A. FRAX assessment in people ageing with HIV. *HIV Med.* **2022**, *23*, 103–108. [CrossRef] [PubMed]
9. Pereira, B.; Mazzitelli, M.; Milinkovic, A.; Moyle, G.; Mandalia, S.; Al-Hussaini, A.; Boffito, M. Short Communication: Predictive Value of HIV-Related Versus Traditional Risk Factors for Coronary Atherosclerosis in People Aging with HIV. *AIDS Res. Hum. Retroviruses* **2022**, *38*, 80–86. [CrossRef]
10. Mazzitelli, M.; Fusco, P.; Brogna, M.; Vallone, A.; D'argenio, L.; Beradelli, G.; Foti, G.; Mangano, C.; Carpentieri, M.S.; Cosco, L.; et al. Weight of Clinical and Social Determinants of Metabolic Syndrome in People Living with HIV. *Viruses* **2022**, *14*, 1339. [CrossRef]
11. Mazzitelli, M.; Pereira, B.I.; Moyle, G.; Asboe, D.; Pozniak, A.; Boffito, M.; Milinkovic, A. Factors associated with overweight/obesity in a cohort of people living with HIV over 50 years of age. *AIDS Care* **2022**, *34*, 542–544. [CrossRef] [PubMed]
12. Micali, C.; Russotto, Y.; Celesia, B.M.; Santoro, L.; Marino, A.; Pellicanò, G.F.; Nunnari, G.; Rullo, E.V. Thyroid Diseases and Thyroid Asymptomatic Dysfunction in People Living with HIV. *Infect. Dis. Rep.* **2022**, *14*, 655–667. [CrossRef] [PubMed]
13. Moore, R.D.; Keruly, J.C. CD4+ Cell Count 6 Years after Commencement of Highly Active Antiretroviral Therapy in Persons with Sustained Virologic Suppression. *Clin. Infect. Dis.* **2007**, *44*, 441–446. [CrossRef] [PubMed]
14. Kelley, C.F.; Kitchen, C.M.; Hunt, P.W.; Rodriguez, B.; Hecht, F.M.; Kitahata, M.; Crane, H.M.; Willig, J.; Mugavero, M.; Saag, M.; et al. Incomplete peripheral CD4+ cell count restoration in HIV-infected patients receiving long-term antiretroviral treatment. *Clin. Infect. Dis.* **2009**, *48*, 787–794. [CrossRef] [PubMed]
15. Liu, J.; Wang, L.; Hou, Y.; Zhao, Y.; Dou, Z.; Ma, Y.; Zhang, D.; Wu, Y.; Zhao, D.; Liu, Z.; et al. Immune restoration in HIV-1-infected patients after 12 years of antiretroviral therapy: A real-world observational study. *Emerg. Microbes Infect.* **2020**, *9*, 2550–2561. [CrossRef] [PubMed]
16. De Vito, A.; Ricci, E.; Menzaghi, B.; Orofino, G.; Martinelli, C.V.; Squillace, N.; Taramasso, L.; De Socio, G.V.; Molteni, C.; Valsecchi, L.; et al. Causes of HIV Treatment Interruption during the Last 20 Years: A Multi-Cohort Real-Life Study. *Viruses* **2023**, *15*, 720. [CrossRef]
17. Madeddu, G.; Fois, A.G.; Calia, G.M.; Babudieri, S.; Soddu, V.; Becciu, F.; Fiori, M.L.; Spada, V.; Lovigu, C.; Mannazzu, M.; et al. Chronic obstructive pulmonary disease: An emerging comorbidity in HIV-infected patients in the HAART era? *Infection* **2012**, *41*, 347–353. [CrossRef]
18. Rosenbloom, M.J.; Sullivan, E.V.; Pfefferbaum, A. Focus on the brain: HIV infection and alcoholism comorbidity effects on brain structure and function. *Alcohol Res. Health* **2010**, *33*, 247–257.
19. Ghattas, M.; Dwivedi, G.; Lavertu, M.; Alameh, M.-G. Vaccine Technologies and Platforms for Infectious Diseases: Current Progress, Challenges, and Opportunities. *Vaccines* **2021**, *9*, 1490. [CrossRef]
20. Mascola, J.R.; Fauci, A.S. Novel vaccine technologies for the 21st century. *Nat. Rev. Immunol.* **2019**, *20*, 87–88. [CrossRef]
21. European AIDS Clinical Society. EACS Guidelines 11.0. 2021. Available online: https://www.eacsociety.org/media/final2021eacsguidelinesv11.0_oct2021.pdf (accessed on 28 February 2023).
22. BHIVA. British HIV Association Guidelines on Immunisation for Adults with HIV: SARS-CoV-2 (COVID-19). 2021. Available online: https://www.bhiva.org/SARS-CoV-2-vaccine-advice-for-adults-living-with-HIV-plain-english-version-update (accessed on 28 February 2023).
23. NIH. Guidelines for the Prevention and Treatment of Opportunistic Infections in Adults and Adolescents with HIV How to Cite the Adult and Adolescent Opportunistic Infection Guidelines: Panel on Guidelines for the Prevention and Treatment of Opportunistic Infections in Adults and Adolescents with HIV. Guidelines for the Prevention and Treatment of Opportunistic Infections in Adults and Adolescents. 2022. Available online: https://clinicalinfo.hiv.gov/en/ (accessed on 28 February 2023).
24. EACS GUIDELINES Version 11.1—October 2022. Available online: https://www.eacsociety.org/media/guidelines-11.1_final_09-10.pdf (accessed on 28 February 2023).
25. Pozniak, A.; Hospital, W.; Alison Rodger, L. British HIV Association Guidelines on the Use of Vaccines in HIV-Positive Adults 2015 BHIVA Guidelines on the Use of Vaccines in Hiv—Positive Adults 2015. Available online: www.nice.org.uk/accreditation (accessed on 28 February 2023).
26. World Health Organization. *Consolidated Guidelines on HIV Prevention, Testing, Treatment, Service Delivery and Monitoring: Recommendations for a Public Health Approach*; WHO: Geneva, Switzerland, 2021.
27. SIMIT (Società Italiana di Malattie Infettive e Tropicali). Linee Guida Italiane sull'utilizzo della Terapia Antiretrovirale e la Gestione Diagnostico-Clinica delle Persone con Infezione da HIV-1 -Edizione 2017. 2017, pp. 135–136. Available online: www.simit.org (accessed on 28 February 2023).
28. Rapicetta, M.; Monarca, R.; Kondili, L.A.; Chionne, P.; Madonna, E.; Madeddu, G.; Soddu, A.; Candido, A.; Carbonara, S.; Mura, M.S.; et al. Hepatitis E virus and hepatitis A virus exposures in an apparently healthy high-risk population in Italy. *Infection* **2012**, *41*, 69–76. [CrossRef] [PubMed]
29. Lin, K.-Y.; Chen, G.-J.; Lee, Y.-L.; Huang, Y.-C.; Cheng, A.; Sun, H.-Y.; Chang, S.-Y.; Liu, C.-E.; Hung, C.-C. Hepatitis A virus infection and hepatitis A vaccination in human immunodeficiency virus-positive patients: A review. *World J. Gastroenterol.* **2017**, *23*, 3589–3606. [CrossRef] [PubMed]
30. Laurence, J.C. Hepatitis A and B immunizations of individuals infected with human immunodeficiency virus. *Am. J. Med.* **2005**, *118*, 75–83. [CrossRef] [PubMed]

31. Antonini, T.M.; Sebagh, M.; Roque-Afonso, A.M.; Teicher, E.; Roche, B.; Sobesky, R.; Coilly, A.; Vaghefi, P.; Adam, R.; Vittecoq, D.; et al. Fibrosing Cholestatic Hepatitis in HIV/HCV Co-Infected Transplant Patients—Usefulness of Early Markers After Liver Transplantation. *Am. J. Transplant.* **2011**, *11*, 1686–1695. [CrossRef]
32. Doulberis, M.; Kotronis, G.; Gialamprinou, D.; Özgüler, O.; Exadaktylos, A.K.; Oikonomou, V.; Katsinelos, P.; Romiopoulos, I.; Polyzos, S.; Tzivras, D. Acute Liver Failure: From Textbook to Emergency Room and Intensive Care Unit with Concomitant Established and Modern Novel Therapies. *J. Clin. Gastroenterol.* **2019**, *53*, 89–101. [CrossRef]
33. Vidor, E.; Fritzell, B.; Plotkin, S. Clinical development of a new inactivated hepatitis a vaccine. *Infection* **1996**, *24*, 447–458. [CrossRef]
34. Mena, G.; García-Basteiro, A.; Bayas, J. Hepatitis B and A vaccination in HIV-infected adults: A review. *Hum. Vaccines Immunother.* **2015**, *11*, 2582–2598. [CrossRef]
35. Chen, G.-J.; Sun, H.-Y.; Lin, K.-Y.; Cheng, A.; Huang, Y.-C.; Hsieh, S.-M.; Sheng, W.-H.; Liu, W.-C.; Hung, C.-C.; Chang, S.-C. Serological responses to revaccination with hepatitis A virus (HAV) vaccines among HIV-positive individuals whose anti-HAV antibody waned after primary vaccination. *Liver Int.* **2018**, *38*, 1198–1205. [CrossRef]
36. Jabłonowska, E.; Kuydowicz, J. Durability of response to vaccination against viral hepatitis A in HIV-infected patients: A 5-year observation. *Int. J. STD AIDS* **2014**, *25*, 745–750. [CrossRef]
37. Midthun, K.; Ellerbeck, E.; Gershman, K.; Calandra, G.; Krah, D.; McCaughtry, M.; Nalin, D.; Provost, P. Safety and Immunogenicity of a Live Attenuated Hepatitis A Virus Vaccine in Seronegative Volunteers. *J. Infect. Dis.* **1991**, *163*, 735–739. [CrossRef]
38. Crisinel, P.A.; Posfay-Barbe, K.M.; Aebi, C.; Cheseaux, J.-J.; Kahlert, C.; Rudin, C.; Nadal, D.; Siegrist, C.-A. Determinants of Hepatitis A Vaccine Immunity in a Cohort of Human Immunodeficiency Virus-Infected Children Living in Switzerland. *Clin. Vaccine Immunol.* **2012**, *19*, 1751–1757. [CrossRef] [PubMed]
39. Kourkounti, S.; Paparizos, V.; Leuow, K.; Paparizou, E.; Antoniou, C. Adherence to hepatitis A virus vaccination in HIV-infected men who have sex with men. *Int. J. STD AIDS* **2015**, *26*, 852–856. [CrossRef] [PubMed]
40. Sulkowski, M.S. Viral hepatitis and HIV coinfection. *J. Hepatol.* **2008**, *48*, 353–367. [CrossRef] [PubMed]
41. Bruguera, M.; Cremades, M.; Salinas, R.; Costa, J.; Grau, M.; Sans, J. Impaired Response to Recombinant Hepatitis B Vaccine in HIV-Infected Persons. *J. Clin. Gastroenterol.* **1992**, *14*, 27–30. [CrossRef]
42. Sagnelli, E.; Stroffolini, T.; Sagnelli, C.; Smedile, A.; Morisco, F.; Furlan, C.; Babudieri, S.; Brancaccio, G.; Coppola, N.; Gaeta, G.B.; et al. Epidemiological and clinical scenario of chronic liver diseases in Italy: Data from a multicenter nationwide survey. *Dig. Liver Dis.* **2016**, *48*, 1066–1071. [CrossRef]
43. Tavoschi, L.; Vroling, H.; Madeddu, G.; Babudieri, S.; Monarca, R.; Noordegraaf-Schouten, M.V.; Beer, N.; Dias, J.G.; O'moore, E.; Hedrich, D.; et al. Active Case Finding for Communicable Diseases in Prison Settings: Increasing Testing Coverage and Uptake among the Prison Population in the European Union/European Economic Area. *Epidemiol. Rev.* **2018**, *40*, 105–120. [CrossRef]
44. Thio, C.L.; Seaberg, E.C.; Skolasky, R., Jr.; Phair, J.; Visscher, B.; Muñoz, A.; Thomas, D.L. HIV-1, hepatitis B virus, and risk of liver-related mortality in the Multicenter Cohort Study (MACS). *Lancet* **2002**, *360*, 1921–1926. [CrossRef]
45. Walter, S.R.; Thein, H.H.; Amin, J.; Gidding, H.F.; Ward, K.; Law, M.G.; George, J.; Dore, G.J. Trends in mortality after diagnosis of hepatitis B or C infection: 1992–2006. *J. Hepatol.* **2011**, *54*, 879–886. [CrossRef]
46. Hadler, S.C.; Judson, F.N.; O'Malley, P.M.; Altman, N.L.; Penley, K.; Buchbinder, S.; Schable, C.A.; Coleman, P.J.; Ostrow, D.N.; Francis, D.R. Outcome of Hepatitis B Virus Infection in Homosexual Men and Its Relation to Prior Human Immunodeficiency Virus Infection. *J. Infect. Dis.* **1991**, *163*, 454–457. [CrossRef]
47. Micali, C.; Russotto, Y.; Caci, G.; Ceccarelli, M.; Marino, A.; Celesia, B.M.; Pellicanò, G.F.; Nunnari, G.; Rullo, E.V. Loco-Regional Treatments for Hepatocellular Carcinoma in People Living with HIV. *Infect. Dis. Rep.* **2022**, *14*, 43–55. [CrossRef]
48. Mazzitelli, M.; Greco, G.; Serapide, F.; Scaglione, V.; Morrone, H.; Marascio, N.; Giancotti, A.; Liberto, M.; Matera, G.; Trecarichi, E.; et al. Outcome of HBV screening and vaccination in a migrant population in southern Italy. *Infez. Med.* **2021**, *29*, 236–241.
49. Serraino, R.; Mazzitelli, M.; Greco, G.; Serapide, F.; Scaglione, V.; Marascio, N.; Trecarichi, E.M.; Torti, C. Risk factors for hepatitis B and C among healthy population: A community-based survey from four districts of Southern Italy. *Infez. Med.* **2020**, *28*, 223–226. [PubMed]
50. Farooq, P.D.; Sherman, K.E. Hepatitis B Vaccination and Waning Hepatitis B Immunity in Persons Living with HIV. *Curr. HIV/AIDS Rep.* **2019**, *16*, 395–403. [CrossRef] [PubMed]
51. Mohareb, A.M.; Kouamé, G.M.; Gabassi, A.; Gabillard, D.; Moh, R.; Badje, A.; Emième, A.; Maylin, S.; Ménan, H.; Hyle, E.P.; et al. Mortality in relation to hepatitis B virus (HBV) infection status among HIV-HBV co-infected patients in sub-Saharan Africa after immediate initiation of antiretroviral therapy. *J. Viral Hepat.* **2021**, *28*, 621–629. [CrossRef] [PubMed]
52. Mohareb, A.M.; Kim, A.Y. Hepatitis B vaccination in people living with HIV: If at first you don't succeed, try again. *JAMA Netw. Open* **2021**, *4*, e2121281. [CrossRef] [PubMed]
53. CDC. Availability of Hepatitis B Vaccine That Does Not Contain Thimerosal as a Preservative. 1999. Available online: https://www.cdc.gov/mmwr/preview/mmwrhtml/mm4835a3.htm (accessed on 28 February 2023).
54. Sablan, B.P.; Kim, D.J.; Barzaga, N.G.; Chow, W.C.; Cho, M.; Ahn, S.H.; Hwang, S.G.; Lee, J.H.; Namini, H.; Heyward, W.L. Demonstration of safety and enhanced seroprotection against hepatitis B with investigational HBsAg-1018 ISS vaccine compared to a licensed hepatitis B vaccine. *Vaccine* **2012**, *30*, 2689–2696. [CrossRef] [PubMed]

55. Halperin, S.A.; Ward, B.; Cooper, C.; Predy, G.; Diaz-Mitoma, F.; Dionne, M.; Embree, J.; McGeer, A.; Zickler, P.; Moltz, K.-H.; et al. Comparison of safety and immunogenicity of two doses of investigational hepatitis B virus surface antigen co-administered with an immunostimulatory phosphorothioate oligodeoxyribonucleotide and three doses of a licensed hepatitis B vaccine in healthy adults 18–55 years of age. *Vaccine* **2012**, *30*, 2556–2563. [CrossRef]
56. HEPLISAV-B® Safely and Effectively. 2019. Available online: www.vaers.hhs.gov (accessed on 28 February 2023).
57. TWINRIX Information Sheet. Available online: https://ca.gsk.com/media/6262/twinrix.pdf (accessed on 28 February 2023).
58. Corcorran, M.A.; Kim, N. Chronic hepatitis B and HIV coinfection. *Top Antivir Med.* **2023**, *31*, 14–22.
59. de Vries-Sluijs, T.E.M.S.; Hansen, B.E.; van Doornum, G.J.J.; Kauffmann, R.H.; Leyten, E.M.S.; Mudrikova, T.; Brinkman, K.; den Hollander, J.G.; Kroon, F.P.; Janssen, H.L.A.; et al. A Randomized Controlled Study of Accelerated Versus Standard Hepatitis B Vaccination in HIV-Positive Patients. *J. Infect. Dis.* **2011**, *203*, 984–991. [CrossRef]
60. Cornejo-Juárez, P.; Volkow-Fernández, P.; Escobedo-López, K.; Vilar-Compte, D.; Ruiz-Palacios, G.; Soto-Ramírez, L.E. Randomized controlled trial of Hepatitis B virus vaccine in HIV-1-infected patients comparing two different doses. *AIDS Res. Ther.* **2006**, *3*, 9. [CrossRef]
61. Fonseca, M.O.; Pang, L.W.; Cavalheiro, N.D.P.; Barone, A.A.; Lopes, M.H. Randomized trial of recombinant hepatitis B vaccine in HIV-infected adult patients comparing a standard dose to a double dose. *Vaccine* **2005**, *23*, 2902–2908. [CrossRef] [PubMed]
62. Launay, O.; van der Vliet, D.; Rosenberg, A.R.; Michel, M.-L.; Piroth, L.; Rey, D.; de Verdière, N.C.; Slama, L.; Martin, K.; Lortholary, O.; et al. Safety and Immunogenicity of 4 Intramuscular Double Doses and 4 Intradermal Low Doses vs Standard Hepatitis B Vaccine Regimen in Adults with HIV-1: A Randomized Controlled Trial. *JAMA* **2011**, *305*, 1432–1440. [CrossRef] [PubMed]
63. Chaiklang, K.; Wipasa, J.; Chaiwarith, R.; Praparattanapan, J.; Supparatpinyo, K. Comparison of Immunogenicity and Safety of Four Doses and Four Double Doses vs. Standard Doses of Hepatitis B Vaccination in HIV-Infected Adults: A Randomized, Controlled Trial. *PLoS ONE* **2013**, *8*, e80409. [CrossRef]
64. Ni, J.D.; Xiong, Y.Z.; Wang, X.J.; Xiu, L.C. Does increased hepatitis B vaccination dose lead to a better immune response in HIV-infected patients than standard dose vaccination: A meta-analysis? *Int. J. STD AIDS* **2013**, *24*, 117–122. [CrossRef] [PubMed]
65. Conseil de la Santé Publique, H. Vaccination des Personnes Immunodéprimées ou Aspléniques Recommandations Collection Avis et Rapports 2 e Édition. Available online: www.hcsp.fr (accessed on 28 February 2023).
66. Psevdos, G.; Kim, J.H.; Groce, V.; Sharp, V. Efficacy of Double-Dose Hepatitis B Rescue Vaccination in HIV-Infected Patients. *AIDS Patient Care STDS* **2010**, *24*, 403–407. [CrossRef]
67. Rey, D.; Piroth, L.; Wendling, M.-J.; Miailhes, P.; Michel, M.-L.; Dufour, C.; Haour, G.; Sogni, P.; Rohel, A.; Ajana, F.; et al. Safety and immunogenicity of double-dose versus standard-dose hepatitis B revaccination in non-responding adults with HIV-1 (ANRS HB04 B-BOOST): A multicentre, open-label, randomised controlled trial. *Lancet Infect. Dis.* **2015**, *15*, 1283–1291. [CrossRef] [PubMed]
68. Vargas, J.I.; Jensen, D.; Martínez, F.; Sarmiento, V.; Peirano, F.; Acuña, P.; Provoste, F.; Bustos, V.; Cornejo, F.; Fuster, A.; et al. Comparative Efficacy of a High-Dose vs Standard-Dose Hepatitis B Revaccination Schedule among Patients with HIV: A Randomized Clinical Trial. *JAMA Netw. Open* **2021**, *4*, e2120929. [CrossRef]
69. Pallawela, S.N.S.; Sonnex, C.; Mabayoje, D.; Bloch, E.; Chaytor, S.; Johnson, M.A.; Carne, C.; Webster, D.P. Positive hepatitis B virus core antibody in HIV infection-false positive or evidence of previous infection? *J. Med. Virol.* **2015**, *87*, 208–212. [CrossRef]
70. Witt, M.D.; Lewis, R.J.; Rieg, G.; Seaberg, E.C.; Rinaldo, C.R.; Thio, C.L. Predictors of the Isolated Hepatitis B Core Antibody Pattern in HIV-Infected and -Uninfected Men in the Multicenter AIDS Cohort Study. *Clin. Infect. Dis.* **2013**, *56*, 606–612. [CrossRef]
71. Tassachew, Y.; Abebe, T.; Belyhun, Y.; Teffera, T.; Shewaye, A.B.; Desalegn, H.; Andualem, H.; Kinfu, A.; Mulu, A.; Mihret, A.; et al. Prevalence of HIV and Its Co-Infection with Hepatitis B/C Virus among Chronic Liver Disease Patients in Ethiopia. *Hepatic Med.* **2022**, *14*, 67–77. [CrossRef]
72. Khamduang, W.; Ngo-Giang-Huong, N.; Gaudy-Graffin, C.; Jourdain, G.; Suwankornsakul, W.; Jarupanich, T.; Chalermpolprapa, V.; Nanta, S.; Puarattana-Aroonkorn, N.; Tonmat, S.; et al. Prevalence, Risk Factors, and Impact of Isolated Antibody to Hepatitis B Core Antigen and Occult Hepatitis B Virus Infection in HIV-1–Infected Pregnant Women. *Clin. Infect. Dis.* **2013**, *56*, 1704–1712. [CrossRef] [PubMed]
73. Landrum, M.L.; Roediger, M.P.; Fieberg, A.M.; Weintrob, A.C.; Okulicz, J.F.; Crum-Cianflone, N.F.; Ganesan, A.; Lalani, T.; Macalino, G.E.; Chun, H.M. Development of chronic hepatitis B virus infection in hepatitis B surface antigen negative HIV/HBV co-infected adults: A rare opportunistic illness. *J. Med. Virol.* **2011**, *83*, 1537–1543. [CrossRef] [PubMed]
74. Gandhi, R.T.; Wurcel, A.; Lee, H.; McGovern, B.; Shopis, J.; Geary, M.; Sivamurthy, R.; Sax, P.E.; Ukomadu, C. Response to Hepatitis B Vaccine in HIV-1–Positive Subjects Who Test Positive for Isolated Antibody to Hepatitis B Core Antigen: Implications for Hepatitis B Vaccine Strategies. *J. Infect. Dis.* **2005**, *191*, 1435–1441. [CrossRef] [PubMed]
75. Piroth, L.; Launay, O.; Michel, M.L.; Bourredjem, A.; Miailhes, P.; Ajana, F.; Chirouze, C.; Zucman, D.; Wendling, M.J.; Nazzal, D.; et al. Vaccination Against Hepatitis B Virus (HBV) in HIV-1–Infected Patients with Isolated Anti–HBV Core Antibody: The ANRS HB EP03 CISOVAC Prospective Study. *J. Infect. Dis.* **2016**, *213*, 1735–1742. [CrossRef] [PubMed]
76. Chakvetadze, C.; Bani-Sadr, F.; Le Pendeven, C.; Lescure, F.-X.; Fontaine, C.; Galperine, T.; Slama, L.; Bonnard, P.; Mariot, P.; Soussan, P.; et al. Serologic Response to Hepatitis B Vaccination in HIV-Infected Patients with Isolated Positivity for Antibodies to Hepatitis B Core Antigen. *Clin. Infect. Dis.* **2010**, *50*, 1184–1186. [CrossRef]

77. Kaech, C.; Pache, I.; Bürgisser, P.; Elzi, L.; Darling, K.E.; Cavassini, M. Immune response to hepatitis B vaccination in HIV-positive adults with isolated antibodies to HBV core antigen. *J. Infect.* **2012**, *65*, 157–164. [CrossRef]
78. de Martel, C.; Plummer, M.; Vignat, J.; Franceschi, S. Worldwide burden of cancer attributable to HPV by site, country and HPV type. *Int. J. Cancer* **2017**, *141*, 664–670. [CrossRef]
79. Madeddu, G.; Mameli, G.; Capobianco, G.; Babudieri, S.; Maida, I.; Bagella, P.; Rocca, G.; Cherchi, P.L.; Sechi, L.A.; Zanetti, S.; et al. HPV infection in HIV-positive females: The need for cervical cancer screening including HPV-DNA detection despite successful HAART. *Eur. Rev. Med. Pharmacol. Sci.* **2014**, *18*, 1277–1285.
80. Ceccarelli, M.; Rullo, E.V.; Facciolà, A.; Madeddu, G.; Cacopardo, B.; Taibi, R.; D'Aleo, F.; Pinzone, M.R.; Picerno, I.; di Rosa, M.; et al. Head and neck squamous cell carcinoma and its correlation with human papillomavirus in people living with HIV: A systematic review. *Oncotarget* **2018**, *9*, 17171–17180. [CrossRef]
81. Lacey, C.J. HPV vaccination in HIV infection. *Papillomavirus Res.* **2019**, *8*, 100174. [CrossRef]
82. Ceccarelli, M.; Rullo, E.V.; Marino, M.A.; D'Aleo, F.; Pellicanò, G.F.; D'Andrea, F.; Marino, A.; Cacopardo, B.; Celesia, B.M.; La Rocca, G.; et al. Non-AIDS defining cancers: A comprehensive update on diagnosis and management. *Eur. Rev. Med. Pharmacol. Sci.* **2020**, *24*, 3849–3875.
83. Stelzle, D.; Tanaka, L.F.; Lee, K.K.; Ibrahim Khalil, A.; Baussano, I.; Shah, A.S.V.; McAllister, D.A.; Gottlieb, S.L.; Klug, S.J.; Winkler, A.S.; et al. Estimates of the global burden of cervical cancer associated with HIV. *Lancet Glob. Health* **2021**, *9*, e161–e169. [CrossRef] [PubMed]
84. Denny, L.A.; Franceschi, S.; de Sanjosé, S.; Heard, I.; Moscicki, A.B.; Palefsky, J. Human Papillomavirus, Human Immunodeficiency Virus and Immunosuppression. *Vaccine* **2012**, *30*, F168–F174. [CrossRef] [PubMed]
85. Looker, K.J.; Rönn, M.M.; Brock, P.M.; Brisson, M.; Drolet, M.; Mayaud, P.; Boily, M.C. Evidence of synergistic relationships between HIV and Human Papillomavirus (HPV): Systematic reviews and meta-analyses of longitudinal studies of HPV acquisition and clearance by HIV status, and of HIV acquisition by HPV status. *J. Int. AIDS Soc.* **2018**, *21*, e25110. [CrossRef] [PubMed]
86. Liu, G.; Mugo, N.R.; Bayer, C.; Rao, D.W.; Onono, M.; Mgodi, N.M.; Chirenje, Z.M.; Njoroge, B.W.; Tan, N.; A Bukusi, E.; et al. Impact of catch-up human papillomavirus vaccination on cervical cancer incidence in Kenya: A mathematical modeling evaluation of HPV vaccination strategies in the context of moderate HIV prevalence. *Eclinicalmedicine* **2022**, *45*, 101306. [CrossRef]
87. World Health Organization. Global Strategy to Accelerate the Elimination of Cervical Cancer as a Public Health Problem. Available online: http://apps.who.int/bookorders (accessed on 28 February 2023).
88. Kreimer, A.R.; Herrero, R.; Sampson, J.N.; Porras, C.; Lowy, D.R.; Schiller, J.T.; Schiffman, M.; Rodriguez, A.C.; Chanock, S.; Jimenez, S.; et al. Evidence for single-dose protection by the bivalent HPV vaccine—Review of the Costa Rica HPV vaccine trial and future research studies. *Vaccine* **2018**, *36*, 4774–4782. [CrossRef]
89. Staadegaard, L.; Rönn, M.M.; Soni, N.; Bellerose, M.E.; Bloem, P.; Brisson, M.; Maheu-Giroux, M.; Barnabas, R.V.; Drolet, M.; Mayaud, P.; et al. Immunogenicity, safety, and efficacy of the HPV vaccines among people living with HIV: A systematic review and meta-analysis. *Eclinicalmedicine* **2022**, *52*, 101585. [CrossRef]
90. Brophy, J.; Bitnun, A.; Alimenti, A.; Lapointe, N.; Samson, L.; Read, S.; Karatzios, C.; Dobson, S.; Moses, E.; Blitz, S.; et al. Immunogenicity and Safety of the Quadrivalent Human Papillomavirus Vaccine in Girls Living with HIV. *Pediatr. Infect. Dis. J.* **2018**, *37*, 595–597. [CrossRef]
91. Kahn, J.A.; Xu, J.; Kapogiannis, B.G.; Rudy, B.; Gonin, R.; Liu, N.; Wilson, C.M.; Worrell, C.; Squires, K.E. Immunogenicity and Safety of the Human Papillomavirus 6, 11, 16, 18 Vaccine in HIV-Infected Young Women. *Clin. Infect. Dis.* **2013**, *57*, 735–744. [CrossRef]
92. Money, D.M.; Moses, E.; Blitz, S.; Vandriel, S.M.; Lipsky, N.; Walmsley, S.L.; Loutfy, M.; Trottier, S.; Smaill, F.; Yudin, M.H.; et al. HIV viral suppression results in higher antibody responses in HIV-positive women vaccinated with the quadrivalent human papillomavirus vaccine. *Vaccine* **2016**, *34*, 4799–4806. [CrossRef]
93. Levin, M.J.; Huang, S.; Moscicki, A.-B.; Song, L.-Y.; Read, J.S.; Meyer, W.A.; Saah, A.J.; Richardson, K.; Weinberg, A. Four-year persistence of type-specific immunity after quadrivalent human papillomavirus vaccination in HIV-infected children: Effect of a fourth dose of vaccine. *Vaccine* **2017**, *35*, 1712–1720. [CrossRef] [PubMed]
94. Kojic, E.M.; Kang, M.; Cespedes, M.S.; Umbleja, T.; Godfrey, C.; Allen, R.T.; Firnhaber, C.; Grinsztejn, B.; Palefsky, J.M.; Webster-Cyriaque, J.Y.; et al. Immunogenicity and Safety of the Quadrivalent Human Papillomavirus Vaccine in HIV-1-Infected Women. *Clin. Infect. Dis.* **2014**, *59*, 127–135. [CrossRef] [PubMed]
95. Moscicki, A.-B.; Karalius, B.; Tassiopoulos, K.; Yao, T.-J.; Jacobson, D.L.; Patel, K.; Purswani, M.; Seage, G.R.; Yogev, R.; Sanders, M.A.; et al. Human Papillomavirus Antibody Levels and Quadrivalent Vaccine Clinical Effectiveness in Perinatally Human Immunodeficiency Virus–infected and Exposed, Uninfected Youth. *Clin. Infect. Dis.* **2019**, *69*, 1183–1191. [CrossRef] [PubMed]
96. Faust, H.; Toft, L.; Sehr, P.; Müller, M.; Bonde, J.; Forslund, O.; Østergaard, L.; Tolstrup, M.; Dillner, J. Human Papillomavirus neutralizing and cross-reactive antibodies induced in HIV-positive subjects after vaccination with quadrivalent and bivalent HPV vaccines. *Vaccine* **2016**, *34*, 1559–1565. [CrossRef] [PubMed]
97. Cooper, C.L.; Angel, J.B.; Seguin, I.; Davis, H.L.; Cameron, B. CPG 7909 Adjuvant plus Hepatitis B Virus Vaccination in HIV-Infected Adults Achieves Long-Term Seroprotection for Up to 5 Years. *Clin. Infect. Dis.* **2008**, *46*, 1310–1314. [CrossRef]
98. Gilca, V.; Sauvageau, C.; Panicker, G.; De Serres, G.; Ouakki, M.; Unger, E.R. Immunogenicity and safety of a mixed vaccination schedule with one dose of nonavalent and one dose of bivalent HPV vaccine versus two doses of nonavalent vaccine—A randomized clinical trial. *Vaccine* **2018**, *36*, 7017–7024. [CrossRef] [PubMed]

99. Ceccarelli, M.; Berretta, M.; Rullo, E.V.; Nunnari, G.; Cacopardo, B. Differences and similarities between Severe Acute Respiratory Syndrome (SARS)-CoronaVirus (CoV) and SARS-CoV-2. Would a rose by another name smell as sweet? *Eur. Rev. Med. Pharmacol. Sci.* **2020**, *24*, 2781–2783.
100. World Health Organization. Influenza (Seasonal). Available online: https://www.who.int/news-room/fact-sheets/detail/influenza-(seasonal) (accessed on 11 February 2023).
101. World Health Organization. Global Influenza Surveillance and Response System (GISRS). Available online: https://www.who.int/initiatives/global-influenza-surveillance-and-response-system (accessed on 11 February 2023).
102. Geretti, A.M.; Brook, G.; Cameron, C.; Chadwick, D.; French, N.; Heyderman, R.; Ho, A.; Hunter, M.; Ladhani, S.; Lawton, M.; et al. British HIV Association Guidelines on the Use of Vaccines in HIV-Positive Adults 2015. *HIV Med.* **2016**, *17*, s2–s81. [CrossRef]
103. Caldera, F.; Mercer, M.; Samson, S.I.; Pitt, J.M.; Hayney, M.S. Influenza vaccination in immunocompromised populations: Strategies to improve immunogenicity. *Vaccine* **2021**, *39* (Suppl. S1), A15–A23. [CrossRef]
104. Breitschwerdt, S.; Schwarze-Zander, C.; Al Tayy, A.; Mutevelli, J.; Wasmuth, J.C.; Rockstroh, J.K.; Boesecke, C. Implementation of EACS vaccination recommendations among people living with HIV. *Infection* **2022**, *50*, 1491–1497. [CrossRef]
105. Remschmidt, C.; Wichmann, O.; Harder, T. Influenza vaccination in HIV-infected individuals: Systematic review and assessment of quality of evidence related to vaccine efficacy, effectiveness and safety. *Vaccine* **2014**, *32*, 5585–5592. [CrossRef] [PubMed]
106. Pallikkuth, S.; De Armas, L.R.; Pahwa, R.; Rinaldi, S.; George, V.K.; Sanchez, C.M.; Pan, L.; Dickinson, G.; Rodriguez, A.; Fischl, M.; et al. Impact of aging and HIV infection on serologic response to seasonal influenza vaccination. *AIDS* **2018**, *32*, 1085–1094. [CrossRef] [PubMed]
107. Pallikkuth, S.; De Armas, L.R.; Rinaldi, S.; George, V.K.; Pan, L.; Arheart, K.L.; Pahwa, R.; Pahwa, S. Dysfunctional peripheral T follicular helper cells dominate in people with impaired influenza vaccine responses: Results from the FLORAH study. *PLoS Biol.* **2019**, *17*, e3000257. [CrossRef] [PubMed]
108. Pepin, S.; Nicolas, J.-F.; Szymanski, H.; Leroux-Roels, I.; Schaum, T.; Bonten, M.; Icardi, G.; Shrestha, A.; Tabar, C. The QHD00011 study team Immunogenicity and safety of a quadrivalent high-dose inactivated influenza vaccine compared with a standard-dose quadrivalent influenza vaccine in healthy people aged 60 years or older: A randomized Phase III trial. *Hum. Vaccines Immunother.* **2021**, *17*, 5475–5486. [CrossRef] [PubMed]
109. Liu, X.; Park, J.; Xia, S.; Liang, B.; Yang, S.; Wang, Y.; Syrkina, O.; Lavis, N.; Liu, S.; Zhao, C.; et al. Immunological non-inferiority and safety of a quadrivalent inactivated influenza vaccine versus two trivalent inactivated influenza vaccines in China: Results from two studies. *Hum. Vaccines Immunother.* **2022**, *18*, 2132798. [CrossRef]
110. Zanetti, A.R.; Amendola, A.; Besana, S.; Boschini, A.; Tanzi, E. Safety and immunogenicity of influenza vaccination in individuals infected with HIV. *Vaccine* **2002**, *20*, B29–B32. [CrossRef] [PubMed]
111. Kaplan, L.J.; Daum, R.S.; Smaron, M.; McCarthy, C.A. Severe Measles in Immunocompromised Patients. *JAMA* **1992**, *267*, 1237–1241. [CrossRef]
112. Rodriguez, C.; Gouilh, M.A.; Weiss, N.; Stroer, S.; Mokhtari, K.; Seilhean, D.; Mathon, B.; Demontant, V.; N'debi, M.; Gricourt, G.; et al. Fatal Measles Inclusion-Body Encephalitis in Adult with Untreated AIDS, France. *Emerg. Infect. Dis.* **2020**, *26*, 2231–2234. [CrossRef]
113. Dubey, S.; Chakraborty, A.P.; Ray, A.; Mukherjee, D.; Gupta, S.; Pandit, A. Subacute measles encephalitis in a case of late presenting congenital HIV with epilepsia partialis continua as the first manifestation: A case report. *J. Fam. Med. Prim. Care* **2021**, *10*, 3502. [CrossRef]
114. Moss, W.J.; Fisher, C.; Scott, S.; Monze, M.; Ryon, J.J.; Quinn, T.C.; Griffin, D.E.; Cutts, F.T. HIV Type 1 Infection Is a Risk Factor for Mortality in Hospitalized Zambian Children with Measles. *Clin. Infect. Dis.* **2008**, *46*, 523–527. [CrossRef]
115. Bechini, A.; Boccalini, S.; Ninci, A.; Zanobini, P.; Sartor, G.; Bonaccorsi, G.; Grazzini, M.; Bonanni, P. Childhood vaccination coverage in Europe: Impact of different public health policies. *Expert Rev. Vaccines* **2019**, *18*, 693–701. [CrossRef] [PubMed]
116. Facciola, A.; D'Andrea, G.; Cuffari, R.; Pellicano, G.; Visalli, G.; Di Pietro, A. Measles, Mumps, Rubella and Chickenpox epidemic and vaccination in Eastern Sicily: An epidemiologic study on seroconversion. *Infect. Dis. Trop. Med.* **2019**, *5*, e571.
117. Mehtani, N.J.; Rosman, L.; Moss, W.J. Immunogenicity and Safety of the Measles Vaccine in HIV-infected Children: An Updated Systematic Review. *Am. J. Epidemiol.* **2019**, *188*, 2240–2251. [CrossRef] [PubMed]
118. Mutsaerts, E.A.; Nunes, M.C.; van Rijswijk, M.N.; Klipstein-Grobusch, K.; Grobbee, D.E.; Madhi, S.A. Safety and Immunogenicity of Measles Vaccination in HIV-Infected and HIV-Exposed Uninfected Children: A Systematic Review and Meta-Analysis. *Eclinicalmedicine* **2018**, *1*, 28–42. [CrossRef] [PubMed]
119. Bruzzese, E.; Pagano, F.; Diana, A.; Punzi, L.; Guarino, A. Protection of Vaccine Preventable Diseases in a Population of HIV-Infected Children: A 3 Years Prospective Study. *Vaccines* **2021**, *9*, 1331. [CrossRef]
120. Loevinsohn, G.; Rosman, L.; Moss, W.J. Measles Seroprevalence and Vaccine Responses in Human Immunodeficiency Virus–infected Adolescents and Adults: A Systematic Review. *Clin. Infect. Dis.* **2018**, *69*, 836–844. [CrossRef]
121. Measles Pneumonitis Following Measles-Mumps-Rubella Vaccination of a Patient with HIV Infection. 1993. Available online: https://www.cdc.gov/mmwr/preview/mmwrhtml/00043110.htm (accessed on 17 December 2022).
122. Rearigh, L.; O'neill, J.; Kubat, M.; Sayles, H.; Swindells, S.; Bares, S.H. Surprisingly Low Levels of Measles Immunity in Persons with HIV: A Seroprevalence Survey in a United States HIV Clinic. *Open Forum Infect. Dis.* **2020**, *7*, 1–6. [CrossRef]

123. Candevir, A.; Kuşcu, F.; Yildirim, F.; Kömür, S.; Şentürk, G.; Inal, A.S.; Eser, F.; Çetiner, S.; Kurtaran, B.; Taşova, Y. Low immunity against vaccine preventable diseases in Turkish HIV cohort. *Turk. J. Med. Sci.* **2021**, *51*, 2311–2317. [CrossRef]
124. Lefebvre, M.; Secher, S.; Bouchez, S.; Vandamme, Y.-M.; Fialaire, P.; Leautez, S.; Blanchi, S.; Michau, C.; Coste-Burel, M.; Brunet-Cartier, C.; et al. Measles seroprevalence in human immunodeficiency virus-infected adults born in the era of measles vaccination. *AIDS* **2022**, *36*, 1273–1278. [CrossRef]
125. Di Giulio, D.B.; Eckburg, P.B. Human monkeypox: An emerging zoonosis. *Lancet Infect. Dis.* **2004**, *4*, 15–25. [CrossRef]
126. Ladnyj, I.D.; Ziegler, P.; Kima, E. A human infection caused by monkeypox virus in Basankusu Territory, Democratic Republic of the Congo. *Bull. World Health Organ.* **1972**, *46*, 593–597. [PubMed]
127. Reed, K.D.; Melski, J.W.; Graham, M.B.; Regnery, R.L.; Sotir, M.J.; Wegner, M.V.; Kazmierczak, J.J.; Stratman, E.J.; Li, Y.; Fairley, J.A.; et al. The Detection of Monkeypox in Humans in the Western Hemisphere. *N. Engl. J. Med.* **2004**, *350*, 342–350. [CrossRef] [PubMed]
128. World Health Organization. Multi-Country Monkeypox Outbreak in Non-Endemic Countries. Available online: https://www.who.int/emergencies/disease-outbreak-news/item/2022-DON385 (accessed on 11 February 2023).
129. Minhaj, F.S.; Ogale, Y.P.; Whitehill, F.; Schultz, J.; Foote, M.; Davidson, W.; Hughes, C.M.; Wilkins, K.; Bachmann, L.; Chatelain, R.; et al. Monkeypox Outbreak—Nine States, May 2022. *MMWR Morb. Mortal Wkly. Rep.* **2022**, *71*, 764–769. [CrossRef] [PubMed]
130. Thornhill, J.P.; Barkati, S.; Walmsley, S.; Rockstroh, J.; Antinori, A.; Harrison, L.B.; Palich, R.; Nori, A.; Reeves, I.; Habibi, M.S.; et al. Monkeypox Virus Infection in Humans across 16 Countries—April–June 2022. *N. Engl. J. Med.* **2022**, *387*, 679–691. [CrossRef]
131. Yinka-Ogunleye, A.; Aruna, O.; Dalhat, M.; Ogoina, D.; McCollum, A.; Disu, Y.; Mamadu, I.; Akinpelu, A.; Ahmad, A.; Burga, J.; et al. Outbreak of human monkeypox in Nigeria in 2017–18: A clinical and epidemiological report. *Lancet Infect. Dis.* **2019**, *19*, 872–879. [CrossRef]
132. Antinori, A.; Mazzotta, V.; Vita, S.; Carletti, F.; Tacconi, D.; Lapini, L.E.; D'abramo, A.; Cicalini, S.; Lapa, D.; Pittalis, S.; et al. Epidemiological, clinical and virological characteristics of four cases of monkeypox support transmission through sexual contact, Italy, May 2022. *Eurosurveillance* **2022**, *27*, 2200421. [CrossRef]
133. Food and Drug Administration. Monkeypox Update: FDA Authorizes Emergency Use of JYNNEOS Vaccine to Increase Vaccine Supply | FDA. Available online: https://www.fda.gov/news-events/press-announcements/monkeypox-update-fda-authorizes-emergency-use-jynneos-vaccine-increase-vaccine-supply (accessed on 13 February 2023).
134. Greenberg, R.N.; Overton, E.T.; Haas, D.W.; Frank, I.; Goldman, M.; Von Krempelhuber, A.; Virgin, G.; Bädeker, N.; Vollmar, J.; Chaplin, P. Safety, Immunogenicity, and Surrogate Markers of Clinical Efficacy for Modified Vaccinia Ankara as a Smallpox Vaccine in HIV-Infected Subjects. *J. Infect. Dis.* **2012**, *207*, 749–758. [CrossRef]
135. Overton, E.T.; Lawrence, S.J.; Stapleton, J.T.; Weidenthaler, H.; Schmidt, D.; Koenen, B.; Silbernagl, G.; Nopora, K.; Chaplin, P. A randomized phase II trial to compare safety and immunogenicity of the MVA-BN smallpox vaccine at various doses in adults with a history of AIDS. *Vaccine* **2020**, *38*, 2600–2607. [CrossRef]
136. Pugliese, P.; Arvieux, C.; Huleux, T.; Pialoux, G.; Vignier, N. Proposal of the French HIV Society on the CD4 threshold below which patients living with HIV who wish to be vaccinated against Monkeypox should receive a 3-dose regimen. *Infect. Dis. Now* **2022**, *52*, 459–460. [CrossRef]
137. Agunbiade, S.; Burton, F.; Muirhead, J.; Whitlock, G.G.; Girometti, N. Clinical characteristics of mpox infection in individuals who received a first dose of modified vaccinia Ankara immunisation. *Sex. Transm. Infect.* **2023**, *99*, 198–199. [CrossRef]
138. MMWR. Recommendations for Using Smallpox Vaccine in a Pre-Event Vaccination Program: Supplemental Recommendations of the Advisory Committee on Immunization Practices (ACIP) and the Healthcare Infection Control Practices Advisory Committee (HICPAC). Available online: https://www.cdc.gov/mmwr/preview/mmwrhtml/rr5207a1.htm (accessed on 13 February 2023).
139. Tasker, S.A.; Schnepf, G.A.; Lim, M.; Caraviello, H.E.; Armstrong, A.; Bavaro, M.; Agan, B.K.; Delmar, J.; Aronson, N.; Wallace, M.R.; et al. Unintended Smallpox Vaccination of HIV-1–Infected Individuals in the United States Military. *Clin. Infect. Dis.* **2004**, *38*, 1320–1322. [CrossRef] [PubMed]
140. Redfield, R.R.; Wright, D.C.; James, W.D.; Jones, T.S.; Brown, C.; Burke, D.S. Disseminated Vaccinia in a Military Recruit with Human Immunodeficiency Virus (HIV) Disease. *N. Engl. J. Med.* **1987**, *316*, 673–676. [CrossRef]
141. O'Shea, J.; Filardo, T.D.; Morris, S.B.; Weiser, J.; Petersen, B.; Brooks, J.T. Interim Guidance for Prevention and Treatment of Monkeypox in Persons with HIV Infection—United States, August 2022. *Morb. Mortal. Wkly. Rep.* **2022**, *71*, 1023. [CrossRef] [PubMed]
142. Gorbalenya, A.E.; Baker, S.C.; Baric, R.S.; de Groot, R.J.; Drosten, C.; Gulyaeva, A.A.; Haagmans, B.L.; Lauber, C.; Leontovich, A.M.; Neuman, B.W.; et al. The species Severe acute respiratory syndrome-related coronavirus: Classifying 2019-nCoV and naming it SARS-CoV-2. *Nat. Microbiol.* **2020**, *5*, 536–544.
143. De Vito, A.; Geremia, N.; Fiore, V.; Princic, E.; Babudieri, S.; Madeddu, G. Clinical features, laboratory findings and predictors of death in hospitalized patients with COVID-19 in Sardinia, Italy. *Eur. Rev. Med. Pharmacol. Sci.* **2020**, *24*, 7861–7868. [PubMed]
144. Guarneri, C.; Rullo, E.V.; Pavone, P.; Berretta, M.; Ceccarelli, M.; Natale, A.; Nunnari, G. Silent COVID-19: What your skin can reveal. *Lancet Infect. Dis.* **2020**, *21*, 24–25. [CrossRef]
145. Singh, H.; Kaur, H.; Singh, K.; Sen, C.K. Cutaneous Manifestations of COVID-19: A Systematic Review. *Adv. Wound Care* **2021**, *10*, 51–80. [CrossRef] [PubMed]
146. Geremia, N.; De Vito, A.; Gunnella, S.; Fiore, V.; Princic, E.; Panu Napodano, C.; Madeddu, G.; Babudieri, S. A Case of Vasculitis-Like Skin Eruption Associated with COVID-19. *Infect. Dis. Clin. Pract.* **2020**, *28*, e30–e31. [CrossRef]

147. De Vito, A.; Fiore, V.; Princic, E.; Geremia, N.; Napodano, C.M.P.; Muredda, A.A.; Maida, I.; Madeddu, G.; Babudieri, S. Predictors of infection, symptoms development, and mortality in people with SARS-CoV-2 living in retirement nursing homes. *PLoS ONE* **2021**, *16*, e0248009. [CrossRef]
148. Vaira, L.A.; Hopkins, C.; Salzano, G.; Petrocelli, M.; Melis, A.; Cucurullo, M.; Ferrari, M.; Gagliardini, L.; Pipolo, C.; Deiana, G.; et al. Olfactory and gustatory function impairment in COVID-19 patients: Italian objective multicenter-study. *Head Neck* **2020**, *42*, 1560–1569. [CrossRef]
149. Vaira, L.A.; De Vito, A.; Deiana, G.; Pes, C.; Giovanditto, F.; Fiore, V.; Lechien, J.R.; Saussez, S.; Policicchio, D.; Boccaletti, R.; et al. Systemic inflammatory markers and psychophysical olfactory scores in coronavirus disease 2019 patients: Is there any correlation? *J. Laryngol. Otol.* **2021**, *135*, 723–738. [CrossRef]
150. Kimball, A.; Hatfield, K.M.; Arons, M.; James, A.; Taylor, J.; Spicer, K.; Bardossy, A.C.; Oakley, L.P.; Tanwar, S.; Chisty, Z.; et al. Asymptomatic and Presymptomatic SARS-CoV-2 Infections in Residents of a Long-Term Care Skilled Nursing Facility—King County, Washington, March 2020. *MMWR Morb. Mortal. Wkly. Rep.* **2020**, *69*, 377–381. [CrossRef] [PubMed]
151. De Vito, A.; Geremia, N.; Princic, E.; Fanelli, C.; Panu Napodano, C.M.; Muredda, A.A.; Fiore, V.; Maida, I.; Fois, A.G.; Babudieri, S.; et al. Does Angiotensin II receptor blockers increase the risk of SARS-CoV-2 infection? A real-life experience. *Eur. Rev. Med. Pharmacol. Sci.* **2021**, *25*, 523–526. [PubMed]
152. Lodigiani, C.; Iapichino, G.; Carenzo, L.; Cecconi, M.; Ferrazzi, P.; Sebastian, T.; Kucher, N.; Studt, J.D.; Sacco, C.; Bertuzzi, A.; et al. Venous and arterial thromboembolic complications in COVID-19 patients admitted to an academic hospital in Milan, Italy. *Thromb. Res.* **2020**, *191*, 9–14. [CrossRef] [PubMed]
153. Geng, Y.-J.; Wei, Z.-Y.; Qian, H.-Y.; Huang, J.; Lodato, R.; Castriotta, R.J. Pathophysiological characteristics and therapeutic approaches for pulmonary injury and cardiovascular complications of coronavirus disease 2019. *Cardiovasc. Pathol.* **2020**, *47*, 107228. [CrossRef]
154. Trunfio, M.; Portesani, F.; Vicinanza, S.; Nespoli, P.; Traverso, F.; Cortese, G.; Bonora, S.; Calcagno, A.; Di Perri, G. Real-life Evidence of Lower Lung Virulence in COVID-19 Inpatients Infected with SARS-CoV-2 Omicron Variant Compared to Wild-Type and Delta SARS-CoV-2 Pneumonia. *Lung* **2022**, *200*, 573–577. [CrossRef]
155. Zinellu, A.; De Vito, A.; Scano, V.; Paliogiannis, P.; Fiore, V.; Madeddu, G.; Maida, I.; Zinellu, E.; Mangoni, A.A.; Arru, L.B.; et al. The PaO_2/FiO_2 ratio on admission is independently associated with prolonged hospitalization in COVID-19 patients. *J. Infect. Dev. Ctries* **2021**, *15*, 353–359. [CrossRef]
156. Cooper, T.J.; Woodward, B.; Alom, S.; Harky, A. Coronavirus disease 2019 (COVID-19) outcomes in HIV/AIDS patients: A systematic review. *HIV Med.* **2020**, *21*, 567–577. [CrossRef]
157. Tesoriero, J.M.; Swain, C.-A.E.; Pierce, J.L.; Zamboni, L.; Wu, M.; Holtgrave, D.R.; Gonzalez, C.J.; Udo, T.; Morne, J.E.; Hart-Malloy, R.; et al. COVID-19 Outcomes among Persons Living with or without Diagnosed HIV Infection in New York State. *JAMA Netw. Open* **2021**, *4*, e2037069. [CrossRef]
158. Gagliardini, R.; Vergori, A.; Lorenzini, P.; Cicalini, S.; Pinnetti, C.; Mazzotta, V.; Mondi, A.; Mastrorosa, I.; Camici, M.; Lanini, S.; et al. Characteristics and Outcomes of COVID-19-Related Hospitalization among PLWH. *J. Clin. Med.* **2022**, *11*, 1546. [CrossRef]
159. De Vito, A.; Colpani, A.; Bitti, A.; Zauli, B.; Meloni, M.C.; Fois, M.; Denti, L.; Bacciu, S.; Marcia, C.; Maida, I.; et al. Safety and efficacy of molnupiravir in SARS-CoV-2-infected patients: A real-life experience. *J. Med. Virol.* **2022**, *94*, 5582–5588. [CrossRef]
160. De Vito, A.; Colpani, A.; Saderi, L.; Puci, M.; Zauli, B.; Fiore, V.; Fois, M.; Meloni, M.C.; Bitti, A.; Di Castri, C.; et al. Impact of Early SARS-CoV-2 Antiviral Therapy on Disease Progression. *Viruses* **2023**, *15*, 71. [CrossRef] [PubMed]
161. Dallocchio Rn Dessì, A.; De Vito, A.; Delogu, G.; Serra Pa Madeddu, G. Early combination treatment with existing HIV antivirals: An effective treatment for COVID-19? *Eur. Rev. Med. Pharmacol. Sci.* **2021**, *25*, 2435–2448.
162. Chien, M.; Anderson, T.K.; Jockusch, S.; Tao, C.; Li, X.; Kumar, S.; Russo, J.J.; Kirchdoerfer, R.N.; Ju, J. Nucleotide Analogues as Inhibitors of SARS-CoV-2 Polymerase, a Key Drug Target for COVID-19. *J. Proteome Res.* **2020**, *19*, 4690–4697. [CrossRef] [PubMed]
163. Del Amo, J.; Polo, R.; Moreno, S.; Martínez, E.; Cabello, A.; Iribarren, J.A.; Curran, A.; Macías, J.; Montero, M.; Dueñas, C.; et al. Tenofovir disoproxil fumarate/emtricitabine and severity of coronavirus disease 2019 in people with HIV infection. *AIDS* **2022**, *36*, 2171–2179. [CrossRef]
164. Del Amo, J.; Polo, R.; Moreno, S.; Jarrin, I.; Hernan, M.A. SARS-CoV-2 infection and coronavirus disease 2019 severity in persons with HIV on antiretroviral treatment. *AIDS* **2022**, *36*, 161–168. [CrossRef] [PubMed]
165. Tanriover, M.D.; Doğanay, H.L.; Akova, M.; Güner, H.R.; Azap, A.; Akhan, S.; Köse, Ş.; Erdinç, F.Ş.; Akalın, E.H.; Tabak, Ö.F.; et al. Efficacy and safety of an inactivated whole-virion SARS-CoV-2 vaccine (CoronaVac): Interim results of a double-blind, randomised, placebo-controlled, phase 3 trial in Turkey. *Lancet* **2021**, *398*, 213–222. [CrossRef]
166. Xia, S.; Zhang, Y.; Wang, Y.; Wang, H.; Yang, Y.; Gao, G.F.; Tan, W.; Wu, G.; Xu, M.; Lou, Z.; et al. Safety and immunogenicity of an inactivated SARS-CoV-2 vaccine, BBIBP-CorV: A randomised, double-blind, placebo-controlled, phase 1/2 trial. *Lancet Infect. Dis.* **2021**, *21*, 39–51. [CrossRef]
167. Ella, R.; Reddy, S.; Blackwelder, W.; Potdar, V.; Yadav, P.; Sarangi, V.; Aileni, V.K.; Kanungo, S.; Rai, S.; Reddy, P.; et al. Efficacy, safety, and lot-to-lot immunogenicity of an inactivated SARS-CoV-2 vaccine (BBV152): Interim results of a randomised, double-blind, controlled, phase 3 trial. *Lancet* **2021**, *398*, 2173–2184. [CrossRef] [PubMed]

168. Falsey, A.R.; Sobieszczyk, M.E.; Hirsch, I.; Sproule, S.; Robb, M.L.; Corey, L.; Neuzil, K.M.; Hahn, W.; Hunt, J.; Mulligan, M.J.; et al. Phase 3 Safety and Efficacy of AZD1222 (ChAdOx1 nCoV-19) COVID-19 Vaccine. *N. Engl. J. Med.* **2021**, *385*, 2348–2360. [CrossRef]
169. Sadoff, J.; Gray, G.; Vandebosch, A.; Cárdenas, V.; Shukarev, G.; Grinsztejn, B.; Goepfert, P.A.; Truyers, C.; Fennema, H.; Spiessens, B.; et al. Safety and Efficacy of Single-Dose Ad26.COV2.S Vaccine against COVID-19. *N. Engl. J. Med.* **2021**, *384*, 2187–2201. [CrossRef]
170. Li, J.; Hou, L.; Guo, X.; Jin, P.; Wu, S.; Zhu, J.; Pan, H.; Wang, X.; Song, Z.; Wan, J.; et al. Heterologous AD5-nCOV plus CoronaVac versus homologous CoronaVac vaccination: A randomized phase 4 trial. *Nat. Med.* **2022**, *28*, 401–409. [CrossRef] [PubMed]
171. Polack, F.P.; Thomas, S.J.; Kitchin, N.; Absalon, J.; Gurtman, A.; Lockhart, S.; Perez, J.L.; Pérez Marc, G.; Moreira, E.D.; Zerbini, C.; et al. Safety and efficacy of the BNT162b2 mRNA COVID-19 vaccine. *N. Engl. J. Med.* **2020**, *383*, 2603–2615. [CrossRef]
172. Baden, L.R.; El Sahly, H.M.; Essink, B.; Kotloff, K.; Frey, S.; Novak, R.; Diemert, D.; Spector, S.A.; Rouphael, N.; Creech, C.B.; et al. Efficacy and Safety of the mRNA-1273 SARS-CoV-2 Vaccine. *N. Engl. J. Med.* **2021**, *384*, 403–416. [CrossRef] [PubMed]
173. Mallory, R.M.; Formica, N.; Pfeiffer, S.; Wilkinson, B.; Marcheschi, A.; Albert, G.; McFall, H.; Robinson, M.; Plested, J.S.; Zhu, M.; et al. Safety and immunogenicity following a homologous booster dose of a SARS-CoV-2 recombinant spike protein vaccine (NVX-CoV2373): A secondary analysis of a randomised, placebo-controlled, phase 2 trial. *Lancet Infect. Dis.* **2022**, *22*, 1565–1576. [CrossRef]
174. Merza, M.; Abdulah, D.; Malo, D.; Haleem, D.; Atrushi, D. Current status of COVID-19 infection and vaccination coverage, and factors associated with infection acquisition and vaccine uptake. *Infect. Dis. Trop. Med.* **2023**, *9*, e1062.
175. Ochoa-Azze, R.; Chang-Monteagudo, A.; Climent-Ruiz, Y.; Macías-Abraham, C.; Valenzuela-Silva, C.; de Los Ángeles García-García, M.; Jerez-Barceló, Y.; Triana-Marrero, Y.; Ruiz-Villegas, L.; Dairon Rodríguez-Prieto, L.; et al. Safety and immunogenicity of the FINLAY-FR-1A vaccine in COVID-19 convalescent participants: An open-label phase 2a and double-blind, randomised, placebo-controlled, phase 2b, seamless, clinical trial. *Lancet Respir. Med.* **2022**, *10*, 785–795. [CrossRef]
176. Folegatti, P.M.; Ewer, K.J.; Aley, P.K.; Angus, B.; Becker, S.; Belij-Rammerstorfer, S.; Bellamy, D.; Bibi, S.; Bittaye, M.; Clutterbuck, E.A.; et al. Safety and immunogenicity of the ChAdOx1 nCoV-19 vaccine against SARS-CoV-2: A preliminary report of a phase 1/2, single-blind, randomised controlled trial. *Lancet* **2020**, *396*, 467–478. [CrossRef] [PubMed]
177. Madhi, S.A.; Koen, A.L.; Izu, A.; Fairlie, L.; Cutland, C.L.; Baillie, V.; Padayachee, S.D.; Dheda, K.; Barnabas, S.L.; Bhorat, Q.E.; et al. Safety and immunogenicity of the ChAdOx1 nCoV-19 (AZD1222) vaccine against SARS-CoV-2 in people living with and without HIV in South Africa: An interim analysis of a randomised, double-blind, placebo-controlled, phase 1B/2A trial. *Lancet HIV* **2021**, *8*, e568–e580. [CrossRef]
178. Schmidt, K.G.; Harrer, E.G.; Tascilar, K.; Kübel, S.; El Kenz, B.; Hartmann, F.; Simon, D.; Schett, G.; Nganou-Makamdop, K.; Harrer, T. Characterization of Serum and Mucosal SARS-CoV-2-Antibodies in HIV-1-Infected Subjects after BNT162b2 mRNA Vaccination or SARS-CoV-2 Infection. *Viruses* **2022**, *14*, 651. [CrossRef]
179. Heftdal, L.D.; Knudsen, A.D.; Hamm, S.R.; Hansen, C.B.; Møller, D.L.; Pries-Heje, M.; Fogh, K.; Hasselbalch, R.B.; Jarlhelt, I.; Pérez-Alós, L.; et al. Humoral response to two doses of BNT162b2 vaccination in people with HIV. *J. Intern. Med.* **2021**, *291*, 513–518. [CrossRef] [PubMed]
180. Xu, X.; Vesterbacka, J.; Aleman, S.; Nowak, P. High seroconversion rate after vaccination with mRNA BNT162b2 vaccine against SARS-CoV-2 among people with HIV—But HIV viremia matters? *AIDS* **2022**, *36*, 479–481. [CrossRef] [PubMed]
181. Cossu, M.V.; Mileto, D.; Giacomelli, A.; Oreni, L.; Bracchitta, F.; Pellicciotta, M.; Salari, F.; Petri, F.; Meraviglia, P.; Antinori, S.; et al. Comorbidity Burden and Suboptimal Immunological Responses to Coronavirus Disease 2019 Vaccination in People Living with Human Immunodeficiency Virus. *J. Infect. Dis.* **2022**, *227*, 733–735. [CrossRef]
182. Jedicke, N.; Stankov, M.V.; Cossmann, A.; Dopfer-Jablonka, A.; Knuth, C.; Ahrenstorf, G.; Ramos, G.M.; Behrens, G.M.N. Humoral immune response following prime and boost BNT162b2 vaccination in people living with HIV on antiretroviral therapy. *HIV Med.* **2021**, *23*, 558–563. [CrossRef]
183. Pourcher, V.; Belin, L.; Soulie, C.; Rosenzwajg, M.; Marot, S.; Lacombe, K.; Valin, N.; Pialoux, G.; Calin, R.; Palacios, C.; et al. High seroconversion rate and SARS-CoV-2 Delta neutralization in people with HIV vaccinated with BNT162b2. *AIDS* **2022**, *36*, 1545–1552. [CrossRef] [PubMed]
184. Hassold, N.; Brichler, S.; Ouedraogo, E.; Leclerc, D.; Carroue, S.; Gater, Y.; Alloui, C.; Carbonnelle, E.; Bouchaud, O.; Mechai, F.; et al. Impaired antibody response to COVID-19 vaccination in advanced HIV infection. *AIDS* **2022**, *36*, F1–F5. [CrossRef] [PubMed]
185. Gianserra, L.; Donà, M.G.; Giuliani, E.; Stingone, C.; Pontone, M.; Buonomini, A.R.; Giuliani, M.; Pimpinelli, F.; Morrone, A.; Latini, A. Immunogenicity and Safety of BNT162b2 Homologous Booster Vaccination in People Living with HIV under Effective cART. *Vaccines* **2022**, *10*, 1243. [CrossRef] [PubMed]
186. Lapointe, H.R.; Mwimanzi, F.; Cheung, P.K.; Sang, Y.; Yaseen, F.; Umviligihozo, G.; Kalikawe, R.; Speckmaier, S.; Moran-Garcia, N.; Datwani, S.; et al. People with Human Immunodeficiency Virus Receiving Suppressive Antiretroviral Therapy Show Typical Antibody Durability After Dual Coronavirus Disease 2019 Vaccination and Strong Third Dose Responses. *J. Infect. Dis.* **2022**, *4*, 14. [CrossRef] [PubMed]
187. Portillo, V.; Fedeli, C.; Ustero Alonso, P.; Petignat, I.; Mereles Costa, E.C.; Sulstarova, A.; Jaksic, C.; Yerly, S.; Calmy, A. Impact on HIV-1 RNA Levels and Antibody Responses Following SARS-CoV-2 Vaccination in HIV-Infected Individuals. *Front. Immunol.* **2021**, *12*, 820126. [CrossRef]

188. Khan, K.; Lustig, G.; Bernstein, M.; Archary, D.; Cele, S.; Karim, F.; Smith, M.; Ganga, Y.; Jule, Z.; Reedoy, K.; et al. Immunogenicity of Severe Acute Respiratory Syndrome Coronavirus 2 (SARS-CoV-2) Infection and Ad26.CoV2.S Vaccination in People Living with Human Immunodeficiency Virus (HIV). *Clin. Infect. Dis.* **2021**, *75*, e857–e864. [CrossRef]
189. Netto, L.C.; Ibrahim, K.Y.; Picone, C.M.; Alves, A.P.P.S.; Aniceto, E.V.; Santiago, M.R.; Parmejani, P.S.S.; E Aikawa, N.; Medeiros-Ribeiro, A.C.; Pasoto, S.G.; et al. Safety and immunogenicity of CoronaVac in people living with HIV: A prospective cohort study. *Lancet HIV* **2022**, *9*, e323–e331. [CrossRef] [PubMed]
190. Zeng, G.; Xu, L.; Feng, S.; Tang, J.; Wang, X.; Li, G.; Gan, Y.; Zheng, C.; Zhao, J.; Yang, Z. IgG Antibody Responses and Immune Persistence of Two Doses of BBIBP-CorV Vaccine or CoronaVac Vaccine in People Living with HIV (PLWH) in Shenzhen, China. *Vaccines* **2022**, *10*, 880. [CrossRef]
191. Liu, Y.; Han, J.; Li, X.; Chen, D.; Zhao, X.; Qiu, Y.; Zhang, L.; Xiao, J.; Li, B.; Zhao, H. COVID-19 Vaccination in People Living with HIV (PLWH) in China: A Cross Sectional Study of Vaccine Hesitancy, Safety, and Immunogenicity. *Vaccines* **2021**, *9*, 1458. [CrossRef] [PubMed]
192. Zou, S.; Guo, W.; Wu, S.; Ming, F.; Tan, Y.; Wu, M.; Tang, W.; Liang, K. Six-month humoral immune response to inactivated COVID-19 vaccine among people living with HIV. *Front. Immunol.* **2022**, *13*, 6329. [CrossRef]
193. Gushchin, V.A.; Tsyganova, E.V.; Ogarkova, D.A.; Adgamov, R.R.; Shcheblyakov, D.V.; Glukhoedova, N.V.; Zhilenkova, A.S.; Kolotii, A.G.; Zaitsev, R.D.; Logunov, D.Y.; et al. Sputnik V protection from COVID-19 in people living with HIV under antiretroviral therapy. *EClinicalMedicine* **2022**, *46*, 101360. [CrossRef] [PubMed]
194. Chaabouni, H.; Smaoui, F.; Hammami, F.; Rekik, K.; Chakroun, A.; Marrakchi, C.; Koubaa, M.; Jemaa, M.B. Herpetic meningoencephalitis following inactivated COVID-19 vaccine: A coexistence or coincidence? *Infect. Dis. Trop. Med.* **2022**, *8*, e838.
195. Atiyat, R.; Elias, S.; Kiwan, C.; Shaaban, H.S.; Slim, J. Varicella-Zoster Virus Reactivation in AIDS Patient After Pfizer-BioNTech COVID-19 Vaccine. *Cureus* **2021**, *13*, e20145. [CrossRef]
196. Patil, A.; Goldust, M.; Wollina, U. *Herpes zoster*: A Review of Clinical Manifestations and Management. *Viruses* **2022**, *14*, 192. [CrossRef]
197. Moanna, A.; Rimland, D. Decreasing Incidence of Herpes Zoster in the Highly Active Antiretroviral Therapy Era. *Clin. Infect. Dis.* **2013**, *57*, 122–125. [CrossRef]
198. McKay, S.L.; Guo, A.; A Pergam, S.; Dooling, K. Herpes Zoster Risk in Immunocompromised Adults in the United States: A Systematic Review. *Clin. Infect. Dis.* **2019**, *71*, e125–e134. [CrossRef]
199. Kim, J.; Kim, M.K.; Choi, G.J.; Shin, H.Y.; Kim, B.G.; Kang, H. Pharmacological and non-pharmacological strategies for preventing postherpetic neuralgia: A systematic review and network meta-analysis. *Korean J. Pain* **2021**, *34*, 509–533. [CrossRef]
200. The WHO Strategic Advisory Group of Experts on Immunisation (SAGE). Systematic Review of Available Evidence on Effectiveness and Duration of Protection of Varicella Vaccines—DocsLib. 2013. Available online: https://docslib.org/doc/4103059/systematic-review-of-available-evidence-on-effectiveness-and-duration-of-protection-of-varicella-vaccines (accessed on 2 December 2022).
201. Purswani, M.U.; Karalius, B.; Yao, T.-J.; Schmid, D.S.; Burchett, S.K.; Siberry, G.K.; Patel, K.; Van Dyke, R.B.; Yogev, R. Prevalence and Persistence of Varicella Antibodies in Previously Immunized Children and Youth with Perinatal HIV-1 Infection. *Clin. Infect. Dis.* **2015**, *62*, 106–114. [CrossRef] [PubMed]
202. Weinberg, A.; Levin, M.J.; MacGregor, R.R. Safety and immunogenicity of a live attenuated varicella vaccine in VZV-seropositive HIV-infected adults. *Hum. Vaccines* **2010**, *6*, 318–321. [CrossRef] [PubMed]
203. Taweesith, W.; Puthanakit, T.; Kowitdamrong, E.; Bunupuradah, T.; Wongngam, W.; Phasomsap, C.; Apornpong, T.; Bouko, C.; Pancharoen, C. The Immunogenicity and Safety of Live Attenuated Varicella-zoster Virus Vaccine in Human Immunodeficiency Virus-infected Children. *Pediatr. Infect. Dis. J.* **2011**, *30*, 320–324. [CrossRef]
204. Mullane, K.M.; Winston, D.J.; Wertheim, M.S.; Betts, R.F.; Poretz, D.M.; Camacho, L.H.; Pergam, S.A.; Mullane, M.R.; Stek, J.E.; Sterling, T.M.; et al. Safety and Immunogenicity of Heat-Treated Zoster Vaccine (ZVHT) in Immunocompromised Adults. *J. Infect. Dis.* **2013**, *208*, 1375–1385. [CrossRef]
205. Benson, C.A.; Andersen, J.W.; Macatangay, B.J.C.; Mailliard, R.B.; Rinaldo, C.R.; Read, S.; Bozzolo, D.R.; Purdue, L.; Jennings, C.; Keefer, M.C.; et al. Safety and Immunogenicity of Zoster Vaccine Live in Human Immunodeficiency Virus–Infected Adults with CD4+ Cell Counts >200 Cells/mL Virologically Suppressed on Antiretroviral Therapy. *Clin. Infect. Dis.* **2018**, *67*, 1712–1719. [CrossRef]
206. Chlibek, R.; Smetana, J.; Pauksens, K.; Rombo, L.; Hoek, J.A.R.V.D.; Richardus, J.H.; Plassmann, G.; Schwarz, T.F.; Ledent, E.; Heineman, T.C. Safety and immunogenicity of three different formulations of an adjuvanted varicella-zoster virus subunit candidate vaccine in older adults: A phase II, randomized, controlled study. *Vaccine* **2014**, *32*, 1745–1753. [CrossRef]
207. Chlibek, R.; Bayas, J.M.; Collins, H.; De La Pinta, M.L.R.; Ledent, E.; Mols, J.F.; Heineman, T.C. Erratum to: Safety and Immunogenicity of an AS01-adjuvanted Varicella-zoster Virus Subunit Candidate Vaccine Against Herpes Zoster in Adults ≥50 Years of Age. *J. Infect. Dis.* **2013**, *208*, 1953–1961. [CrossRef]
208. Leroux-Roels, I.; Leroux-Roels, G.; Clement, F.; Vandepapelière, P.; Vassilev, V.; Ledent, E.; Heineman, T.C. A phase 1/2 clinical trial evaluating safety and immunogenicity of a varicella zoster glycoprotein e subunit vaccine candidate in young and older adults. *J. Infect. Dis.* **2012**, *206*, 1280–1290. [CrossRef]

209. Berkowitz, E.M.; Moyle, G.; Stellbrink, H.J.; Schürmann, D.; Kegg, S.; Stoll, M.; El Idrissi, M.; Oostvogels, L.; Heineman, T.C.; Zoster-015 HZ/su Study Group. Safety and immunogenicity of an adjuvanted herpes zoster subunit candidate vaccine in HIV-infected adults: A phase 1/2a randomized, placebo-controlled study. *J. Infect. Dis.* **2015**, *211*, 1279–1287. [CrossRef]
210. López-Fauqued, M.; der Mee, M.C.-V.; Bastidas, A.; Beukelaers, P.; Dagnew, A.F.; Garcia, J.J.F.; Schuind, A.; Tavares-Da-Silva, F. Safety Profile of the Adjuvanted Recombinant Zoster Vaccine in Immunocompromised Populations: An Overview of Six Trials. *Drug Saf.* **2021**, *44*, 811–823. [CrossRef]
211. Izurieta, H.S.; Wu, X.; Forshee, R.; Lu, Y.; Sung, H.-M.; Agger, P.E.; Chillarige, Y.; Link-Gelles, R.; Lufkin, B.; Wernecke, M.; et al. Recombinant Zoster Vaccine (Shingrix): Real-World Effectiveness in the First 2 Years Post-Licensure. *Clin. Infect. Dis.* **2021**, *73*, 941–948. [CrossRef]
212. Rouphael, N.G.; Stephens, D.S. Neisseria meningitidis: Biology, microbiology, and epidemiology. *Methods Mol. Biol.* **2012**, *799*, 1–20.
213. ECDC. Invasive Meningococcal Disease Annual Epidemiological Report for 2018 Key Facts. 2018. Available online: https://www.ecdc.europa.eu/sites/default/files/documents/AER-Invasive-meningococcal-disease-2018.pdf (accessed on 10 December 2022).
214. Carter, E.; McGill, F. The management of acute meningitis: An update. *Clin. Med.* **2022**, *22*, 396–400. [CrossRef]
215. Sharda, S.; Sachdeva, A.; Ahuja, C.; Bhatia, M. Diagnostic accuracy of point-of-care cerebrospinal fluid leucocyte esterase dipstick test for bacterial meningitis in the Emergency Department. *Infect. Dis. Trop. Med.* **2022**, *8*, e1028.
216. Miller, L.; Arakaki, L.; Ramautar, A.; Bodach, S.; Braunstein, S.L.; Kennedy, J.; Steiner-Sichel, L.; Ngai, S.; Shepard, C.; Weiss, D. Elevated Risk for Invasive Meningococcal Disease among Persons with HIV. *Ann. Intern. Med.* **2014**, *160*, 30–37. [CrossRef]
217. Cohen, C.; Singh, E.; Wu, H.M.; Martin, S.; de Gouveia, L.; Klugman, K.P.; Meiring, S.; Govender, N.; von Gottberg, A. Increased incidence of meningococcal disease in HIV-infected individuals associated with higher case-fatality ratios in South Africa. *AIDS* **2010**, *24*, 1351–1360. [CrossRef]
218. Riccardi, N.; Ungaro, R.; Marchese, A.; Di Biagio, A. Neisseria meningitidis serogroup C bacteremia causes of single petechiae in a immunocompetent patient. *Infect. Dis. Trop. Med.* **2018**, *4*, e503.
219. Dull, P.M.; McIntosh, E.D. Meningococcal vaccine development—From glycoconjugates against MenACWY to proteins against MenB—Potential for broad protection against meningococcal disease. *Vaccine* **2012**, *30*, B18–B25. [CrossRef]
220. Sanofi Pasteur. Menactra® Meningococcal (Groups A, C, Y and W-135) Polysaccharide Diphtheria Toxoid Conjugate Vaccine Solution for Injection Active Immunizing Agent for the Prevention of Meningococcal Disease. 2017. Available online: https://products.sanofi.ca/en/menactra.pdf (accessed on 22 December 2022).
221. CHMP. Menveo, INN-Meningococcal Group A, C, W135 and Y Conjugate Vaccine. Available online: https://www.ema.europa.eu/en/documents/product-information/menveo-epar-product-information_en.pdf (accessed on 10 December 2022).
222. Huston, J.; Galicia, K.; Egelund, E.F. MenQuadfi (MenACWY-TT): A New Vaccine for Meningococcal Serogroups ACWY. *Ann. Pharmacother.* **2022**, *56*, 727–735. [CrossRef]
223. Gandhi, A.; Balmer, P.; York, L.J. Characteristics of a new meningococcal serogroup B vaccine, bivalent rLP2086 (MenB-FHbp; Trumenba®). *Postgrad. Med.* **2016**, *128*, 548–556. [CrossRef]
224. Vernikos, G.; Medini, D. Bexsero® chronicle. *Ann. Trop. Med. Parasitol.* **2014**, *108*, 305–316. [CrossRef]
225. Siberry, G.K.; Williams, P.L.; Lujan-Zilbermann, J.; Warshaw, M.G.; Spector, S.A.; Decker, M.; Heckman, B.E.; Demske, E.F.; Read, J.S.; Jean-Philippe, P.; et al. Phase I/II, Open-Label Trial of Safety and Immunogenicity of Meningococcal (Groups A, C, Y, and W-135) Polysaccharide Diphtheria Toxoid Conjugate Vaccine in Human Immunodeficiency Virus-Infected Adolescents. *Pediatr. Infect. Dis. J.* **2010**, *29*, 391–396. [CrossRef]
226. Lujan-Zilbermann, J.; Warshaw, M.G.; Williams, P.L.; Spector, S.A.; Decker, M.D.; Abzug, M.J.; Heckman, B.; Manzella, A.; Kabat, B.; Jean-Philippe, P.; et al. Immunogenicity and Safety of 1 vs 2 Doses of Quadrivalent Meningococcal Conjugate Vaccine in Youth Infected with Human Immunodeficiency Virus. *J. Pediatr.* **2012**, *161*, 676–681.e2. [CrossRef]
227. Frota, A.C.; Milagres, L.G.; Harrison, L.H.; Ferreira, B.; Barreto, D.M.; Pereira, G.S.; Cruz, A.C.; Manfro, W.; de Oliveira, R.H.; Abreu, T.F.; et al. Immunogenicity and Safety of Meningococcal C Conjugate Vaccine in Children and Adolescents Infected and Uninfected with HIV in Rio de Janeiro, Brazil. *Pediatr. Infect. Dis. J.* **2015**, *34*, e113–e118. [CrossRef]
228. Frota, A.C.C.; Ferreira, B.; Harrison, L.H.; Pereira, G.S.; Pereira-Manfro, W.; Machado, E.S.; de Oliveira, R.H.; Abreu, T.F.; Milagres, L.G.; Hofer, C.B. Safety and immune response after two-dose meningococcal C conjugate immunization in HIV-infected children and adolescents in Rio de Janeiro, Brazil. *Vaccine* **2017**, *35*, 7042–7048. [CrossRef]
229. Raccagni, A.R.; Galli, L.; Spagnuolo, V.; Bruzzesi, E.; Muccini, C.; Bossolasco, S.; Ranzenigo, M.; Gianotti, N.; Lolatto, R.; Castagna, A.; et al. Meningococcus B Vaccination Effectiveness against Neisseria gonorrhoeae Infection in People Living with HIV: A Case-control Study. *Sex. Transm. Dis.* **2023**, *50*, 247–251. [CrossRef]
230. Petousis-Harris, H.; Paynter, J.; Morgan, J.; Saxton, P.; McArdle, B.; Goodyear-Smith, F.; Black, S. Effectiveness of a group B outer membrane vesicle meningococcal vaccine against gonorrhoea in New Zealand: A retrospective case-control study. *Lancet* **2017**, *390*, 1603–1610. [CrossRef]
231. Paynter, J.; Goodyear-Smith, F.; Morgan, J.; Saxton, P.; Black, S.; Petousis-Harris, H. Effectiveness of a Group B Outer Membrane Vesicle Meningococcal Vaccine in Preventing Hospitalization from Gonorrhea in New Zealand: A Retrospective Cohort Study. *Vaccines* **2019**, *7*, 5. [CrossRef]
232. Donisi, A.; Colpani, A.; Zauli, B.; De Vito, A.; Fiore, V.; Babudieri, S.; Madeddu, G. Sexually Transmitted Infections Prevalence and Cascade of Care among Undocumented Sex Workers: A Twenty-Year-Long Experience. *Life* **2023**, *13*, 606. [CrossRef]

233. Alkan, S.; Evlice, O. Bibliometric analysis of global gonorrhea research. *Infect. Dis. Trop. Med.* **2022**, *8*, e876.
234. Ghaswalla, P.K.; Marshall, G.S.; Bengtson, L.G.S.; Buikema, A.R.; Bancroft, T.; Koep, E.; Novy, P.; Hogea, C.S. Meningococcal Vaccination Rates among People with a New Diagnosis of HIV Infection in the US. *JAMA Netw. Open* **2022**, *5*, e228573. [CrossRef]
235. De Vito, A.; Colpani, A.; Zauli, B.; Meloni, M.C.; Fois, M.; Fiore, V.; Pintus, G.A.; Nardi, V.G.; Babudieri, S.; Madeddu, G. How Little Do We Know about HIV and STIs Prevention? Results from a Web-Based Survey among the General Population. *Healthcare* **2022**, *10*, 1059. [CrossRef]
236. Kiedrzynski, T.; Bissielo, A.; Suryaprakash, M.; Bandaranayake, D. Whooping cough—Where are we now? A review. *N. Z. Med. J.* **2015**, *128*, 21–27.
237. Troy, S.B.; Rossheim, A.E.-B.; Hilliard, D.D.; Cunningham, T.D. Seroprevalence of Pertussis Infection in HIV-Infected Adults in the United States. *J. Acquir. Immune Defic. Syndr.* **2016**, *73*, 282. [CrossRef]
238. Colebunders, R.; Vael, C.; Blot, K.; Van Meerbeeck, J.; Ende, J.V.D.; Ieven, M. Bordetella pertussis as a cause of chronic respiratory infection in an AIDS patient. *Eur. J. Clin. Microbiol. Infect. Dis.* **1994**, *13*, 313–315. [CrossRef]
239. Doebbeling, B.N.; Feilmeier, M.L.; Herwaldt, L.A. Pertussis in an Adult Man Infected with the Human Immunodeficiency Virus. *J. Infect. Dis.* **1990**, *161*, 1296–1298. [CrossRef]
240. Truelove, S.A.; Keegan, L.T.; Moss, W.J.; Chaisson, L.H.; Macher, E.; Azman, A.; Lessler, J. Clinical and Epidemiological Aspects of Diphtheria: A Systematic Review and Pooled Analysis. *Clin. Infect. Dis.* **2019**, *71*, 89–97. [CrossRef]
241. Bonetti, T.C.; Succi, R.C.; Weckx, L.Y.; Tavares-Lopes, L.; de Moraes-Pinto, M. Tetanus and diphtheria antibodies and response to a booster dose in Brazilian HIV-1-infected women. *Vaccine* **2004**, *22*, 3707–3712. [CrossRef]
242. Kroon, F.P.; Van Dissel, J.T.; Labadie, J.; Van Loon, A.M.; Van Furth, R. Antibody Response to Diphtheria, Tetanus, and Poliomyelitis Vaccines in Relation to the Number of CD4+ T Lymphocytes in Adults Infected with Human Immunodeficiency Virus. *Clin. Infect. Dis.* **1995**, *21*, 1197–1203. [CrossRef]
243. Dafallah, M.A.; Ragab, E.A.; Elawad, O.A.M.A. Experience with Tetanus in a Tertiary Care Hospital in Sudan: A Retrospective Review. *Emerg. Med. Int.* **2021**, *2021*, 4818312. [CrossRef]
244. Simani, O.E.; Izu, A.; Nunes, M.C.; Violari, A.; Cotton, M.F.; Van Niekerk, N.; Adrian, P.V.; Madhi, S.A. Effect of HIV exposure and timing of antiretroviral therapy initiation on immune memory responses to diphtheria, tetanus, whole cell pertussis and hepatitis B vaccines. *Expert Rev. Vaccines* **2018**, *18*, 95–104. [CrossRef]
245. Choudhury, S.A.; Matin, F. Subnormal and waning immunity to tetanus toxoid in previously vaccinated HIV-infected children and response to booster doses of the vaccine. *Int. J. Infect. Dis.* **2013**, *17*, e1249–e1251. [CrossRef]
246. Dieye, T.N.; Sow, P.S.; Simonart, T.; Guèye-Ndiaye, A.; Popper, S.J.; Delforge, M.-L.; Dieye, A.; Sarr, A.D.; Crusiaux, A.; Van Vooren, J.-P.; et al. Immunologic and virologic response after tetanus toxoid booster among HIV-1- and HIV-2-infected Senegalese individuals. *Vaccine* **2001**, *20*, 905–913. [CrossRef]
247. Dauby, N.; Gobert, C.; Benslimane, A.; Nagant, C.; Necsoi, C.; Wijngaert, S.V.D.; Corrazza, F.; Delforge, M.; De Wit, S. Durability of tetanus seroprotection in people living with HIV. *AIDS* **2022**, *36*, 1135–1139. [CrossRef]
248. Varon, E.; Mainardi, J.; Gutmann, L. *Streptococcus pneumoniae*: Still a major pathogen. *Clin. Microbiol. Infect.* **2010**, *16*, 401. [CrossRef]
249. Henriques-Normark, B.; Tuomanen, E.I. The Pneumococcus: Epidemiology, Microbiology, and Pathogenesis. *Cold Spring Harb. Perspect. Med.* **2013**, *3*, a010215. [CrossRef]
250. Klugman, K.P.; Madhi, S.A.; Feldman, C. HIV and pneumococcal disease. *Curr. Opin. Infect. Dis.* **2007**, *20*, 11–15. [CrossRef]
251. Jordano, Q.; Falcó, V.; Almirante, B.; Planes, A.M.; Del Valle, O.; Ribera, E.; Len, O.; Pigrau, C.; Pahissa, A. Invasive Pneumococcal Disease in Patients Infected with HIV: Still a Threat in the Era of Highly Active Antiretroviral Therapy. *Clin. Infect. Dis.* **2004**, *38*, 1623–1628. [CrossRef]
252. Lee, K.-Y.; Tsai, M.-S.; Kuo, K.-C.; Tsai, J.-C.; Sun, H.-Y.; Cheng, A.C.; Chang, S.-Y.; Lee, C.-H.; Hung, C.-C. Pneumococcal vaccination among HIV-infected adult patients in the era of combination antiretroviral therapy. *Hum. Vaccines Immunother.* **2014**, *10*, 3700–3710. [CrossRef]
253. Kobayashi, M.; Farrar, J.L.; Gierke, R.; Britton, A.; Childs, L.; Leidner, A.J.; Campos-Outcalt, D.; Morgan, R.L.; Long, S.S.; Talbot, H.K.; et al. Use of 15-Valent Pneumococcal Conjugate Vaccine and 20-Valent Pneumococcal Conjugate Vaccine among U.S. Adults: Updated Recommendations of the Advisory Committee on Immunization Practices—United States, 2022. *MMWR. Morb. Mortal. Wkly. Rep.* **2022**, *71*, 109–117. [CrossRef]
254. Garmpi, A.; Damaskos, C.; Garmpis, N.; Patsouras, A.; Savvanis, S.; Gravvanis, N.; Diamantis, E. Pneumococcal Vaccination Strategies among HIV-infected Adult Patients: A Review of the Literature. *In Vivo* **2019**, *33*, 1425–1430. [CrossRef]
255. Lesprit, P.; Pédrono, G.; Molina, J.-M.; Goujard, C.; Girard, P.-M.; Sarrazin, N.; Katlama, C.; Yéni, P.; Morineau, P.; Delfraissy, J.-F.; et al. Immunological efficacy of a prime-boost pneumococcal vaccination in HIV-infected adults. *AIDS* **2007**, *21*, 2425–2434. [CrossRef]
256. Feikin, D.R.; Elie, C.M.; Goetz, M.B.; Lennox, J.L.; Carlone, G.M.; Romero-Steiner, S.; Holder, P.F.; O'brien, W.A.; Whitney, C.G.; Butler, J.C.; et al. Randomized trial of the quantitative and functional antibody responses to a 7-valent pneumococcal conjugate vaccine and/or 23-valent polysaccharide vaccine among HIV-infected adults. *Vaccine* **2001**, *20*, 545–553. [CrossRef]
257. French, N.; Gordon, S.B.; Mwalukomo, T.; White, S.A.; Mwafulirwa, G.; Longwe, H.; Mwaiponya, M.; Zijlstra, E.E.; Molyneux, M.E.; Gilks, C.F. A Trial of a 7-Valent Pneumococcal Conjugate Vaccine in HIV-Infected Adults. *N. Engl. J. Med.* **2010**, *362*, 812–822. [CrossRef]

258. Adongo, C.A.; Amenumey, E.K.; Kumi-Kyereme, A.; Dubé, E. Beyond fragmentary: A proposed measure for travel vaccination concerns. *Tour. Manag.* **2021**, *83*, 104180. [CrossRef]
259. Frew, G.; McGeorge, E.; Grant, S.; de Wildt, G. Hepatitis B: A cross-sectional survey of knowledge, attitudes and practices amongst backpackers in Thailand. *Travel Med. Infect. Dis.* **2016**, *15*, 57–62. [CrossRef]
260. Larson, H.J.; De Figueiredo, A.; Xiahong, Z.; Schulz, W.S.; Verger, P.; Johnston, I.G.; Cook, A.R.; Jones, N.S. The State of Vaccine Confidence 2016: Global Insights Through a 67-Country Survey. *EBioMedicine* **2016**, *12*, 295–301. [CrossRef]
261. Poulos, C.; Curran, D.; Anastassopoulou, A.; De Moerlooze, L. German travelers' preferences for travel vaccines assessed by a discrete choice experiment. *Vaccine* **2018**, *36*, 969–978. [CrossRef]
262. Bedford, H.; Attwell, K.; Danchin, M.; Marshall, H.; Corben, P.; Leask, J. Vaccine hesitancy, refusal and access barriers: The need for clarity in terminology. *Vaccine* **2018**, *36*, 6556–6558. [CrossRef]
263. von Seidlein, L.; Wang, X.Y.; Macuamule, A.; Mondlane, C.; Puri, M.; Hendriksen, I.; Deen, J.L.; Chaignat, C.L.; Clemens, J.D.; Ansaruzzaman, M.; et al. Is HIV infection associated with an increased risk for cholera? Findings from a case-control study in Mozambique. *Trop. Med. Int. Health* **2008**, *13*, 683–688. [CrossRef]
264. Perry, R.T.; Plowe, C.V.; Koumaré, B.; Bougoudogo, F.; Kotloff, K.L.; A Losonsky, G.; Wasserman, S.S.; Levine, M.M. A single dose of live oral cholera vaccine CVD 103-HgR is safe and immunogenic in HIV-infected and HIV-noninfected adults in Mali. *Bull. World Health Organ.* **1998**, *76*, 63–71.
265. Lewis, D.J.; Gilks, C.F.; Ojoo, S.; Castello-Branco, L.R.; Dougan, G.; Evans, M.R.; McDermott, S.; Griffin, G.E. Immune response following oral administration of cholera toxin B subunit to HIV-1-infected UK and Kenyan subjects. *AIDS* **1994**, *8*, 779–786. [CrossRef]
266. Wang, S.-Y.; Cheng, X.-H.; Li, J.-X.; Li, X.-Y.; Zhu, F.-C.; Liu, P. Comparing the immunogenicity and safety of 3 Japanese encephalitis vaccines in Asia-Pacific area: A systematic review and meta-analysis. *Hum. Vaccines Immunother.* **2015**, *11*, 1418–1425. [CrossRef]
267. Thisyakorn, U.; Pancharoen, C.; Ruxrungtham, K.; Ubolyam, S.; Khawplod, P.; Tantawichien, T.; Phanuphak, P.; Wilde, H. Safety and Immunogenicity of Preexposure Rabies Vaccination in Children Infected with Human Immunodeficiency Virus Type 1. *Clin. Infect. Dis.* **2000**, *30*, 218. [CrossRef]
268. Tantawichien, T.; Jaijaroensup, W.; Khawplod, P.; Sitprija, V. Failure of Multiple-Site Intradermal Postexposure Rabies Vaccination in Patients with Human Immunodeficiency Virus with Low $CD4^{+}T$ Lymphocyte Counts. *Clin. Infect. Dis.* **2001**, *33*, e122–e124. [CrossRef]
269. Troy, S.B.; Musingwini, G.; Halpern, M.S.; Huang, C.; Stranix-Chibanda, L.; Kouiavskaia, D.; Shetty, A.K.; Chumakov, K.; Nathoo, K.; Maldonado, Y.A. Vaccine Poliovirus Shedding and Immune Response to Oral Polio Vaccine in HIV-Infected and -Uninfected Zimbabwean Infants. *J. Infect. Dis.* **2013**, *208*, 672–678. [CrossRef]
270. Chitsike, I.; Van Furth, R. Paralytic poliomyelitis associated with live oral poliomyelitis vaccine in child with HIV infection in Zimbabwe: Case report. *BMJ* **1999**, *318*, 841–843. [CrossRef]
271. Zumla, A.; Raviglione, M.; Hafner, R.; von Reyn, C.F. Tuberculosis. *N. Engl. J. Med.* **2013**, *368*, 745–755. [CrossRef]
272. Olamilekan Adesola, R.; Ayomide Adebowale, E. Mycobacterium tuberculosis: Mechanisms and interactions between drug resistance mutations with fitness costs and the drug resistance phenotypes. *Infect. Dis. Trop. Med.* **2022**, *8*, e1044.
273. Abubakar, I.; Pimpin, L.; Ariti, C.; Beynon, R.; Mangtani, P.; Sterne, J.; Fine, P.; Smith, P.; Lipman, M.; Elliman, D.; et al. Systematic review and meta-analysis of the current evidence on the duration of protection by bacillus Calmette–Guérin vaccination against tuberculosis. *Health Technol. Assess.* **2013**, *17*, 1–372. [CrossRef] [PubMed]
274. Date, K.A.; Bentsi-Enchill, A.; Marks, F.; Fox, K. Typhoid fever vaccination strategies. *Vaccine* **2015**, *33* (Suppl. S3), C55–C61. [CrossRef] [PubMed]
275. Monath, T.P. Review of the risks and benefits of yellow fever vaccination including some new analyses. *Expert Rev. Vaccines* **2012**, *11*, 427–448. [CrossRef] [PubMed]
276. Khromava, A.Y.; Eidex, R.B.; Weld, L.; Kohl, K.S.; Bradshaw, R.D.; Chen, R.T.; Cetron, M.S. Yellow fever vaccine: An updated assessment of advanced age as a risk factor for serious adverse events. *Vaccine* **2005**, *23*, 3256–3263. [CrossRef] [PubMed]
277. Barte, H.; Horvath, T.H.; Rutherford, G.W. Yellow fever vaccine for patients with HIV infection. *Cochrane Database Syst. Rev.* **2014**, *1*, CD010929. [CrossRef]

vaccines

MDPI

Systematic Review

How Well the Constructs of Health Belief Model Predict Vaccination Intention: A Systematic Review on COVID-19 Primary Series and Booster Vaccines

Yam B. Limbu [1,*] and Rajesh K. Gautam [2]

1 Feliciano School of Business, Montclair State University, 1 Normal Ave., Montclair, NJ 07043, USA
2 Department of Anthropology, Dr. Harisingh Gour Central University, Sagar 470003, MP, India; rkgautam@dhsgsu.edu.in
* Correspondence: limbuy@montclair.edu; Tel.: +1-973-655-3361; Fax: +1-973-655-7673

Abstract: This systematic review synthesizes the findings of quantitative studies examining the relationships between Health Belief Model (HBM) constructs and COVID-19 vaccination intention. We searched PubMed, Medline, CINAHL, Web of Science, and Scopus using the Preferred Reporting Items for Systematic Reviews and Meta-Analyses (PRISMA) guidelines and identified 109 eligible studies. The overall vaccination intention rate was 68.19%. Perceived benefits, perceived barriers, and cues to action were the three most frequently demonstrated predictors of vaccination intention for both primary series and booster vaccines. For booster doses, the influence of susceptibility slightly increased, but the impact of severity, self-efficacy, and cues to action on vaccination intention declined. The impact of susceptibility increased, but severity's effect declined sharply from 2020 to 2022. The influence of barriers slightly declined from 2020 to 2021, but it skyrocketed in 2022. Conversely, the role of self-efficacy dipped in 2022. Susceptibility, severity, and barriers were dominant predictors in Saudi Arabia, but self-efficacy and cues to action had weaker effects in the USA. Susceptibility and severity had a lower impact on students, especially in North America, and barriers had a lower impact on health care workers. However, cues to action and self-efficacy had a dominant influence among parents. The most prevalent modifying variables were age, gender, education, income, and occupation. The results show that HBM is useful in predicting vaccine intention.

Keywords: health belief model; HBM; COVID-19; vaccination intention; primary series vaccines; boosters; systematic review

1. Introduction

The outbreak of COVID-19 has affected the world severely. As of 9 March 2023, over 759 million global cases and over 6.8 million deaths have been reported [1]. The virus still poses serious health threats, especially to older adults and those with underlying comorbidities. People's acceptability and demand for COVID-19 vaccines and their intentions to take the COVID vaccine are slowly fading away, and this trend is even worse in the case of booster doses.

Since vaccination intention is pivotal to the success of mass vaccination campaigns as well as to the attaining of herd immunity, it is essential to understand the health beliefs that influence vaccination intention against COVID-19. Some reviews have been conducted focusing on the factors associated with COVID-19 vaccination intention. These reviews analyzed COVID-19 vaccination intentions across genders [2] and healthcare workers [3], and between healthcare workers and the general adult population [4]. Two studies conducted rapid reviews, a simplified approach to systematic reviews [5,6]. Two studies performed scoping reviews to explore broad factors such as demographic, social, and contextual factors that influenced the intention to use COVID-19 vaccines [7,8]. Wang et al. [9] and Chen et al. [10] estimated the COVID-19 vaccine acceptance rate and identified predictors associated with COVID-19 vaccine acceptance. However, these studies did not focus on the health belief model (HBM) and its constructs (i.e., perceived susceptibility, perceived severity, perceived benefits, perceived barriers). To date, only one study has systematically reviewed the extant literature on HBM [11], but it focused on vaccine hesitancy. In conclusion, prior systematic reviews have focused on narrow topics and rapid and scoping reviews. As of yet, no systematic review has addressed HBM's utility in predicting COVID-19 vaccination intention.

Hence, the purpose of the current systematic review was to analyze the research that used the HBM as a theoretical framework for understanding vaccination intention against COVID-19. We reported the prevalence of HBM constructs influencing COVID-19 vaccination intention. These results were further broken down by vaccine type (primary series versus booster doses), data collection year, country, continent, and sample type. In addition, we provided an up-to-date and comprehensive review of the literature by including articles published during 2020–2023, and those studies covering booster/third dose and parents' or caregivers' vaccination intention to vaccinate their young children for COVID-19. Finally, we reported the prevalence of HBM modifying variables, including demographic variables (e.g., age, gender, race, ethnicity, education, income, marital status) and structural variables (e.g., knowledge about a given disease, prior contact with the disease) that were significantly associated with COVID-19 vaccination intention.

2. Methodology

This systematic review was carried out in accordance with the guidelines of the Preferred Reporting Items for Systematic Review and Meta-Analysis (PRISMA) [12,13]. The ROBIS (Risk of Bias in Systematic Reviews) tool [14] was used to evaluate the quality of included studies and the risk of bias.

2.1. Eligibility

2.1.1. Inclusion Criteria

We included quantitative studies that used the HBM framework and statistical methods to examine associations between HBM constructs and COVID-19 vaccination intention for both primary series and booster doses. To ensure the quality of scientific investigation, we included only studies published in peer-reviewed journals. Other inclusion criteria were articles published in English between December 2019 and February 2023.

2.1.2. Exclusion Criteria

We excluded (1) studies that reported only vaccination intention against COVID-19 without applying HBM constructs; (2) studies that reported vaccination intention against COVID-19 with HBM constructs but which did not perform a quantitative analysis; (3) qualitative studies, non-peer reviewed studies, and conference proceedings; (4) reviews, comments, case reports, editorials and letters; and (5) grey literature.

2.2. Search Strategy

A comprehensive search for published literature was conducted in the selected databases: PubMed, Web of Science, CINAHL, and Scopus using various key words such as "health belief model" or "HBM", "vaccination intention" or "vaccine acceptance", "COVID-19" or "coronavirus" or "SARS-CoV-2", "first or second dose" or "primary series", "booster shot or dose" or "third dose".

The search was conducted from 1 January 2022 to 28 February 2023. Full length papers published between December 2019 and February 2023 were retrieved for analysis. Initially, the titles and abstracts of all articles identified by the search were screened by two researchers independently in line with the inclusion criteria; any disagreements were resolved by consensus. The titles and abstracts of non-quantitative studies and studies that did not apply the health belief model framework to predict vaccination intention were excluded. Full-text articles were obtained for studies whose titles and abstracts met inclusion criteria. All full-text articles were then evaluated to confirm if they reported necessary statistics of HBM constructs–vaccination intention relationships.

A PRISMA flow diagram was drawn to demonstrate the study selection process, the number of records identified, screened, and excluded, and the reasons for exclusion (see Figure 1). A total of 539 records were retrieved from the four electronic databases. Of them, 312 records were removed for duplicates, systematic reviews, and studies not using HBM constructs. A total of 82 articles were excluded after screening the abstracts as they were irrelevant or did not study vaccination intention or qualitative studies. The remaining 145 full-text papers were further assessed for eligibility. We included 109 studies that met all inclusion criteria after excluding studies not reporting vaccination intention or acceptance, reporting vaccination uptake (behavior) and hesitancy, not reporting required statistics, or not meeting other criteria.

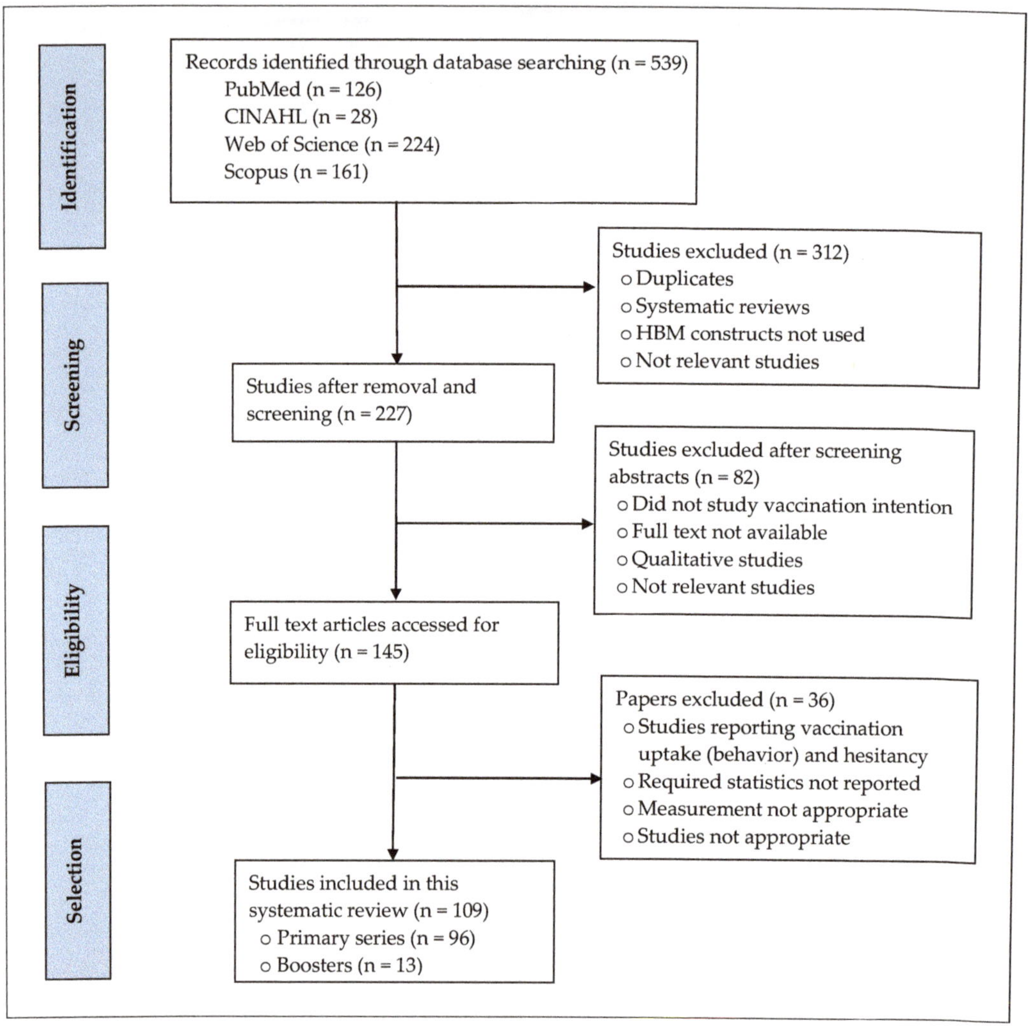

Figure 1. PRISMA flow diagram illustrating literature search.

2.3. Data Extraction and Analysis

The same two researchers extracted data from the studies independently. The information extracted consist of the author's name, data collection year, publication year, study objective, study design, population, sample size, sampling method, measure, statistical analysis technique, the country where the study was conducted, and vaccination rate. We also extracted information on HBM constructs associated with vaccination intention (susceptibility, severity, benefits, barriers, cues to action, self-efficacy, and modifying variables). The outcome variable was COVID-19 vaccination intention.

Data were analyzed using IBM SPSS Statistics 27. First, the characteristics of studies included in the review were summarized using frequencies and percentages. Next, we reported average vaccination intention rates by country, data collection year, and population. Finally, the prevalence of HBM constructs significantly related to vaccination intention was presented by data collection year, population, and geographic locations (country and continent).

2.4. Risk of Bias

To ensure the methodological quality as well as to evaluate the level of bias and to assess specific concerns about potential biases in the database search, selection, data extraction, and synthesis, the ROBIS tool was used as per the guidelines of Whiting et al. [14]. The ratings were used to judge the overall risk of bias. The signaling questions were answered as "yes", "probably yes", "probably no", "no", or "no information". The subsequent level of concern about bias associated with each domain was then judged as "low", "high", or "unclear". If the answers to all signaling questions for a domain were "yes" or "probably yes", the level of concern was judged as low. If any signaling question was answered "no" or "probably no", then bias exists.

The same two researchers independently used the ROBIS tool to evaluate risk of bias and to identify studies to be included in the present investigation. Any disagreements were resolved through discussion or a decision made by an expert, a third umpire. Similarly, the selection of databases or digital libraries was also decided with consensus.

3. Results

3.1. Characteristics of the Included Studies

This systematic review included 109 studies comprising 96 primary series vaccines and 13 booster vaccines. Fifty-seven articles were published in 2022, forty-two in 2021, eight in 2023, and three in 2020 (see Table 1). Thirty-three (33%) were published in *Vaccines*, a peer-reviewed journal, and eight studies appeared in *Human Vaccines & Immunotherapeutics*. Over half of the studies (58/109) collected data in 2021, thirty in 2020, eight in 2022, and eight in 2020–2021. Fifty-nine studies were conducted in Asia, nineteen in North America, fourteen in Europe, and ten in Africa. These studies represent 21 countries, with twenty-one studies from China and eighteen from the USA.

All studies were cross-sectional in design. The studies included in this review consisted of 174,490 respondents with a sample size ranging from 110 to 18,201 (mean = 1601, SD = 2234.20). Sixty-six articles studied general adult populations, fourteen health care workers, nine parents, and nine college students. Other populations included patients, teachers, employees, and travelers. All studies recruited participants aged 18 years and above. The vast majority of the studies (87.16%) used non-random sampling (convenience sampling); the remaining fourteen used random sampling techniques. Except for two studies that conducted experiments, all other studies collected data using the survey method. Forty-nine studies used SPSS to analyze their data, twenty-three used STATA, and seven used R. Most studies (70%) used regression analysis and ten used structural equation modeling.

Table 1. Basic characteristics of the studies included in this systematic review.

Author(s)	Year of Publication	Journal	Country	Vaccine Intention %	Population	Sample Size
Al-Hasan et al. [15]	2021	Frontiers in Public Health	NR*	75	General population	372
Al-Metwali et al. [16]	2021	Journal of Evaluation in Clinical Practice	Iraq	62	HCW	1680
Almalki et al. [17]	2022	Frontier in Public Health	Saudi Arabia	38	Parents	4135
Alobaidi [18]	2021	Journal of Multidisciplinary Healthcare	Saudi Arabia	72	General population	1333
Alobaidi and Hashim [19]	2022	Vaccines	Saudi Arabia	71	HCW	2059
Alobaidi et al. [20]	2023	Vaccines	Saudi Arabia	78	Patients	179
An et al. [21]	2021	Health Services Insights	Vietnam	81	Patients	462
Ao et al. [22]	2022	Vaccines	Malawi	61	General population	758
Apuke and Tunca [23]	2022	Journal of Asian and African Studies	Nigeria	55	General population	385
Arabyat et al. [24]	2023	Research in Social and Administrative Pharmacy	Jordan	-	General population	3116
Banik et al. [25]	2021	BMC Infectious Diseases	Bangladesh	66	General population	682
Barattucci et al. [26]	2022	Vaccines	Italy	84	General population	1095
Berg and Lin [27]	2021	Translational Behavioral Medicine	USA	71	General population	350
Berni et al. [28]	2022	Vaccines	Morocco	71	General population	3800
Burke et al. [29]	2021	Vaccine	Australia, Canada, England, New Zealand, USA	73	General population	4303
Cahapay [30]	2022	Journal of Human Behavior in the Social Environment	Philippine	-	Teachers	1070
Caple et al. [31]	2022	PeerJ	Philippines	63	General population	7193
Chu and Liu [32]	2021	Patient Education and Counseling	USA	80	General population	934
Coe et al. [33]	2022	Research in Social and Administrative Pharmacy	USA	63	General population	1047
Duan et al. [34]	2022	Vaccines	China	80	Patients	645
Dziedzic et al. [35]	2022	Frontiers in Public Health	Poland	75	HCW	443
Ellithorpe et al. [36]	2022	Vaccine	USA	60	Parents	682
Enea et al. [37]	2022	Health Communication	Argentina, Australia, Brazil, Canada, Croatia, France, Germany, Greece, Hungary, Italy, Malaysia, Netherlands, Romania, Russia, South Africa, Spain, Turkey, Ukraine, UK, USA	73	General population	6697
Getachew et al. [38]	2022	Frontier in Public Health	Ethiopia	36	HCW	417
Getachew et al. [39]	2023	BMJ Open	Ethiopia	55	Patient	412
Ghazy et al. [40]	2022	IJERPH	EMR	75	General population	2327
Goffe et al. [41]	2021	HVI	UK	62	General population	1660
Goruntla et al. [42]	2022	Asian Pacific Journal of Tropical Medicine	India	89	General population	2451
Guidry et al. [43]	2021	American Journal of Infection Control	USA	60	General population	788
Guidry et al. [44]	2022	International Journal of Environmental Research and Public Health	USA	80	Evangelicals	531

Table 1. *Cont.*

Author(s)	Year of Publication	Journal	Country	Vaccine Intention %	Population	Sample Size
Guillon and Kergall [45]	2021	Public Health	France	31	General population	1146
Handebo et al. [46]	2021	PLOS ONE	Ethiopia	67	Teachers	301
Hawlader et al. [47]	2022	International Journal of Infectious Diseases	Bangladesh, India, Pakistan, Nepal	68	General population	18,201
Hossian et al. [48]	2022	PLOS ONE	Pakistan	73	Students	2865
Hu et al. [49]	2022	Vaccines	China	84	General population	898
Huang et al. [50]	2023	Journal of Environmental and Public Health	China	92	General population	525
Huynh et al. [51]	2022	Asian Pacific Journal of Tropical Medicine	Vietnam	76	HCW	410
Iacob et al. [52]	2021	Frontiers in Psychology	Romania	45	General population	864
Jahanshahi-Amjazi et al. [53]	2022	JEHP	Iran	72	General population	2365
Jiang et al. [54]	2021	HVI	China	72	HCW	1039
Jin et al. [55]	2021	Vaccines	Pakistan		General population	320
Kasting et al. [56]	2022	JMIR Public Health and Surveillance	USA	80	General population	1643
Khalafalla et al. [57]	2022	Vaccines	Saudi Arabia	84	General population	1039
Kabir et al. [58]	2021	Vaccines	Bangladesh	69	General population	697
Lai et al. [59]	2021	Vaccines	China	85	General population	1145
Le An et al. [60]	2021	HVI	Vietnam	77	Students	854
Le et al. [61]	2022	BMC Public Health	Vietnam	58	HCW	911
Lee et al. [62]	2022	JHCPF	Hong Kong	29	General population	800
Li, J.-B. et al. [63]	2022	Vaccine	Hong Kong	-	Parents	11,141
Li, G. et al. [64]	2022	Health Services Research and Managerial Epidemiology	Thailand	67	HCW	226
Liao et al. [65]	2022	Vaccine	Hong Kong	61	General population	4055
Lin et al. [66]	2020	PLOS Neglected Tropical Diseases	China	83	General population	3541
Lin et al. [5]	2021	HVI	China	78	Parents	2026
Liu et al. [67]	2022	IJERPH	China	63	General population	3389
Lopez-Cepero et al. [68]	2021	HVI	Puerto Rico	83	General population	1911
Lyons et al. [69]	2023	Vaccines	Trinidad	60	Patients	272
Mahmud et al. [70]	2021	Vaccines	Saudi Arabia	58	General population	1387
Mahmud et al. [71]	2022	Vaccines	Jordan	84	General population	2307
Maria et al. [72]	2022	Vaccines	Indonesia	89	HCW	1684
Mercadante and Law [73]	2021	Research in Social and Administrative Pharmacy	USA	67	General population	525
Miyachi et al. [74]	2022	Vaccines	Japan	91	Students	1776
Mohammed et al. [75]	2022	Vaccine	Iraq, Jordan, UAE, Oman, Yemen	56	Parents	1154
Morar et al. [76]	2022	IJERPH	Romania	51	General population	110
Nguyen et al. [77]	2021	Risk Management and Healthcare Policy	Vietnam	78	Students	412
Okai and Abekah-Nkrumah [78]	2022	PLOS ONE	Ghana	63	General population	362
Okmi et al. [79]	2022	Cureus	Saudi Arabia	73	General population	1939

Table 1. *Cont.*

Author(s)	Year of Publication	Journal	Country	Vaccine Intention %	Population	Sample Size
Okuyan et al. [80]	2021	International Journal of Clinical Pharmacy	Turkey	75	HCW	961
Otiti-Sengeri et al. [81]	2022	Vaccines	Uganda	98	HCW	300
Patwary et al. [82]	2021	Vaccines	Bangladesh	85	General population	543
Qin et al. [83]	2022a	Vaccines	China	94	General population	3119
Qin et al. [84]	2022b	Frontiers in Public Health	China	88	Parents	1724
Qin et al. [85]	2022c	Frontiers in Public Health	China	83	60 or older	3321
Qin et al. [86]	2023	HVI	China	81	General population	3224
Quinto et al. [87]	2021	Philippine Journal of Health Research and Development	Philippine	93	Teachers	707
Rabin and Durta [88]	2021	Psychology, Health & Medicine	USA	76	General population	186
Reindl and Catma [89]	2022	Expert Review of Pharmacoeconomics & Outcomes Research	USA	66	Parents	30
Reiter et al. [90]	2020	Vaccine	USA	69	General population	2006
Rosental and Shmueli [91]	2021	Vaccines	Israel	82	Students	628
Rountree and Prentice [92]	2022	Irish Journal of Medical Science	Ireland	32	General population	1995
Seangpraw et al. [93]	2022	Frontiers in Medicine	Thailand		General population	1024
Seboka et al. [94]	2021	Risk Management and Healthcare Policy	Ethiopia	65	General population	1160
Shah et al. [95]	2022	Vaccine	Singapore	-	General population	1009
Shmueli [96]	2021	BMC Public Health	Israel	80	General population	398
Shmueli [97]	2022	Vaccines	Israel	65	General population	461
Short et al. [98]	2022	Families, Systems and Health	USA	37	Students	526
Sieverding et al. [99]	2023	Psychology, Health & Medicine	UK and Germany	88	General population	1425
Spinewine et al. [100]	2021	Vaccines	Belgium	58	General population	1132
Ştefănuţ et al. [101]	2021	Frontiers in Psychology	Romania	45	Students	432
Su et al. [102]	2022	Frontiers in Psychology	China	73	General population	557
Suess et al. [103]	2022	Tourism Management	USA	71	Travelers	1478
Tran et al. [104]	2021	Pharmacy Practice	Russia	42	General population	876
Ung et al. [105]	2022	BMC Infectious Diseases	Macao	62	General population	552
Vatcharavongvan et al. [106]	2023	Vaccine	Thailand	90	Parents	1056
Wagner et al. [107]	2022	Vaccines	USA	38	General population	1012
Walker et al. [108]	2021	Vaccines	China	36	Students	330
Wang [109]	2022	Health Communication	China	80	General population	460
Wang et al. [110]	2021	HVI	China	64	Students	833
Wijesinghe et al. [111]	2021	Asia Pacific Journal of Public Health	Sri Lanka	54	General population	895
Wirawan et al. [112]	2022	Vaccines	Indonesia	56	General population	2674
Wong et al. [113]	2020	HVI	Malaysia	94	General population	1159
Xiao et al. [114]	2021	Vaccines	China	56	General population	2528

Table 1. *Cont.*

Author(s)	Year of Publication	Journal	Country	Vaccine Intention %	Population	Sample Size
Yan et al. [115]	2021	Vaccines	Hong Kong	42	General population	1255
Yang et al. [116]	2022	IJERPH	China	82	General population	621
Youssef et al. [117]	2022	PLOS ONE	Lebanon	58	HCW	1800
Yu et al. [118]	2021	HVI	China	72	HCW	2254
Zakeri et al. [119]	2021	Journal of Pharmaceutical Health Services Research	USA	62	Parents	595
Zampetakis and Melas [120]	2021	Appl Psychol Health Well-Being	Greece	44	Employees	1165
Zhang et al. [121]	2023	Vaccines	China	86	General population	1472
Zhelyazkova et al. [122]	2022	Vaccines	Germany	84	HCW	2555

NR* = Country is not reported, but the regions are (North America, the Middle East, Europe, Asia); HCW = Health care workers; IJERPH = International Journal of Environmental Research and Public Health; HVI = Human Vaccines & Immunotherapeutics; JHCPF = INQUIRY: The Journal of Health Care Organization, Provision, and Financing.

3.2. *Vaccination Intention Rate by Country, Population, and Year*

Overall COVID-19 vaccination intention rate was 68.19% (Std. = 17.58), which ranged from 31% to 97.6%. Average vaccination intention percentages for COVID-19 by country were: Malaysia (94.3%), India (89.3%), Puerto Rico (82.7%), Philippines (77.50%), China (76.34%), Israel (75.72%), UK (74.23%), Vietnam (73.48%), Bangladesh (73.17%), Saudi Arabia (66.18%), USA (65.21%), Ethiopia (55.64%), Sri Lanka (54%), and Romania (46.95%). The overall acceptance rate for the COVID-19 vaccine across all studies increased from 63.68% in 2020 to 70% in 2021 and then remained flat in 2022 (69%). As shown in Figure 2, average vaccination intention rate was highest among teachers (80%), followed by patients (75%), health care workers (72%), and general adults (68%). Only 60% of the parents intended to get their children vaccinated against COVID-19.

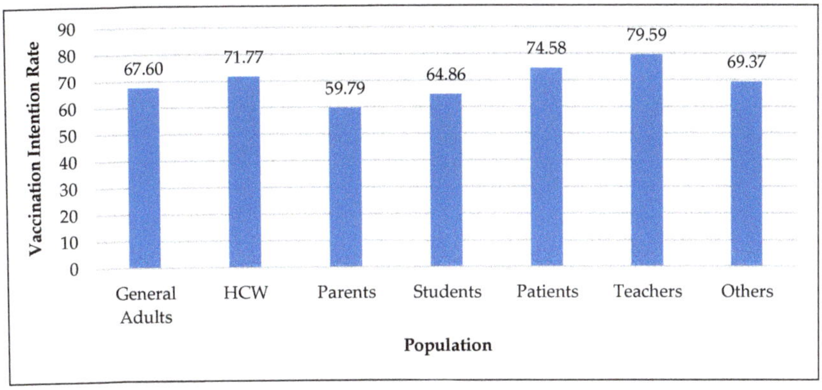

Figure 2. Vaccination intention rate by population.

3.3. *HBM Constructs Associated with Vaccination Intention*

Table 2 presents the studies that reported significant associations between HBM constructs and COVID-19 vaccination intention. As shown in Figure 3, perceived benefits of COVID-19 vaccination, the most commonly demonstrated HBM construct, predicted vaccination intention in eighty-seven studies (90.59%) for primary series vaccines. Perceived barriers to accepting the vaccine against COVID-19 were found to be inversely associated with vaccination intention in seventy-seven studies (85.19%). Cues to action were found to be positively associated with vaccination intention in fifty-eight studies (84.61%), perceived susceptibility to develop COVID-19 infection in fifty-five studies (63.22%), perceived severity of COVID-19 infection in fifty-one studies (56.63%), and self-efficacy in twenty-nine studies (77.78%). Surprisingly, thirty-six studies (43.37%) reported insignificant associations between perceived severity and vaccination intention. Similarly, over one-third of the studies (36.78%) that examined perceived susceptibility and over one-fifth of the studies (22.22%) that examined self-efficacy were not significant predictors of vaccination intention.

Only thirteen articles used the health belief model to explore the predictors of COVID-19 booster vaccination intention. As presented in Figure 4, perceived benefits, the most commonly demonstrated HBM factor, predicted booster vaccination intention in eleven studies (91.67%). Perceived barriers were negatively related to booster vaccination intention in nine studies (81.82%). Susceptibility was positively associated with booster intention in seven studies (70%). On the contrary, Hu et al. [49] found a negative effect of susceptibility on booster acceptance. Of the eleven studies that examined severity, only four reported perceived severity as a significant determinant of booster intention; however, such an effect was not evident in seven articles (63.64%). In addition, self-efficacy was not significantly associated with booster intention in three out of four studies. Similarly, cues to action did not predict booster intention in three studies (42.86%).

Table 2. Health belief model constructs significantly associated with vaccination intention.

HBM Construct	Studies
Perceived susceptibility	[17–19,22,25,26,28,29,31,33,34,37–40,42,43,46–48,50,57–59,62,63,66–68,70–72,75,78–85,87–96,98,100,104,105,109,111,113,115,118,120,122]
Perceived severity	[5,15,17,18,22,24,28,29,31,33–36,38–42,47,48,50,57,58,61,64–68,70,71,74,75,79,80,87,89,90,92,93,97–100,102,107,113,118,120–122]
Perceived benefits	[5,15–22,24,25,28,29,31–35,39,41–55,57–63,66,68–80,82–91,96,97,99–104,106,108–122]
Perceived barriers	[5,15–23,25,27–32,34,35,39,40,42–59,61–63,66,68,70,71,73–75,77–80,82,83,85,87,89,91,92,95,98,99,101,102,104–106,108,110,112–117,119–121]
Self-efficacy	[5,17,21,22,28,34,43,53,55–57,61,71,75,76,79,82,89,90,92,93,95,96,105,109,114,115,118,121]
Cues to action	[15–18,20–24,28,29,31,34,42,45–49,51,54,57,58,60–63,66,68–71,75,77,79,82,83,85–87,89,91–94,96,97,100,104,106,108,110,113,115–119,122]

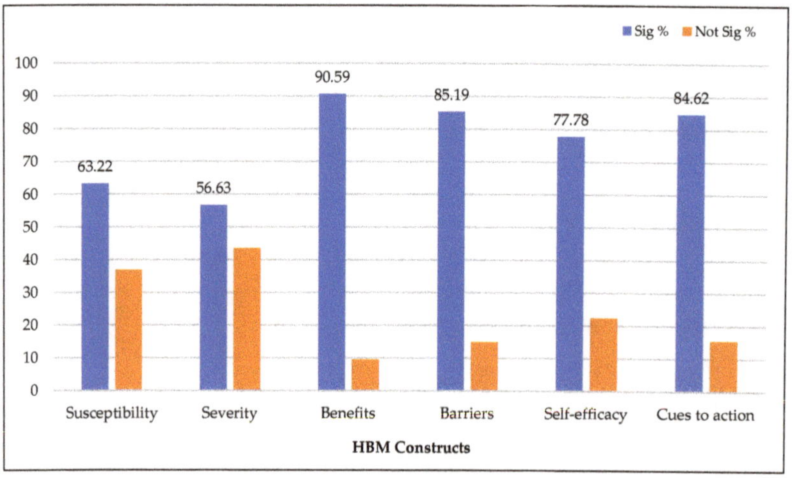

Figure 3. Health belief model constructs predicting primary series vaccination intention.

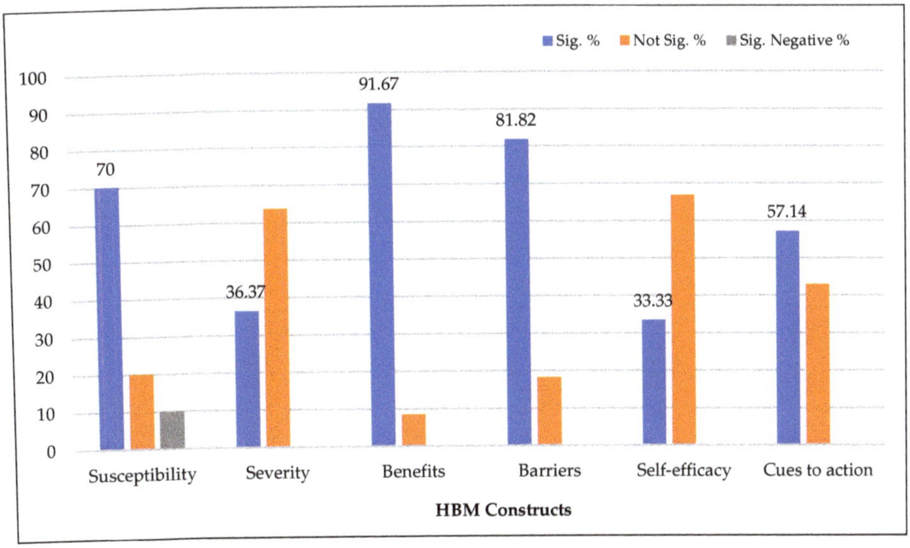

Figure 4. Health belief model constructs predicting booster vaccination intention.

In conclusion, the influence of perceived severity, self-efficacy, and cues to action on vaccination intention declined for boosters. However, the impact of perceived susceptibility slightly increased for boosters.

3.4. Modifying HBM Constructs Associated with Vaccination Intention

As shown in Figure 5, the most prevalent modifying variable significantly associated with COVID-19 vaccination intention was age (39 studies), followed by gender (38), education (31), income (23), occupation (23), region (17), race (13 studies), and marital status (12). Other frequently explored modifying variables significantly influencing vaccination intention were religion, nationality, political leaning, history of flu or COVID-19 vaccination, history of COVID infection, knowledge of disease or COVID-19, trust in healthcare system, science or media, sources of information, and health status.

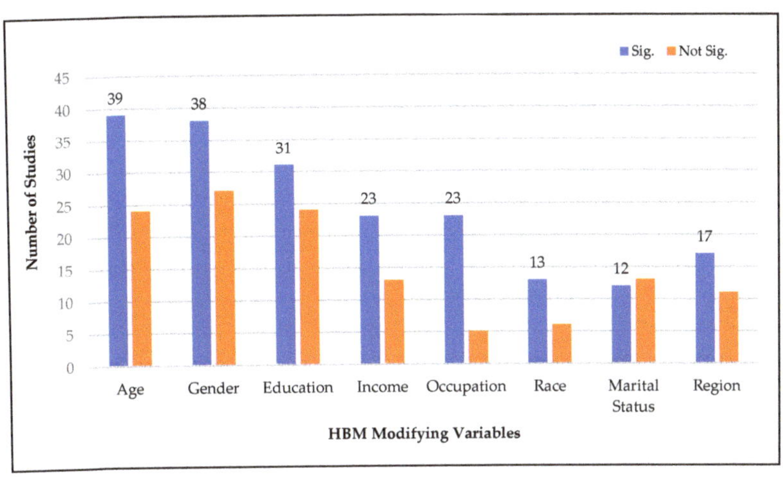

Figure 5. Major HBM modifying variables associated with vaccination intention.

3.5. HBM Constructs Associated with Vaccination Intention by Data Collection Year, Country, Continent, and Sample

3.5.1. Data Collection Year

While the effects of perceived susceptibility on vaccination intention increased significantly from 2020 to 2022, the influence of perceived severity declined sharply (see Figure 6). The significant association of perceived barriers with vaccination intention slightly declined from 2020 to 2021, but it skyrocketed in 2022. Conversely, the effect of self-efficacy dipped in 2022. In addition, the role of perceived benefits declined from 2020 to 2021 but remained flat in 2022. Conversely, the influence of cues to action increased in 2021, but slightly declined in 2022.

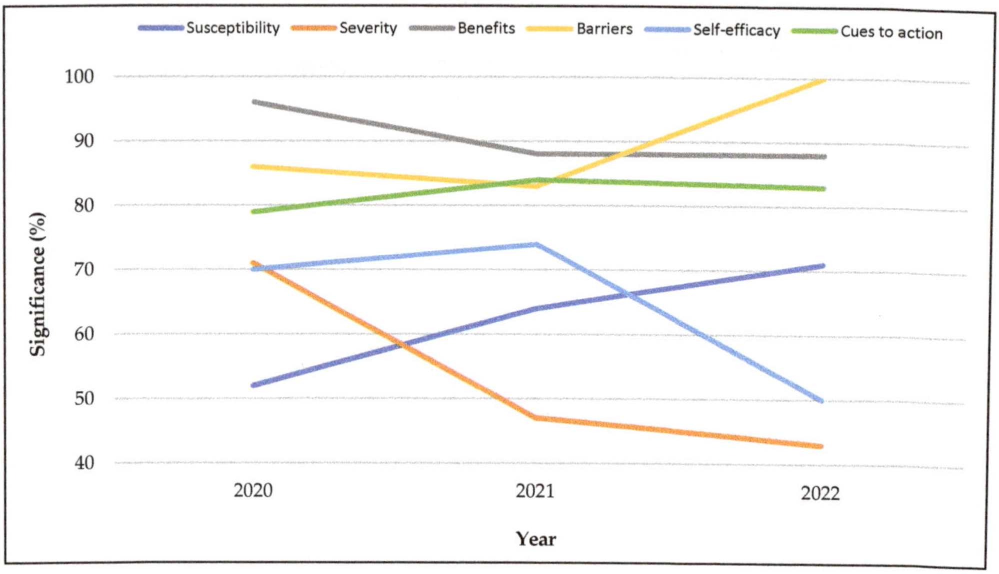

Figure 6. Health belief model constructs associated with vaccination intention by data collection year.

3.5.2. Geographic Location

Figure 7 presents the associations between HBM factors and vaccination intention by continent with five or more studies. All other HBM constructs, except perceived susceptibility, were associated with vaccination intention less frequently in Africa compared to Asia, Europe, and North America. In addition, perceived susceptibility was a less prevalent significant predictor in North America and Europe, compared to Africa and Asia.

Figure 8 presents the relationships between HBM dimensions and vaccination intention by countries with five or more studies. Perceived susceptibility and perceived severity were more common determinants of vaccination intention in Saudi Arabia than in China and the USA. Perceived severity was the least frequently demonstrated predictor of vaccination intention in China. Self-efficacy and cues to action were less frequently demonstrated predictors in the USA than in China, Saudi Arabia, and Vietnam. Perceived barriers were the more dominant factor influencing vaccination intention in Saudi Arabia than in other countries.

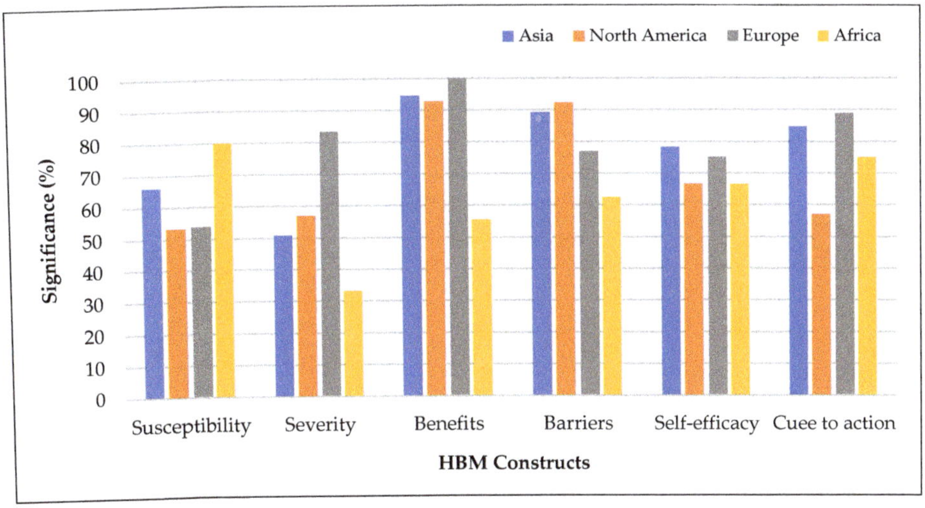

Figure 7. Health belief model constructs associated with vaccination intention by continent with five or more studies.

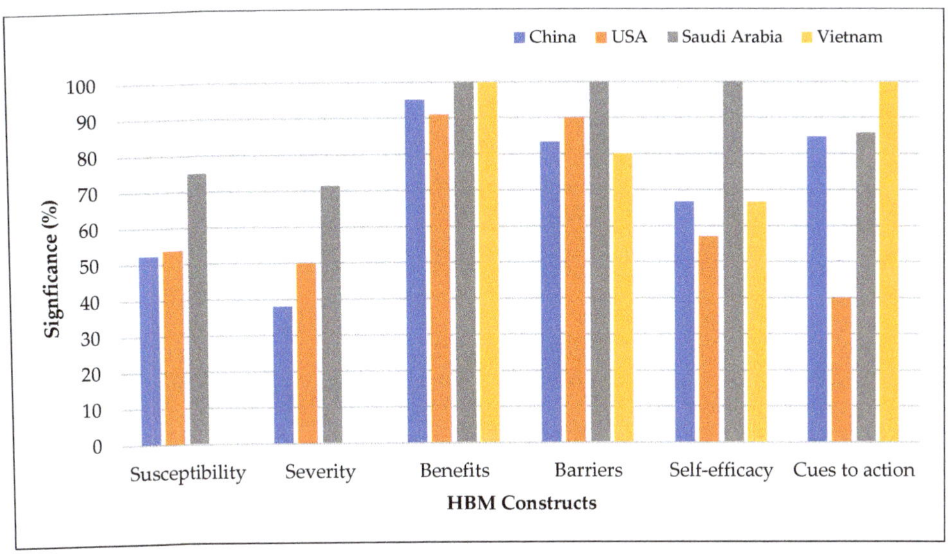

Figure 8. Health belief model constructs associated with vaccination intention by country with five or more studies.

3.5.3. Study Population

Figure 9 shows the associations between HBM constructs and vaccination intention by the study population. The effects of perceived susceptibility and perceived severity on vaccination intention were lower among students. Perceived barriers were the least frequently demonstrated predictor among health care workers. Cues to action and self-efficacy had a dominant influence among parents.

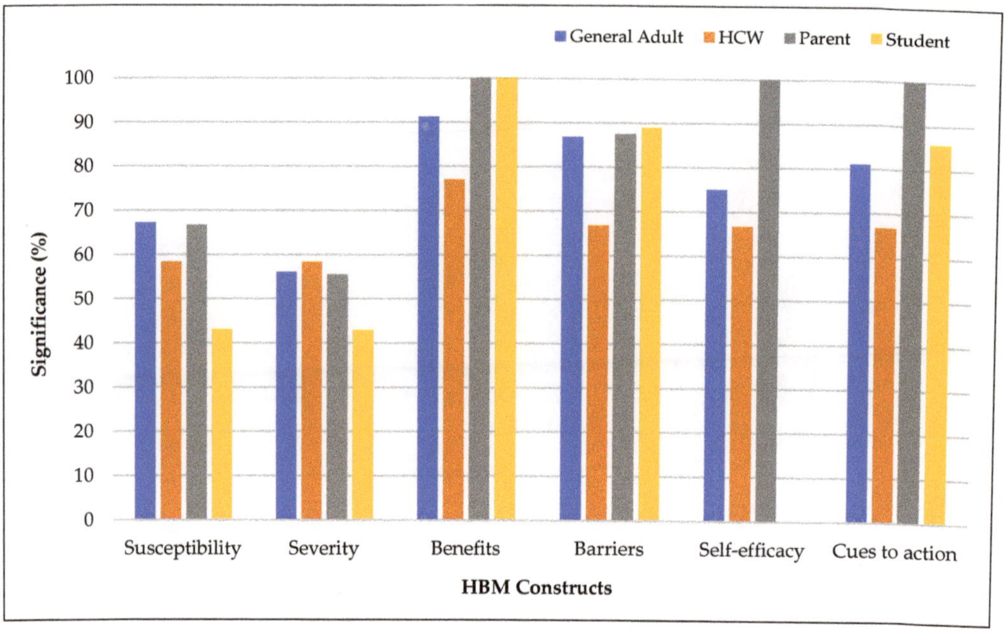

Figure 9. Health belief model constructs associated with vaccination intention by study population.

4. Discussion and Implications

The results suggest that perceived benefits of receiving the COVID-19 vaccine was the most common HBM construct predicting vaccination intention. Other dominant HBM constructs were perceived barriers to receiving the vaccine and cues to action (i.e., information, people, and events that guided them to be vaccinated). However, perceived susceptibility to developing COVID-19 infection, perceived severity of COVID-19 infection, and perceived self-efficacy of receiving the COVID-19 vaccine were weaker determinants of vaccination intention. The findings of this systematic review provide some support for the health belief model as a useful framework for understanding the facilitators and barriers to COVID-19 vaccination intention. This finding is consistent with previous studies, which suggested similar evidence in the context of influenza vaccination [123–125].

Our results indicate that perceived benefits, perceived barriers, and cues to action were the three most frequently demonstrated HBM constructs predicting vaccination intention for both primary series and booster vaccines. Hence, COVID-19 vaccine promotional campaigns should emphasize the benefits of vaccinating against COVID-19. Providing truthful and up-to-date information about the benefits of vaccines can encourage individuals to get vaccinated. Therefore, COVID-19 vaccination communication campaigns may need to progressively shift emphasis from addressing risk perceptions and concerns to stressing the benefits of vaccination for the individual and the community [126].

The results also highlight the importance of identifying the barriers to vaccination (e.g., lack of trust in the government or healthcare system, insufficient knowledge about the benefits of vaccines, misinformation about the coronavirus and vaccines, lack of affordability or shortage of vaccines) and ensuring a course of action to overcome them. In addition, making the vaccine easily accessible (e.g., offering walk-in clinics and mobile vaccination units) can reduce barriers to vaccination and increase uptake. Similarly, offering incentives, such as free or discounted products or services, can motivate individuals to accept vaccines.

The results also show that increasing the vaccination cue to action is crucial. For example, vaccine recommendations or reminders by trusted authorities, government agencies, public health officials, and healthcare experts can effectively persuade people to accept vaccines. In addition, social media and the social influence of celebrities, politicians, friends, family members, or community leaders can play a crucial role in educating, persuading, and influencing people's vaccination decisions.

This review reveals that the influence of susceptibility on vaccination intention increased from 2020 to 2022 and was higher for booster doses than for primary series vaccines. On the contrary, severity was a less common predictor of vaccination intention for boosters. These results imply that people were increasingly concerned about being infected by COVID-19. Simultaneously, an increasing number of individuals perceived COVID-19 as a less severe disease. One reason is that the virus might have infected several people after receiving primary series vaccines, and they might have experienced mild systems, similar to traditional viruses such as the common cold and influenza. These counterintuitive beliefs pose a significant obstacle to vaccination. Therefore, the government and other concerned parties promoting vaccines should focus on increasing people's perceptions of the seriousness of COVID infections.

In conclusion, to combat the ongoing pandemic and to increase vaccine uptake against COVID-19, agencies such as the government, policymakers, and the WHO should take account of health beliefs when designing interventions and public health campaigns encouraging vaccination. However, such initiatives should take into account not only the HBM constructs but also geographic (e.g., country, regions), socioeconomic status (e.g., income, education), and other demographic (e.g., age, gender, and occupation) factors that can influence an individual's vaccination decision.

5. Directions for Future Research

This systematic review synthesized the literature that investigated the relationships between HBM constructs and vaccine intention against COVID-19. However, the findings are mixed. Several studies reported strong correlations between HBM constructs and vaccination intention, but others did not; this is true for both primary series and booster doses. These contradictory results may have been due to several limitations (e.g., research design, study population, data collection approach, measures, analytical approach, and theoretical frameworks) that can be addressed by future studies.

Our results show that the vast majority of studies that utilized theoretical models were based on HBM and the Theory of Planned Behavior. Hence, future research can examine the applicability of other theories such as the Theory of Reasoned Action, Protection Motivation Theory, Social Cognitive Theory, Self-Determination Theory, Information–Motivation–Behavioral Skills Model, Cognitive Behavioral Theory, Theory of Triadic Influence, Social Network Theory, Diffusion of Innovation Theory, and Social Support Theory.

All the studies included in this systematic review used cross-sectional data. Thus, future research should apply a longitudinal approach because people's opinions and health beliefs on COVID-19 and vaccines may change over time [127].

Furthermore, this review shows that the vast majority of the studies included in this review used a descriptive/correlational study design and relied on survey methodology. Hence, we recommend causal research and experiments to establish cause-and-effect relationships between the predictors and outcomes. In addition, machine learning techniques and secondary data can be utilized. Finally, qualitative methods such as focus group studies, in-depth interviews, and case studies can provide important insights into vaccine hesitancy and help understand the nuances of vaccination intention across different populations and geographic regions [128].

The studies included in this review used various measures to assess people's intentions and hesitancy using a slider or a Likert scale. Some of them were dichotomized into vaccine intention and hesitancy. These measures can be misleading and unreliable as they can oversimplify complex attitudes and behaviors related to vaccination against COVID-19. In addition, these measures may not capture the nuances of individuals' vaccine intentions and hesitancy. Hence, alternative measures (e.g., multiple-item scales that assess different aspects of vaccination attitudes and behaviors) can be developed and used for future research.

A vast majority of studies included in this systematic review used regression analysis, especially logistic regression using dichotomous dependent variables. Thus, we recommend using other statistical analyses (e.g., SEM, linear regression) with a continuous outcome variable.

Our results indicate that the HBM has been primarily applied to study vaccine intentions of the general adult population, parents, students, and health care workers. Future research should focus on specific and under-represented populations such as deprived communities, ethnic and racial minorities, rural and aged populations, and people with multiple chronic conditions. Likewise, more research is needed to explore understudied regions or countries, especially Australia, Oceania, South America, and African countries. Similarly, comparing high-income versus low-income countries, Western versus non-Western countries, and developed versus developing regions/countries may provide additional insights into the conflicting literature.

Finally, it is also essential to consider the cultural and social context in which vaccine intention and hesitancy are assessed. Different cultures and social groups may have unique beliefs, values, and experiences related to COVID-19 and vaccination, and these factors can influence attitudes and behaviors towards vaccination. Therefore, it is crucial to use culturally sensitive and culturally appropriate measures when assessing vaccine intention and hesitancy.

6. Conclusions

This systematic review synthesizes the findings of quantitative studies examining the associations between HBM constructs and vaccination intention against COVID-19. Our results indicate that perceived benefits, perceived barriers, and cues to action are the most common determinants of vaccination intention. However, perceived susceptibility to developing COVID-19 infection, perceived severity of COVID-19 infection, and perceived self-efficacy of receiving the COVID-19 vaccine were weaker predictors of vaccination intention. In addition, the associations between HBM factors and vaccination intention differed across vaccine type, study year, geographic location, and study population. The results show that the health belief model can be helpful for understanding the facilitators and barriers to COVID-19 vaccination intention.

Author Contributions: Conceptualization, methodology, software, data curation, validation, formal analysis, and writing original draft, Y.B.L. and R.K.G.; investigation, R.K.G.; resources, R.K.G.; writing—review and editing, Y.B.L. and R.K.G.; visualization, R.K.G. and Y.B.L.; supervision, Y.B.L.; project administration, R.K.G. All authors have read and agreed to the published version of the manuscript.

Funding: This research received no external funding.

Institutional Review Board Statement: Not applicable.

Informed Consent Statement: Not applicable.

Data Availability Statement: Data generated in this study is available by contacting the first author, Yam B. Limbu, if requested reasonably.

Conflicts of Interest: The authors declare no conflict of interest.

References

1. World Health Organization. WHO Coronavirus Disease (COVID-19) Dashboard. Available online: https://covid19.who.int (accessed on 12 March 2023).
2. Zintel, S.; Flock, C.; Arbogast, A.L.; Forster, A.; Von Wagner, C.; Sieverding, M. Gender differences in the intention to get vaccinated against COVID-19: A systematic review and meta-analysis. *J. Public Health* **2022**, 1–25. [CrossRef] [PubMed]
3. Galanis, P.; Vraka, I.; Fragkou, D.; Bilali, A.; Kaitelidou, D. Intention of healthcare workers to accept COVID-19 vaccination and related factors: A systematic review and meta-analysis. *Asian Pac. J. Trop. Med.* **2021**, *14*, 543. [CrossRef]

4. Al-Amer, R.; Maneze, D.; Everett, B.; Montayre, J.; Villarosa, A.R.; Dwekat, E.; Salamonson, Y. COVID-19 Vaccination Intention in the First Year of the Pandemic: A Systematic Review. *J. Clin. Nurs.* **2022**, *31*, 62–86. [CrossRef] [PubMed]
5. Lin, Y.; Hu, Z.; Zhao, Q.; Alias, H.; Danaee, M.; Wong, L.P. Chinese Parents' Intentions to Vaccinate Their Children against SARS-CoV-2 Infection and Vaccine Preferences. *Hum. Vaccines Immunother.* **2021**, *17*, 4806–4815. [CrossRef]
6. Wang, Y.; Liu, Y. Multilevel Determinants of COVID-19 Vaccination Hesitancy in the United States: A Rapid Systematic Review. *Prev. Med. Rep.* **2022**, *25*, 101673. [CrossRef]
7. AlShurman, B.A.; Khan, A.F.; Mac, C.; Majeed, M.; Butt, Z.A. What demographic, social, and contextual factors influence the intention to use COVID-19 vaccines: A scoping review. *Int. J. Environ. Res. Public Health* **2021**, *18*, 9342. [CrossRef]
8. Biswas, M.; Alzubaidi, M.S.; Shah, U.; Abd-Alrazaq, A.A.; Shah, Z. A scoping review to find out worldwide COVID-19 vaccine hesitancy and its underlying determinants. *Vaccines* **2021**, *9*, 1243. [CrossRef]
9. Wang, Q.; Yang, L.; Jin, H.; Lin, L. Vaccination against COVID-19: A Systematic Review and Meta-Analysis of Acceptability and Its Predictors. *Prev. Med.* **2021**, *150*, 106694. [CrossRef]
10. Chen, H.; Li, X.; Gao, J.; Liu, X.; Mao, Y.; Wang, R.; Zheng, P.; Xiao, Q.; Jia, Y.; Fu, H.; et al. Health Belief Model Perspective on the Control of COVID-19 Vaccine Hesitancy and the Promotion of Vaccination in China: Web-Based Cross-sectional Study. *J. Med. Internet Res.* **2021**, *23*, e29329. [CrossRef]
11. Limbu, Y.B.; Gautam, R.K.; Pham, L. The Health Belief Model Applied to COVID-19 Vaccine Hesitancy: A Systematic Review. *Vaccines* **2022**, *10*, 973. [CrossRef]
12. Liberati, A.; Altman, D.G.; Tetzlaff, J.; Mulrow, C.; Gøtzsche, P.C.; Ioannidis, J.P.; Clarke, M.; Devereaux, P.J.; Kleijnen, J.; Moher, D. The PRISMA statement for reporting systematic reviews and meta-analyses of studies that evaluate health care interventions: Explanation and elaboration. *J. Clin. Epidemiol.* **2009**, *62*, e1–e34. [CrossRef] [PubMed]
13. Page, M.J.; McKenzie, J.E.; Bossuyt, P.M.; Boutron, I.; Hoffmann, T.C.; Mulrow, C.D.; Shamseer, L.; Tetzlaff, J.M.; Moher, D. Updating guidance for reporting systematic reviews: Development of the PRISMA 2020 statement. *J. Clin. Epidemiol.* **2021**, *134*, 103–112. [CrossRef]
14. Whiting, P.; Savović, J.; Higgins, J.P.; Caldwell, D.M.; Reeves, B.C.; Shea, B.; Davies, P.; Kleijnen, J.; Churchill, R.; ROBIS Group. ROBIS: A new tool to assess risk of bias in systematic reviews was developed. *J. Clin. Epidemiol.* **2016**, *69*, 225–234. [CrossRef] [PubMed]
15. Al-Hasan, A.; Khuntia, J.; Yim, D. Does Seeing What Others Do Through Social Media Influence Vaccine Uptake and Help in the Herd Immunity Through Vaccination? A Cross-Sectional Analysis. *Front. Public Health* **2021**, *9*, 715931. [CrossRef] [PubMed]
16. Al-Metwali, B.Z.; Al-Jumaili, A.A.; Al-Alag, Z.A.; Sorofman, B. Exploring the Acceptance of COVID -19 Vaccine among Healthcare Workers and General Population Using Health Belief Model. *J. Eval. Clin. Pract.* **2021**, *27*, 1112–1122. [CrossRef] [PubMed]
17. Almalki, O.S.; Alfayez, O.M.; Al Yami, M.S.; Asiri, Y.A.; Almohammed, O.A. Parents' Hesitancy to Vaccinate Their 5–11-Year-Old Children Against COVID-19 in Saudi Arabia: Predictors From the Health Belief Model. *Front. Public Health* **2022**, *10*, 842862. [CrossRef]
18. Alobaidi, S. Predictors of Intent to Receive the COVID-19 Vaccination Among the Population in the Kingdom of Saudi Arabia: A Survey Study. *JMDH* **2021**, *14*, 1119–1128. [CrossRef]
19. Alobaidi, S.; Hashim, A. Predictors of the Third (Booster) Dose of COVID-19 Vaccine Intention among the Healthcare Workers in Saudi Arabia: An Online Cross-Sectional Survey. *Vaccines* **2022**, *10*, 987. [CrossRef]
20. Alobaidi, S.; Alsolami, E.; Sherif, A.; Almahdy, M.; Elmonier, R.; Alobaidi, W.Y.; Akl, A. COVID-19 Booster Vaccine Hesitancy among Hemodialysis Patients in Saudi Arabia Using the Health Belief Model: A Multi-Centre Experience. *Vaccines* **2023**, *11*, 95. [CrossRef]
21. An, P.L.; Nguyen, H.T.N.; Dang, H.T.B.; Huynh, Q.N.H.; Pham, B.D.U.; Huynh, G. Integrating Health Behavior Theories to Predict Intention to Get a COVID-19 Vaccine. *Health Serv. Insights* **2021**, *14*, 117863292110601. [CrossRef]
22. Ao, Q.; Egolet, R.O.; Yin, H.; Cui, F. Acceptance of COVID-19 Vaccines among Adults in Lilongwe, Malawi: A Cross-Sectional Study Based on the Health Belief Model. *Vaccines* **2022**, *10*, 760. [CrossRef] [PubMed]
23. Apuke, O.D.; Asude Tunca, E. Modelling the Factors That Predict the Intention to Take COVID-19 Vaccine in Nigeria. *J. Asian Afr. Stud.* **2022**. [CrossRef]
24. Arabyat, R.M.; Nusair, M.B.; Al-Azzam, S.I.; Amawi, H.A.; El-Hajji, F.D. Willingness to Pay for COVID-19 Vaccines: Applying the Health Belief Model. *Res. Soc. Adm. Pharm.* **2023**, *19*, 95–101. [CrossRef]
25. Banik, R.; Islam, M.S.; Pranta, M.U.R.; Rahman, Q.M.; Rahman, M.; Pardhan, S.; Driscoll, R.; Hossain, S.; Sikder, M.T. Understanding the Determinants of COVID-19 Vaccination Intention and Willingness to Pay: Findings from a Population-Based Survey in Bangladesh. *BMC Infect. Dis.* **2021**, *21*, 892. [CrossRef] [PubMed]
26. Barattucci, M.; Pagliaro, S.; Ballone, C.; Teresi, M.; Consoli, C.; Garofalo, A.; De Giorgio, A.; Ramaci, T. Trust in Science as a Possible Mediator between Different Antecedents and COVID-19 Booster Vaccination Intention: An Integration of Health Belief Model (HBM) and Theory of Planned Behavior (TPB). *Vaccines* **2022**, *10*, 1099. [CrossRef] [PubMed]
27. Berg, M.B.; Lin, L. Predictors of COVID-19 Vaccine Intentions in the United States: The Role of Psychosocial Health Constructs and Demographic Factors. *Transl. Behav. Med.* **2021**, *11*, 1782–1788. [CrossRef]
28. Berni, I.; Menouni, A.; Filali Zegzouti, Y.; Kestemont, M.-P.; Godderis, L.; El Jaafari, S. Factors Associated with COVID-19 Vaccine Acceptance in Morocco: Applying the Health Belief Model. *Vaccines* **2022**, *10*, 784. [CrossRef]

29. Burke, P.F.; Masters, D.; Massey, G. Enablers and Barriers to COVID-19 Vaccine Uptake: An International Study of Perceptions and Intentions. *Vaccine* **2021**, *39*, 5116–5128. [CrossRef]
30. Cahapay, M.B. To Get or Not to Get: Examining the Intentions of Philippine Teachers to Vaccinate against COVID-19. *J. Hum. Behav. Soc. Environ.* **2022**, *32*, 325–335. [CrossRef]
31. Caple, A.; Dimaano, A.; Sagolili, M.M.; Uy, A.A.; Aguirre, P.M.; Alano, D.L.; Camaya, G.S.; Ciriaco, B.J.; Clavo, P.J.M.; Cuyugan, D.; et al. Interrogating COVID-19 Vaccine Intent in the Philippines with a Nationwide Open-Access Online Survey. *PeerJ* **2022**, *10*, e12887. [CrossRef]
32. Chu, H.; Liu, S. Integrating Health Behavior Theories to Predict American's Intention to Receive a COVID-19 Vaccine. *Patient Educ. Couns.* **2021**, *104*, 1878–1886. [CrossRef] [PubMed]
33. Coe, A.B.; Elliott, M.H.; Gatewood, S.B.S.; Goode, J.-V.R.; Moczygemba, L.R. Perceptions and Predictors of Intention to Receive the COVID-19 Vaccine. *Res. Soc. Adm. Pharm.* **2022**, *18*, 2593–2599. [CrossRef]
34. Duan, L.; Wang, Y.; Dong, H.; Song, C.; Zheng, J.; Li, J.; Li, M.; Wang, J.; Yang, J.; Xu, J. The COVID-19 Vaccination Behavior and Correlates in Diabetic Patients: A Health Belief Model Theory-Based Cross-Sectional Study in China, 2021. *Vaccines* **2022**, *10*, 659. [CrossRef] [PubMed]
35. Dziedzic, A.; Issa, J.; Hussain, S.; Tanasiewicz, M.; Wojtyczka, R.; Kubina, R.; Konwinska, M.D.; Riad, A. COVID-19 Vaccine Booster Hesitancy (VBH) of Healthcare Professionals and Students in Poland: Cross-Sectional Survey-Based Study. *Front. Public Health* **2022**, *10*, 938067. [CrossRef] [PubMed]
36. Ellithorpe, M.E.; Aladé, F.; Adams, R.B.; Nowak, G.J. Looking Ahead: Caregivers' COVID-19 Vaccination Intention for Children 5 Years Old and Younger Using the Health Belief Model. *Vaccine* **2022**, *40*, 1404–1412. [CrossRef]
37. Enea, V.; Eisenbeck, N.; Carreno, D.F.; Douglas, K.M.; Sutton, R.M.; Agostini, M.; Bélanger, J.J.; Gützkow, B.; Kreienkamp, J.; Abakoumkin, G.; et al. Intentions to Be Vaccinated Against COVID-19: The Role of Prosociality and Conspiracy Beliefs across 20 Countries. *Health Commun.* **2022**, 1–10. [CrossRef]
38. Getachew, T.; Lami, M.; Eyeberu, A.; Balis, B.; Debella, A.; Eshetu, B.; Degefa, M.; Mesfin, S.; Negash, A.; Bekele, H.; et al. Acceptance of COVID-19 Vaccine and Associated Factors among Health Care Workers at Public Hospitals in Eastern Ethiopia Using the Health Belief Model. *Front. Public Health* **2022**, *10*, 957721. [CrossRef]
39. Getachew, T.; Negash, A.; Degefa, M.; Lami, M.; Balis, B.; Debela, A.; Gemechu, K.; Shiferaw, K.; Nigussie, K.; Bekele, H.; et al. COVID-19 Vaccine Acceptance and Associated Factors among Adult Clients at Public Hospitals in Eastern Ethiopia Using the Health Belief Model: Multicentre Cross-Sectional Study. *BMJ Open* **2023**, *13*, e070551. [CrossRef]
40. Ghazy, R.M.; Abdou, M.S.; Awaidy, S.; Sallam, M.; Elbarazi, I.; Youssef, N.; Fiidow, O.A.; Mehdad, S.; Hussein, M.F.; Adam, M.F.; et al. Acceptance of COVID-19 Vaccine Booster Doses Using the Health Belief Model: A Cross-Sectional Study in Low-Middle- and High-Income Countries of the East Mediterranean Region. *Int. J. Environ. Res. Public Health* **2022**, *19*, 12136. [CrossRef]
41. Goffe, L.; Antonopoulou, V.; Meyer, C.J.; Graham, F.; Tang, M.Y.; Lecouturier, J.; Grimani, A.; Bambra, C.; Kelly, M.P.; Sniehotta, F.F. Factors Associated with Vaccine Intention in Adults Living in England Who Either Did Not Want or Had Not yet Decided to Be Vaccinated against COVID-19. *Hum. Vaccines Immunother.* **2021**, *17*, 5242–5254. [CrossRef]
42. Goruntla, N.; Chintamani, S.; Bhanu, P.; Samyuktha, S.; Veerabhadrappa, K.; Bhupalam, P.; Ramaiah, J. Predictors of Acceptance and Willingness to Pay for the COVID-19 Vaccine in the General Public of India: A Health Belief Model Approach. *Asian Pac. J. Trop. Med.* **2021**, *14*, 165. [CrossRef]
43. Guidry, J.P.D.; Laestadius, L.I.; Vraga, E.K.; Miller, C.A.; Perrin, P.B.; Burton, C.W.; Ryan, M.; Fuemmeler, B.F.; Carlyle, K.E. Willingness to Get the COVID-19 Vaccine with and without Emergency Use Authorization. *Am. J. Infect. Control* **2021**, *49*, 137–142. [CrossRef]
44. Guidry, J.P.D.; Miller, C.A.; Perrin, P.B.; Laestadius, L.I.; Zurlo, G.; Savage, M.W.; Stevens, M.; Fuemmeler, B.F.; Burton, C.W.; Gültzow, T.; et al. Between Healthcare Practitioners and Clergy: Evangelicals and COVID-19 Vaccine Hesitancy. *Int. J. Environ. Res. Public Health* **2022**, *19*, 11120. [CrossRef] [PubMed]
45. Guillon, M.; Kergall, P. Factors Associated with COVID-19 Vaccination Intentions and Attitudes in France. *Public Health* **2021**, *198*, 200–207. [CrossRef] [PubMed]
46. Handebo, S.; Wolde, M.; Shitu, K.; Kassie, A. Determinant of Intention to Receive COVID-19 Vaccine among School Teachers in Gondar City, Northwest Ethiopia. *PLoS ONE* **2021**, *16*, e0253499. [CrossRef] [PubMed]
47. Hawlader, M.D.H.; Rahman, M.L.; Nazir, A.; Ara, T.; Haque, M.M.A.; Saha, S.; Barsha, S.Y.; Hossian, M.; Matin, K.F.; Siddiquea, S.R.; et al. COVID-19 Vaccine Acceptance in South Asia: A Multi-Country Study. *Int. J. Infect. Dis.* **2022**, *114*, 1–10. [CrossRef]
48. Hossian, M.; Khan, M.A.S.; Nazir, A.; Nabi, M.H.; Hasan, M.; Maliha, R.; Hossain, M.A.; Rashid, M.U.; Itrat, N.; Hawlader, M.D.H. Factors Affecting Intention to Take COVID-19 Vaccine among Pakistani University Students. *PLoS ONE* **2022**, *17*, e0262305. [CrossRef]
49. Hu, D.; Liu, Z.; Gong, L.; Kong, Y.; Liu, H.; Wei, C.; Wu, X.; Zhu, Q.; Guo, Y. Exploring the Willingness of the COVID-19 Vaccine Booster Shots in China Using the Health Belief Model: Web-Based Online Cross-Sectional Study. *Vaccines* **2022**, *10*, 1336. [CrossRef]
50. Huang, C.; Yan, D.; Liang, S. The Relationship between Information Dissemination Channels, Health Belief, and COVID-19 Vaccination Intention: Evidence from China. *J. Environ. Public Health* **2023**, *2023*, 6915125. [CrossRef]
51. Huynh, G.; Tran, T.; Nguyen, H.N.; Pham, L. COVID-19 Vaccination Intention among Healthcare Workers in Vietnam. *Asian Pac. J. Trop. Med.* **2021**, *14*, 159. [CrossRef]

52. Iacob, C.I.; Ionescu, D.; Avram, E.; Cojocaru, D. COVID-19 Pandemic Worry and Vaccination Intention: The Mediating Role of the Health Belief Model Components. *Front. Psychol.* **2021**, *12*, 674018. [CrossRef] [PubMed]
53. Jahanshahi-Amjazi, R.; Rezaeian, M.; Abdolkarimi, M.; Nasirzadeh, M. Predictors of the Intention to Receive the COVID 19 Vaccine by Iranians 18–70 Year Old: Application of Health Belief Model. *J. Edu. Health Promot.* **2022**, *11*, 175. [CrossRef]
54. Jiang, T.; Zhou, X.; Wang, H.; Dong, S.; Wang, M.; Akezhuoli, H.; Zhu, H. COVID-19 Vaccination Intention and Influencing Factors among Different Occupational Risk Groups: A Cross-Sectional Study. *Hum. Vaccines Immunother.* **2021**, *17*, 3433–3440. [CrossRef] [PubMed]
55. Jin, Q.; Raza, S.H.; Yousaf, M.; Zaman, U.; Siang, J.M.L.D. Can Communication Strategies Combat COVID-19 Vaccine Hesitancy with Trade-Off between Public Service Messages and Public Skepticism? Experimental Evidence from Pakistan. *Vaccines* **2021**, *9*, 757. [CrossRef]
56. Kasting, M.L.; Macy, J.T.; Grannis, S.J.; Wiensch, A.J.; Lavista Ferres, J.M.; Dixon, B.E. Factors Associated With the Intention to Receive the COVID-19 Vaccine: Cross-Sectional National Study. *JMIR Public Health Surveill.* **2022**, *8*, e37203. [CrossRef]
57. Khalafalla, H.E.; Tumambeng, M.Z.; Halawi, M.H.A.; Masmali, E.M.A.; Tashari, T.B.M.; Arishi, F.H.A.; Shadad, R.H.M.; Alfaraj, S.Z.A.; Fathi, S.M.A.; Mahfouz, M.S. COVID-19 Vaccine Hesitancy Prevalence and Predictors among the Students of Jazan University, Saudi Arabia Using the Health Belief Model: A Cross-Sectional Study. *Vaccines* **2022**, *10*, 289. [CrossRef]
58. Kabir, R.; Mahmud, I.; Chowdhury, M.T.H.; Vinnakota, D.; Jahan, S.S.; Siddika, N.; Isha, S.N.; Nath, S.K.; Hoque Apu, E. COVID-19 Vaccination Intent and Willingness to Pay in Bangladesh: A Cross-Sectional Study. *Vaccines* **2021**, *9*, 416. [CrossRef]
59. Lai, X.; Zhu, H.; Wang, J.; Huang, Y.; Jing, R.; Lyu, Y.; Zhang, H.; Feng, H.; Guo, J.; Fang, H. Public Perceptions and Acceptance of COVID-19 Booster Vaccination in China: A Cross-Sectional Study. *Vaccines* **2021**, *9*, 1461. [CrossRef]
60. Le An, P.; Nguyen, H.T.N.; Nguyen, D.D.; Vo, L.Y.; Huynh, G. The Intention to Get a COVID-19 Vaccine among the Students of Health Science in Vietnam. *Hum. Vaccines Immunother.* **2021**, *17*, 4823–4828. [CrossRef]
61. Le, C.N.; Nguyen, U.T.T.; Do, D.T.H. Predictors of COVID-19 vaccine acceptability among health professions students in Vietnam. *BMC Public Health* **2022**, *22*, 854. [CrossRef]
62. Lee, L.Y.; Chu, K.; Chan, M.H.; Wong, C.T.; Leung, H.P.; Chan, I.C.; Ng, C.K.; Wong, R.Y.; Pun, A.L.; Ng, Y.H.; et al. Living in a Region With a Low Level of COVID-19 Infection: Health Belief Toward COVID-19 Vaccination and Intention to Receive a COVID-19 Vaccine in Hong Kong Individuals. *INQUIRY* **2022**, *59*, 004695802210827. [CrossRef]
63. Li, J.-B.; Lau, E.Y.H.; Chan, D.K.C. Why Do Hong Kong Parents Have Low Intention to Vaccinate Their Children against COVID-19? Testing Health Belief Model and Theory of Planned Behavior in a Large-Scale Survey. *Vaccine* **2022**, *40*, 2772–2780. [CrossRef]
64. Li, G.; Zhong, Y.; Htet, H.; Luo, Y.; Xie, X.; Wichaidit, W. COVID-19 Vaccine Acceptance and Associated Factors among Unvaccinated Workers at a Tertiary Hospital in Southern Thailand. *Health Serv. Res. Manag. Epidemiol.* **2022**, *9*, 233339282210830. [CrossRef]
65. Liao, Q.; Cowling, B.J.; Xiao, J.; Yuan, J.; Dong, M.; Ni, M.Y.; Fielding, R.; Lam, W.W.T. Priming with social benefit information of vaccination to increase acceptance of COVID-19 vaccines. *Vaccine* **2022**, *40*, 1074–1081. [CrossRef] [PubMed]
66. Lin, Y.; Hu, Z.; Zhao, Q.; Alias, H.; Danaee, M.; Wong, L.P. Understanding COVID-19 Vaccine Demand and Hesitancy: A Nationwide Online Survey in China. *PLoS Negl. Trop. Dis.* **2020**, *14*, e0008961. [CrossRef]
67. Liu, R.; Huang, Y.-H.C.; Sun, J.; Lau, J.; Cai, Q. A Shot in the Arm for Vaccination Intention: The Media and the Health Belief Model in Three Chinese Societies. *Int. J. Environ. Res. Public Health* **2022**, *19*, 3705. [CrossRef]
68. López-Cepero, A.; Cameron, S.; Negrón, L.E.; Colón-López, V.; Colón-Ramos, U.; Mattei, J.; Fernández-Repollet, E.; Pérez, C.M. Uncertainty and Unwillingness to Receive a COVID-19 Vaccine in Adults Residing in Puerto Rico: Assessment of Perceptions, Attitudes, and Behaviors. *Hum. Vaccines Immunother.* **2021**, *17*, 3441–3449. [CrossRef]
69. Lyons, N.; Bhagwandeen, B.; Edwards, J. Factors Affecting COVID-19 Vaccination Intentions among Patients Attending a Large HIV Treatment Clinic in Trinidad Using Constructs of the Health Belief Model. *Vaccines* **2022**, *11*, 4. [CrossRef]
70. Mahmud, I.; Kabir, R.; Rahman, M.A.; Alradie-Mohamed, A.; Vinnakota, D.; Al-Mohaimeed, A. The Health Belief Model Predicts Intention to Receive the COVID-19 Vaccine in Saudi Arabia: Results from a Cross-Sectional Survey. *Vaccines* **2021**, *9*, 864. [CrossRef] [PubMed]
71. Mahmud, I.; Al Imam, M.H.; Vinnakota, D.; Kheirallah, K.A.; Jaber, M.F.; Abalkhail, A.; Alasqah, I.; Alslamah, T.; Kabir, R. Vaccination Intention against COVID-19 among the Unvaccinated in Jordan during the Early Phase of the Vaccination Drive: A Cross-Sectional Survey. *Vaccines* **2022**, *10*, 1159. [CrossRef] [PubMed]
72. Maria, S.; Pelupessy, D.C.; Koesnoe, S.; Yunihastuti, E.; Handayani, D.O.T.L.; Siddiq, T.H.; Mulyantini, A.; Halim, A.R.V.; Wahyuningsih, E.S.; Widhani, A.; et al. COVID-19 Booster Vaccine Intention by Health Care Workers in Jakarta, Indonesia: Using the Extended Model of Health Behavior Theories. *Trop. Med.* **2022**, *7*, 323. [CrossRef]
73. Mercadante, A.R.; Law, A.V. Will they, or Won't they? Examining patients' vaccine intention for flu and COVID-19 using the Health Belief Model. *Res. Soc. Adm. Pharm.* **2021**, *17*, 1596–1605. [CrossRef] [PubMed]
74. Miyachi, T.; Sugano, Y.; Tanaka, S.; Hirayama, J.; Yamamoto, F.; Nomura, K. COVID-19 Vaccine Intention and Knowledge, Literacy, and Health Beliefs among Japanese University Students. *Vaccines* **2022**, *10*, 893. [CrossRef]
75. Mohammed, A.H.; Hassan, B.A.R.; Wayyes, A.M.; Gadhban, A.Q.; Blebil, A.; Alhija, S.A.; Darwish, R.M.; Al-Zaabi, A.T.; Othman, G.; Jaber, A.A.S.; et al. Parental Health Beliefs, Intention, and Strategies about COVID-19 Vaccine for Their Children: A Cross-Sectional Analysis from Five Arab Countries in the Middle East. *Vaccine* **2022**, *40*, 6549–6557. [CrossRef]

76. Morar, C.; Tiba, A.; Jovanovic, T.; Valjarević, A.; Ripp, M.; Vujičić, M.D.; Stankov, U.; Basarin, B.; Ratković, R.; Popović, M.; et al. Supporting Tourism by Assessing the Predictors of COVID-19 Vaccination for Travel Reasons. *Int. J. Environ. Res. Public Health* **2022**, *19*, 918. [CrossRef]
77. Nguyen, V.T.; Nguyen, M.Q.; Le, N.T.; Nguyen, T.N.H.; Huynh, G. Predictors of Intention to Get a COVID-19 Vaccine of Health Science Students: A Cross-Sectional Study. *RMHP* **2021**, *14*, 4023–4030. [CrossRef]
78. Okai, G.A.; Abekah-Nkrumah, G. The Level and Determinants of COVID-19 Vaccine Acceptance in Ghana. *PLoS ONE* **2022**, *17*, e0270768. [CrossRef]
79. Okmi, E.A.; Almohammadi, E.; Alaamri, O.; Alfawaz, R.; Alomari, N.; Saleh, M.; Alsuwailem, S.; Moafa, N.J. Determinants of COVID-19 Vaccine Acceptance Among the General Adult Population in Saudi Arabia Based on the Health Belief Model: A Web-Based Cross-Sectional Study. *Cureus* **2022**, *14*, 28326. [CrossRef] [PubMed]
80. Okuyan, B.; Bektay, M.Y.; Demirci, M.Y.; Ay, P.; Sancar, M. Factors Associated with Turkish Pharmacists' Intention to Receive COVID-19 Vaccine: An Observational Study. *Int. J. Clin. Pharm.* **2022**, *44*, 247–255. [CrossRef] [PubMed]
81. Otiti-Sengeri, J.; Andrew, O.B.; Lusobya, R.C.; Atukunda, I.; Nalukenge, C.; Kalinaki, A.; Mukisa, J.; Nakanjako, D.; Colebunders, R. High COVID-19 Vaccine Acceptance among Eye Healthcare Workers in Uganda. *Vaccines* **2022**, *10*, 609. [CrossRef]
82. Patwary, M.M.; Bardhan, M.; Disha, A.S.; Hasan, M.; Haque, M.Z.; Sultana, R.; Hossain, M.R.; Browning, M.H.E.M.; Alam, M.A.; Sallam, M. Determinants of COVID-19 Vaccine Acceptance among the Adult Population of Bangladesh Using the Health Belief Model and the Theory of Planned Behavior Model. *Vaccines* **2021**, *9*, 1393. [CrossRef]
83. Qin, C.; Yan, W.; Du, M.; Liu, Q.; Tao, L.; Liu, M.; Liu, J. Acceptance of the COVID-19 Vaccine Booster Dose and Associated Factors among the Elderly in China Based on the Health Belief Model (HBM): A National Cross-Sectional Study. *Front. Public Health* **2022**, *10*, 986916. [CrossRef] [PubMed]
84. Qin, C.; Wang, R.; Tao, L.; Liu, M.; Liu, J. Acceptance of a Third Dose of COVID-19 Vaccine and Associated Factors in China Based on Health Belief Model: A National Cross-Sectional Study. *Vaccines* **2022**, *10*, 89. [CrossRef] [PubMed]
85. Qin, C.; Wang, R.; Tao, L.; Liu, M.; Liu, J. Association Between Risk Perception and Acceptance for a Booster Dose of COVID-19 Vaccine to Children Among Child Caregivers in China. *Front. Public Health* **2022**, *10*, 834572. [CrossRef]
86. Qin, C.; Du, M.; Wang, Y.; Liu, Q.; Yan, W.; Tao, L.; Liu, M.; Liu, J. Assessing acceptability of the fourth dose against COVID-19 among Chinese adults: A population-based survey. *Hum. Vaccines Immunother.* **2023**, *19*, 2186108. [CrossRef] [PubMed]
87. Quinto, J.C.D.; Balderrama, A.N.C.; Hocson, F.N.Z.; Salanguit, M.B.; Palatino, M.C.; Gregorio, E.R., Jr. Association of knowledge and risk perceptions of Manila City school teachers with COVID-19 vaccine acceptance. *Philipp. J. Health Res. Dev.* **2022**, *25*, 8–18.
88. Rabin, C.; Dutra, S. Predicting Engagement in Behaviors to Reduce the Spread of COVID-19: The Roles of the Health Belief Model and Political Party Affiliation. *Psychol. Health Med.* **2022**, *27*, 379–388. [CrossRef] [PubMed]
89. Reindl, D.; Catma, S. A Pre-Vaccine Analysis Using the Health Belief Model to Explain Parents' Willingness to Vaccinate (WTV) Their Children in the United States: Implications for Vaccination Programs. *Expert Rev. Pharm. Outcomes Res.* **2022**, *22*, 753–761. [CrossRef]
90. Reiter, P.L.; Pennell, M.L.; Katz, M.L. Acceptability of a COVID-19 vaccine among adults in the United States: How many people would get vaccinated? *Vaccine* **2020**, *38*, 6500–6507. [CrossRef]
91. Rosental, H.; Shmueli, L. Integrating Health Behavior Theories to Predict COVID-19 Vaccine Acceptance: Differences between Medical Students and Nursing Students. *Vaccines* **2021**, *9*, 783. [CrossRef]
92. Rountree, C.; Prentice, G. Segmentation of Intentions towards COVID-19 Vaccine Acceptance through Political and Health Behaviour Explanatory Models. *Ir. J. Med. Sci.* **2022**, *191*, 2369–2383. [CrossRef]
93. Seangpraw, K.; Pothisa, T.; Boonyathee, S.; Ong-Artborirak, P.; Tonchoy, P.; Kantow, S.; Auttama, N.; Choowanthanapakorn, M. Using the Health Belief Model to Predict Vaccination Intention Among COVID-19 Unvaccinated People in Thai Communities. *Front. Med.* **2022**, *9*, 890503. [CrossRef] [PubMed]
94. Seboka, B.T.; Yehualashet, D.E.; Belay, M.M.; Kabthymer, R.H.; Ali, H.; Hailegebreal, S.; Demeke, A.D.; Amede, E.S.; Tesfa, G.A. Factors influencing COVID-19 vaccination demand and intent in resource-limited settings: Based on health belief model. *Risk Manag. Healthc. Policy* **2021**, *14*, 2743–2756. [CrossRef] [PubMed]
95. Shah, S.; Gui, H.; Chua, P.E.Y.; Tan, J.-Y.; Suen, L.K.; Chan, S.W.; Pang, J. Factors Associated with COVID-19 Vaccination Intent in Singapore, Australia and Hong Kong. *Vaccine* **2022**, *40*, 2949–2959. [CrossRef] [PubMed]
96. Shmueli, L. Predicting Intention to Receive COVID-19 Vaccine among the General Population Using the Health Belief Model and the Theory of Planned Behavior Model. *BMC Public Health* **2021**, *21*, 804. [CrossRef]
97. Shmueli, L. The Role of Incentives in Deciding to Receive the Available COVID-19 Vaccine in Israel. *Vaccines* **2022**, *10*, 77. [CrossRef]
98. Short, M.B.; Marek, R.J.; Knight, C.F.; Kusters, I.S. Understanding factors associated with intent to receive the COVID-19 vaccine. *Fam. Syst. Health* **2022**, *40*, 160. [CrossRef]
99. Sieverding, M.; Zintel, S.; Schmidt, L.; Arbogast, A.L.; von Wagner, C. Explaining the Intention to Get Vaccinated against COVID-19: General Attitudes towards Vaccination and Predictors from Health Behavior Theories. *Psychol. Health Med.* **2023**, *28*, 161–170. [CrossRef]
100. Spinewine, A.; Pétein, C.; Evrard, P.; Vastrade, C.; Laurent, C.; Delaere, B.; Henrard, S. Attitudes towards COVID-19 Vaccination among Hospital Staff—Understanding What Matters to Hesitant People. *Vaccines* **2021**, *9*, 469. [CrossRef]

101. Ştefănuţ, A.M.; Vintilă, M.; Tomiţă, M.; Treglia, E.; Lungu, M.A.; Tomassoni, R. The Influence of Health Beliefs, of Resources, of Vaccination History, and of Health Anxiety on Intention to Accept COVID-19 Vaccination. *Front. Psychol.* **2021**, *12*, 729803. [CrossRef]
102. Su, L.; Du, J.; Du, Z. Government Communication, Perceptions of COVID-19, and Vaccination Intention: A Multi-Group Comparison in China. *Front. Psychol.* **2022**, *12*, 783374. [CrossRef]
103. Suess, C.; Maddock, J.E.; Dogru, T.; Mody, M.; Lee, S. Using the Health Belief Model to Examine Travelers' Willingness to Vaccinate and Support for Vaccination Requirements Prior to Travel. *Tour. Manag.* **2022**, *88*, 104405. [CrossRef]
104. Tran, V.D.; Pak, T.V.; Gribkova, E.I.; Galkina, G.A.; Loskutova, E.E.; Dorofeeva, V.V.; Dewey, R.S.; Nguyen, K.T.; Pham, D.T. Determinants of COVID-19 Vaccine Acceptance in a High Infection-Rate Country: A Cross-Sectional Study in Russia. *Pharm. Pract.* **2021**, *19*, 2276. [CrossRef] [PubMed]
105. Ung, C.O.L.; Hu, Y.; Hu, H.; Bian, Y. Investigating the Intention to Receive the COVID-19 Vaccination in Macao: Implications for Vaccination Strategies. *BMC Infect. Dis.* **2022**, *22*, 218. [CrossRef] [PubMed]
106. Vatcharavongvan, P.; Boonyanitchayakul, N.; Khampachuea, P.; Sinturong, I.; Prasert, V. Health Belief Model and Parents' Acceptance of the Pfizer-BioNTech and Sinopharm COVID-19 Vaccine for Children Aged 5–18 Years Old: A National Survey. *Vaccine* **2023**, *41*, 1480–1489. [CrossRef]
107. Wagner, A.L.; Wileden, L.; Shanks, T.R.; Goold, S.D.; Morenoff, J.D.; Sheinfeld Gorin, S.N. Mediators of Racial Differences in COVID-19 Vaccine Acceptance and Uptake: A Cohort Study in Detroit, MI. *Vaccines* **2021**, *10*, 36. [CrossRef]
108. Walker, A.N.; Zhang, T.; Peng, X.-Q.; Ge, J.-J.; Gu, H.; You, H. Vaccine Acceptance and Its Influencing Factors: An Online Cross-Sectional Study among International College Students Studying in China. *Vaccines* **2021**, *9*, 585. [CrossRef]
109. Wang, X. Putting Emotions in the Health Belief Model: The Role of Hope and Anticipated Guilt on the Chinese's Intentions to Get COVID-19 Vaccination. *Health Commun.* **2022**, 1–10. [CrossRef]
110. Wang, H.; Zhou, X.; Jiang, T.; Wang, X.; Lu, J.; Li, J. Factors Influencing COVID-19 Vaccination Intention among Overseas and Domestic Chinese University Students: A Cross-Sectional Survey. *Hum. Vaccines Immunother.* **2021**, *17*, 4829–4837. [CrossRef]
111. Wijesinghe, M.S.D.; Weerasinghe, W.M.P.C.; Gunawardana, I.; Perera, S.N.S.; Karunapema, R.P.P. Acceptance of COVID-19 Vaccine in Sri Lanka: Applying the Health Belief Model to an Online Survey. *Asia Pac. J. Public Health* **2021**, *33*, 598–602. [CrossRef]
112. Wirawan, G.B.S.; Harjana, N.P.A.; Nugrahani, N.W.; Januraga, P.P. Health Beliefs and Socioeconomic Determinants of COVID-19 Booster Vaccine Acceptance: An Indonesian Cross-Sectional Study. *Vaccines* **2022**, *10*, 724. [CrossRef]
113. Wong, L.P.; Alias, H.; Wong, P.-F.; Lee, H.Y.; AbuBakar, S. The Use of the Health Belief Model to Assess Predictors of Intent to Receive the COVID-19 Vaccine and Willingness to Pay. *Hum. Vaccines Immunother.* **2020**, *16*, 2204–2214. [CrossRef]
114. Xiao, Q.; Liu, X.; Wang, R.; Mao, Y.; Chen, H.; Li, X.; Liu, X.; Dai, J.; Gao, J.; Fu, H.; et al. Predictors of Willingness to Receive the COVID-19 Vaccine after Emergency Use Authorization: The Role of Coping Appraisal. *Vaccines* **2021**, *9*, 967. [CrossRef] [PubMed]
115. Yan, E.; Lai, D.W.L.; Lee, V.W.P. Predictors of Intention to Vaccinate against COVID-19 in the General Public in Hong Kong: Findings from a Population-Based, Cross-Sectional Survey. *Vaccines* **2021**, *9*, 696. [CrossRef]
116. Yang, X.; Wei, L.; Liu, Z. Promoting COVID-19 Vaccination Using the Health Belief Model: Does Information Acquisition from Divergent Sources Make a Difference? *Int. J. Environ. Res. Public Health* **2022**, *19*, 3887. [CrossRef] [PubMed]
117. Youssef, D.; Abou-Abbas, L.; Berry, A.; Youssef, J.; Hassan, H. Determinants of acceptance of Coronavirus disease-2019 (COVID-19) vaccine among Lebanese health care workers using health belief model. *PLoS ONE* **2022**, *17*, e0264128. [CrossRef]
118. Yu, Y.; Ling, R.H.Y.; Ip, T.K.M.; Luo, S.; Lau, J.T.F. Factors of COVID-19 Vaccination among Hong Kong Chinese Men Who Have Sex with Men during Months 5–8 since the Vaccine Rollout—General Factors and Factors Specific to This Population. *Vaccines* **2022**, *10*, 1763. [CrossRef] [PubMed]
119. Zakeri, M.; Li, J.; Sadeghi, S.D.; Essien, E.J.; Sansgiry, S.S. Strategies to Decrease COVID-19 Vaccine Hesitancy for Children. *J. Pharm. Health Serv. Res.* **2021**, *12*, 539–544. [CrossRef]
120. Zampetakis, L.A.; Melas, C. The Health Belief Model Predicts Vaccination Intentions against COVID-19: A Survey Experiment Approach. *Appl. Psychol. Health Well* **2021**, *13*, 469–484. [CrossRef]
121. Zhang, R.; Yan, J.; Jia, H.; Luo, X.; Liu, Q.; Lin, J. Policy Endorsement and Booster Shot: Exploring Politicized Determinants for Acceptance of a Third Dose of COVID-19 Vaccine in China. *Vaccines* **2023**, *11*, 421. [CrossRef]
122. Zhelyazkova, A.; Kim, S.; Klein, M.; Prueckner, S.; Horster, S.; Kressirer, P.; Choukér, A.; Coenen, M.; Adorjan, K. COVID-19 Vaccination Intent, Barriers and Facilitators in Healthcare Workers: Insights from a Cross-Sectional Study on 2500 Employees at LMU University Hospital in Munich, Germany. *Vaccines* **2022**, *10*, 1231. [CrossRef] [PubMed]
123. Brewer, N.T.; Chapman, G.B.; Gibbons, F.X.; Gerrard, M.; McCaul, K.D.; Weinstein, N. D Meta-analysis of the relationship between risk perception and health behavior: The example of vaccination. *Health Psychol.* **2007**, *26*, 136–145. [CrossRef] [PubMed]
124. Tsutsui, Y.; Benzion, U.; Shahrabani, S. Economic and behavioral factors in an individual's decision to take the influenza vaccination in Japan. *J. Socio Econ.* **2012**, *4*, 594–602. [CrossRef]
125. Shahrabani, S.; Benzion, U. Workplace vaccination and other factors impacting influenza vaccination decision among employees in Israel. *Int. J. Environ. Res. Public Health* **2010**, *7*, 853–869. [CrossRef] [PubMed]
126. Griva, K.; Tan, K.Y.K.; Chan, F.H.F.; Periakaruppan, R.; Ong, B.W.L.; Soh, A.S.E.; Chen, M.I. Evaluating Rates and Determinants of COVID-19 Vaccine Hesitancy for Adults and Children in the Singapore Population: Strengthening Our Community's Resilience against Threats from Emerging Infections (SOCRATEs) Cohort. *Vaccines* **2021**, *9*, 1415. [CrossRef]

127. Limbu, Y.B.; Gautam, R.K.; Zhou, W. Predicting Vaccination Intention against COVID-19 Using Theory of Planned Behavior: A Systematic Review and Meta-Analysis. *Vaccines* **2022**, *10*, 2026. [CrossRef]
128. Limbu, Y.B.; Huhmann, B.A. Why Some People Are Hesitant to Receive COVID-19 Boosters: A Systematic Review. *Trop. Med. Infect. Dis.* **2023**, *8*, 159. [CrossRef]

vaccines

Review

Manufacturing and Financial Evaluation of Peptide-Based Neoantigen Cancer Vaccines for Triple-Negative Breast Cancer in the United Kingdom: Opportunities and Challenges

Adriana Novakova, Stephen A. Morris, Ludovica Vaiarelli * and Stefanie Frank *

Department of Biochemical Engineering, University College London, Bernard Katz Building, Gower Street, London WC1E 6BT, UK; adriana.novakova.20@alumni.ucl.ac.uk (A.N.); stephen.morris@ucl.ac.uk (S.A.M.)
* Correspondence: ludovica.vaiarelli.18@ucl.ac.uk (L.V.); stefanie.frank@ucl.ac.uk (S.F.)

Abstract: This review evaluates the financial burden of current treatments for triple-negative breast cancer (TNBC) and projects potential financial scenarios to assess the feasibility of introducing a peptide-based neoantigen cancer vaccine (NCV) targeting the disease, using the UK as a healthcare system model. TNBC, the most aggressive breast cancer subtype, is associated with poor prognosis, worsened by the lack of personalised treatment options. Neoantigen cancer vaccine therapies present a personalised alternative with the potential to enhance T-cell responses independently of genetic factors, unlike approved immunotherapies for TNBC. Through a systematic literature review, the underlying science and manufacturing processes of NCVs are explored, the direct medical costs of existing TNBC treatments are enumerated, and two contrasting pricing scenarios for NCV clinical adoption are evaluated. The findings indicate that limited immunogenicity is the main scientific barrier to NCV clinical advancement, alongside production inefficiencies. Financial analysis shows that the UK spends approximately GBP 230 million annually on TNBC treatments, ranging from GBP 2200 to GBP 54,000 per patient. A best-case pricing model involving government-sponsored NCV therapy appears financially viable, while a worst-case, privately funded model exceeds the National Institute for Health and Care Excellence (NICE) cost thresholds. This study concludes that while NCVs show potential clinical benefits for TNBC, uncertainties about their standalone efficacy make their widespread adoption in the UK unlikely without further clinical research.

Keywords: neoantigen cancer vaccine; triple-negative breast cancer; cancer vaccine manufacturing; cost analysis; pricing strategy

1. Introduction

Breast cancer represents the most commonly diagnosed cancer in the UK, with an annual incidence of 60,000 cases [1]. The disease is classified into four immunohistochemical subtypes based on receptor expression on the tumour surface. Among these, two express oestrogen and progesterone receptors, while the third subtype expresses human epidermal growth factor receptor 2 (HER2). In contrast, triple-negative breast cancer (TNBC), lacking the expression of hormone receptors, accounts for 15% of breast cancer cases and is known for its aggressive nature, resulting in a poorer prognosis [2]. Specifically, only 10% of metastatic TNBC patients survive beyond 5 years, compared to 30% in other metastatic breast cancer subtypes [3]. Furthermore, TNBC patients are twice as likely to develop metastases compared to non-TNBC subtypes [4]. Limited treatment options contribute to the dismal prognosis, with chemotherapy as the sole standardised approach. However,

https://doi.org/10.3390/vaccines13020144

TNBC exhibits high immunogenicity, making it amenable to cancer immunotherapy strategies [5,6]. Despite the established role of immunotherapy in oncology, the development of TNBC-specific agents, like immune checkpoint inhibitors (ICIs), has been constrained by the complex and heterogeneous nature of TNBC tumours [7]. Consequently, attention has shifted to alternative immunotherapies, notably therapeutic cancer vaccines, aimed at augmenting tumour-specific immune responses [8]. Unlike conventional vaccines that establish prophylactic immune memory by administering pathogenic antigens, cancer vaccines seek to enhance the immune response against pre-existing tumour antigens within the body [9].

Several outcomes are needed to enable the successful rollout of new clinical interventions. The primary is an indication of clinical effectiveness by a clinical trial. But, it is also important to evaluate cost effectiveness and affordability to healthcare systems. The study of these aspects in parallel will help to enable a rapid rollout of clinically effective interventions.

As no personalised neoantigen cancer vaccine has been commercialised to date, this review offers a comprehensive outlook on the prospects and hurdles associated with the therapy.

The principal aim of this review is to analyse the physiological properties and the proposed manufacturing process of a peptide-based neoantigen cancer vaccine (NCV) for TNBC, identify the direct medical costs of TNBC treatments, and project two NCV pricing schemes using the UK as a model healthcare system. Our analysis shows that the potential clinical adoption of an NCV for TNBC is highly contingent upon the successful identification of key neoantigens and the definitive pricing model brought forward. We propose a multi-neoantigen setting with a TLR agonist that ought to be investigated for TNBC. Combination therapies may result in an opportunity to lower the current high TNBC therapy costs by leveraging the positive financial impact that an NCV could bring by enhancing clinical outcomes under such a therapeutic framework.

2. Immunotherapy Indication for Triple-Negative Breast Cancer

TNBC represents a group of heterogeneous tumours and currently lacks specialised treatment options, with chemotherapy representing the standard of care despite several limitations. It was reported that over 27% of breast cancer patients undergoing chemotherapy experience life-threatening adverse events, like severe diarrhoea and shortness of breath [1]. Moreover, TNBC patients frequently develop chemotherapy resistance, underscoring the critical need for novel therapeutic interventions. Prognostic outcomes for TNBC are mainly influenced by breast cancer stage (Table 1). Chemotherapy has been shown to be effective for TNBC in stages I and II, but stage III patients had an average survival time of 40 months, while metastatic patients had only 13 months [10,11] (for cancer stage overview, refer to Table 1). Pogoda et al. [12] observed a 35% recurrence rate within six years among metastatic TNBC patients initially diagnosed in stages II and III. These findings underscore the limited efficacy of chemotherapy in managing TNBC and emphasise the pressing need for targeted, personalised therapeutic strategies over generalised approaches.

Immunotherapy offers promise in customising TNBC therapies, particularly in relation to the distinct features of the tumour microenvironment. Compared to other breast cancer subtypes, TNBC exhibits higher levels of tumour-infiltrating lymphocytes (TILs), programmed cell death-ligand 1 (PD-L1) expression, and increased tumour mutational burden (TMB) [13] (refer to Figure 1).

Table 1. Biological definition of breast cancer stages. The prognosis of breast cancer is influenced by its stage, with advancing stages correlating with poorer outcomes. Created from Srimuninnimit et al. [11] and Pogoda et al. [12].

Stage 0	Stage I	Stage II	Stage III	Stage IV
No tumour cells spread outside the tumour	Localised tumour with some cells escaping the tumour	Lymph nodes affected	Lymph nodes, muscles, and skin affected	Tumour cells have spread to any part of the body

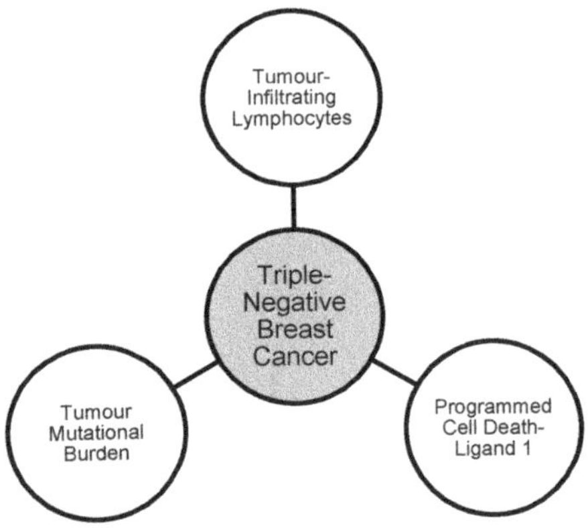

Figure 1. Implications for immunotherapy in TNBC treatment. These three TNBC features (white circles) allow for cancer immunotherapy agents.

Studies have demonstrated a strong association between higher levels of TILs and reduced metastasis [6,14,15], with low TIL levels correlating with higher relapse rates in stage I and II TNBC patients [15]. PD-L1, a protein overexpressed on cells that binds to programmed death protein 1 (PD-1) on immune cells, plays a crucial role in stimulating immune responses. High PD-L1 expression is strongly correlated with improved survival rates in TNBC patients, with TNBC exhibiting the highest PD-L1 expression among all breast cancer subtypes [13,16,17]. Additionally, TNBC's TMB, reflecting the number of antigens presented to immune cells, further drives the exploration of immunotherapy applications. Numerous studies have demonstrated that TNBC cases with high TMB derive greater benefits from immunotherapy [18,19]. The described features of the TNBC tumour microenvironment highlight the significance of immunotherapy in tailoring TNBC therapy options.

Presently, approved immunotherapy agents for TNBC include immune checkpoint inhibitors (ICIs), atezolizumab, and pembrolizumab. For a comprehensive review of ICI therapy for TNBC, refer to Keenan and Tolaney [20]. Atezolizumab is indicated for administration alongside chemotherapy in stage III and IV TNBC, while pembrolizumab, also approved for combination therapy, is prescribed for stage II and III disease [21,22]. Patient eligibility for either agent depends on PD-L1 expression status in TILs. However, studies have shown varying results regarding the prevalence of PD-L1 expression in TNBC patients, ranging from 21% to 53% [23,24]. While the limited patient pool poses a significant constraint on targeted ICI therapy, it also presents an opportunity for alternative cancer immunotherapies that are not reliant on genetic predisposition, such as therapeutic cancer vaccines.

3. Neoantigen Cancer Vaccines

Tumour cells express two types of peptide antigens capable of triggering an immune response: tumour-associated antigens (TAAs) and mutation-derived antigens (neoantigens). TAAs, originating from overexpressed normal cellular proteins, are self-antigens aberrantly expressed in multiple patients [25]. In contrast, neoantigens are patient-specific non-self antigens resulting from unique genetic alterations not shared among patients [26]. Neoantigens are immunogenic peptides representing the key component of peptide-based neoantigen cancer vaccines (NCVs).

Current cancer vaccines are classified into four categories: peptide based, cell based, virus based, and nucleic acid based (Table 2). While all aim to enhance the cancer-immunity cycle (CIC) (refer to Liu et al. [26] for a detailed CIC description), they differ in antigen presentation, irrespective of antigen type. Peptide-based vaccines directly deliver antigen epitopes, initiating the CIC through APC processing. Despite the challenge of weak immunogenicity of peptide-based vaccines, the platform is favoured in research and development (R&D) due to its straightforward manufacturing process correlating with lower vaccine costs [27] and potential for optimisation through the incorporation of adjuvants, offering a practical approach to cancer immunotherapy. Neoantigens formulated in peptide-based cancer vaccines could offer a personalised approach to improve the survival rates of TNBC patients. While there is considerable industry interest in such vaccines, most studies are still in the early stages, with two ongoing investigations focusing on peptide-based NCVs for TNBC (Table A1). However, this platform faces significant challenges in terms of poor immunogenicity, often resulting from the inherently small size of neoantigens [28].

Table 2. Overview of cancer vaccine platforms. While each platform presents distinct advantages and challenges, peptide-based cancer vaccines offer practical optimisation techniques, like adjuvants.

	Peptide Based	Cell Based	Virus Based	Nucleic Acid Based
Main Component	Known or predicted tumour antigen epitopes [27]	DCs containing antigens [29]	Antigen encapsulated in a viral vector [30]	Tumour antigen encoded DNA/ RNA [31]
Antigen Delivery	Tumour antigen epitopes [27]	Autologous antigen-loaded DCs [29]	Antigens in an oncolytic virus [30]	Neoantigens for DNA, TAAs and neoantigens for mRNA [31]
Main Advantage	Ease of production [27]	Broad antigen immune response due to containing whole tumour antigens [29]	Long-lasting immunity [30]	Simple and fast vaccine preparation [31]
Main Disadvantage	Low immunogenicity [28]	Expensive development [32]	Limited multi-dosing regimens [33]	Poor immunogenicity and stability [31]

3.1. Research and Methodology

Research and methodology are organised into three sections: (1) a literature review of the underlying science of peptide-based neoantigen cancer vaccines (NCVs), (2) direct medical cost calculation of TNBC treatment in the UK, and (3) the evaluation of two pricing strategies for the clinical adoption of NCVs in treating this cancer subtype.

3.2. Literature Search

The literature search process shown in Figure 2 was conducted using PubMed and Google Scholar. PubMed was chosen to screen research papers and pre-clinical and clinical study reports, providing a comprehensive view of the neoantigen cancer vaccine (NCV) landscape, and Google Scholar was used to fill in information gaps. EndNote Library was instrumental in categorising publications into folders. The search inclusion criteria were the publication period (2004–2024) and the incorporation of keywords in the titles. The most important primary and secondary keywords used for the search are shown in Figure 2. Any papers published before 2004 were excluded from the review due to the fast-paced nature of the research area. Only peer-reviewed publications were included in this study, and manual quality control checks were carried out to ensure the reliability of data. Clinical trial data were sourced from ClinicalTrials.gov, verifying sources, sponsors, and eligibility criteria to ensure unbiased data. All clinical trial study identification numbers are listed in Table A1.

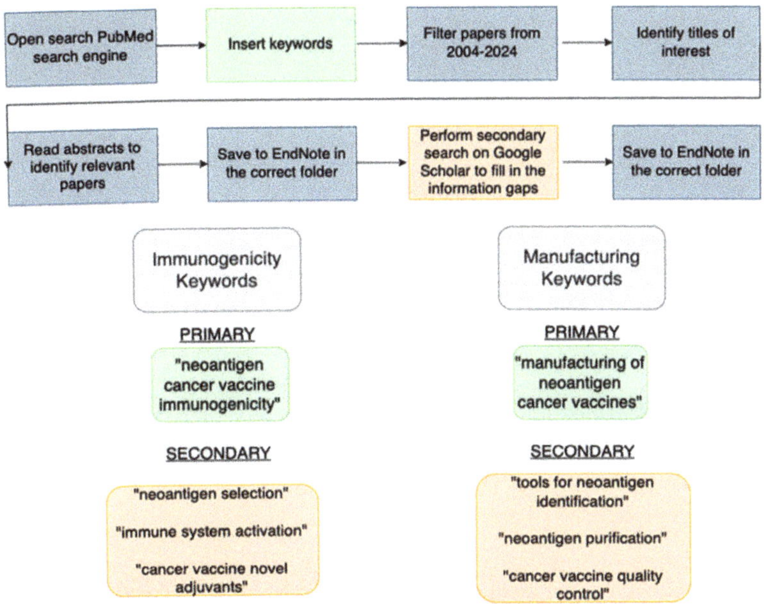

Figure 2. Literature search process and primary and secondary keywords. This method was used to perform a systematic literature review in "Immunogenicity of Neoantigens" and "Proposed Manufacturing of Neoantigen Cancer Vaccines".

3.3. Direct Medical Cost Data Extraction

The first step in calculating direct medical costs was to determine the annual number of TNBC patients diagnosed in the UK, as shown in Figure 3. Data from the National Audit of Breast Cancer Patients (NABCOP) served as the primary source to quantify patients over 50 years, assuming that 15% of all breast cancer cases were TNBC [34,35]. Numbers of stage 0 and metastatic stage breast cancer patients were directly derived from the NABCOP report. The figures were further adjusted to include younger women, considering TNBC's higher prevalence among this demographic, which was not covered in the NABCOP data. A study reporting that only 34% of TNBC patients are above 50 years old was adopted as the status quo to calculate the total number of TNBC patients [4]. The application of Figure 3 is demonstrated in Figure 4, illustrating the distribution across the cancer stages.

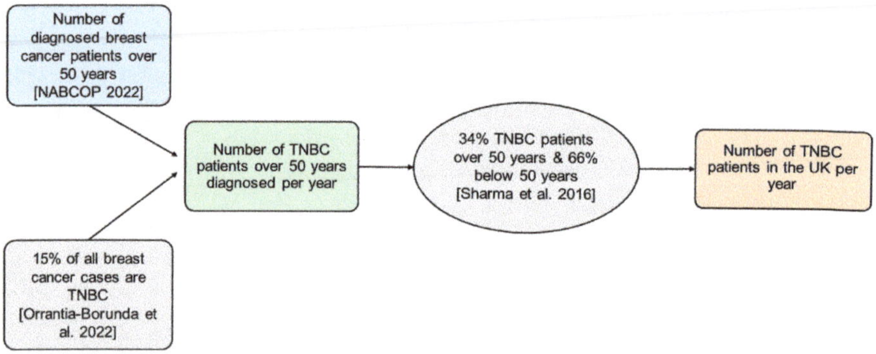

Figure 3. Method for the calculation of annual TNBC patients diagnosed in the UK. Assumptions outlined in the figure were used to calculate the total annual number of TNBC patients [4,34,35].

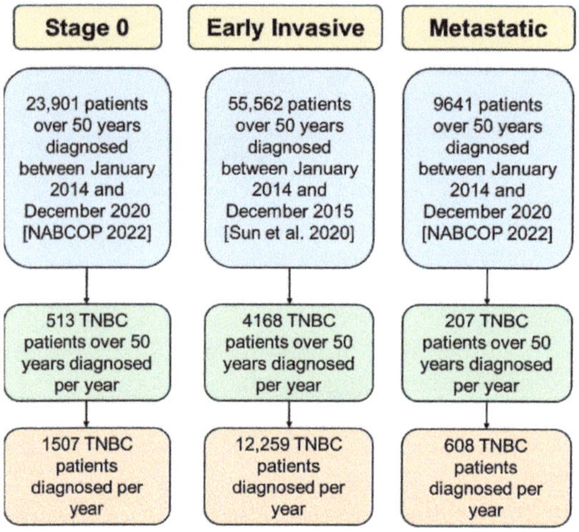

Figure 4. Annual distribution of TNBC patients per cancer stage. The calculation method is applied from Figure 3. The numbers of patients per breast cancer stage were directly derived from the cited sources [35,36]. Stage 0 and metastatic stage patients were adjusted to an annual number of new breast cancer stages, and the values were further adjusted to extract the TNBC proportion of patients. The final number accounted for TNBC patients below 50 years since the primary data did not contain these patients. Notably, the data used to quantify patients in the early-invasive subgroup are limited to the year 2015, compared to more recent data available to quantify patients in stage 0 and metastatic subgroups. This implies a limited degree of accuracy of the estimated numbers.

3.3.1. Conventional Therapies

The costs of conventional therapies for each cancer stage were calculated using various methodologies. Note that all subsequent costs were adjusted to January 2024 Great British Pounds using the UK and US Consumer Price Index. Since no data on stage 0 therapy procedures are publicly reported within the NHS, we calculated the cost per patient following the rationale outlined in Figure 5. An equal distribution between stages I to III was then assumed for the early-invasive stage. Lastly, the known proportions of patients receiving treatment per stage were used to identify the real number of patients requiring treatment presented in Table 3. However, limitations to the process are associated with the assumptions made, as these numbers are not provided by the NHS.

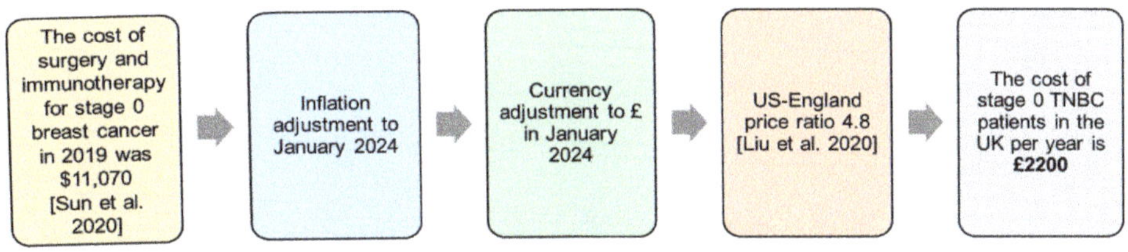

Figure 5. Method for calculating the cost per stage 0 TNBC patient in the UK. This approach was taken due to a lack of stage 0 therapy cost information in the UK [36,37].

Table 3. Proportions of treated TNBC patients. Only certain proportions of patients receive the standardised treatment, and the numbers shown are directly derived from the cited source. Subsequently, the highest percentages were extracted and are shown in this table. N.A. means that a specific therapy option is not provided to the TNBC stage patients. Created from NABCOP [35].

	Stage 0	Early Invasive TNBC	Metastatic TNBC
Total Number of TNBC Patients per Year	1507	12,259	608
Surgery	92% (1387)	89% (10,911)	N.A.
Radiotherapy	58%	87%	N.A.
Chemotherapy	N.A.	53%	25% (152)

The cost values discussed in the financial burden of the triple-negative breast cancer section were adopted from the literature as outlined in Table 4.

Table 4. Cost values per TNBC stage. The referenced values were extracted directly from the cited sources and adjusted to January 2024 Great British Pounds. Equal distribution of early-stage TNBC (stage I–III) numbers of patients was assumed due to no other data being available in the UK.

	Stage 0	Stage I	Stage II	Stage III	Stage IV
Cost per Patient	GBP 2200	GBP 6800	GBP 10,000	GBP 17,500	GBP 22,000
Original Cost Value	USD 11,070 in 2019 [38]	USD 5167 in 2015 [36]	USD 7613 in 2015 [36]	USD 13,330 in 2015 [36]	USD 12,500 in 2014 [39]
Number of Patients	1387	3637	3637	3637	152

3.3.2. Immune Checkpoint Inhibitor Therapy

The direct medical costs for treatment regimens with atezolizumab and pembrolizumab were obtained from publicly available documents (Table 5). Additionally, the number of patients eligible for immune checkpoint inhibitor therapy depends on programmed cell death-ligand 1 expression levels in tumour-infiltrating lymphocytes, with an assumed calculated mean of 37% representing the range of 21% to 53%, as reported in studies [23,24] (Table 6).

Table 5. Administration of cost specifications for atezolizumab and pembrolizumab. Atezolizumab cost was calculated by multiplying its price by 2 to obtain the cost per one cycle and was then multiplied by 6 cycles. Similarly, pembrolizumab costs GBP 2630 × 2 per dose since one dose is 200 mg, multiplied by 4 cycles. Created from NICE [40,41].

Immune Checkpoint Inhibitor	Dosage (mg)	Frequency	Price	Total Cost per Patient
Atezolizumab	840	Day 1 and 5 every 4 weeks, 6 cycles	GBP 2665.38 per 840 mg solution	GBP 32,000
Pembrolizumab	200	Once every 3 weeks, 4 cycles	GBP 2630 per 100 mg solution	GBP 21,000

Table 6. Number of eligible patients for atezolizumab and pembrolizumab. The number of patients per stage was adopted from Table 4. An assumed calculated 37% mean of eligible patients was assumed due to the required genetic predisposition.

Immune Checkpoint Inhibitor	TNBC Stage	Number of Patients	Eligible Patients (37%)
Atezolizumab	III and IV	3789	1402
Pembrolizumab	II and III	7274	2692

3.4. Pricing Scenarios

An identical vaccine formulation and regimen, outlined in Table 7, was assumed for two pricing scenarios—the best-case decentralised government-sponsored therapy model and the worst-case privately owned therapy model with in-house production.

Table 7. Assumed regimen of the neoantigen cancer vaccine administration. A multi-neoantigen formulation in an 11-dose regimen that prolongs a patient's life by 5.6 months was adopted from publications in the table due to the lack of late-stage trials for an NCV for TNBC.

Number of Neoantigens in a Single Vaccine per Patient	5 [42]	
Dose of a Single Peptide in a Single Vaccine	75 µg [43]	
Number of Doses	11 [44]	
Total Amount Required of a Single Peptide per Patient	1 mg	=75 µg × 11 doses
Progression-Free Survival Gained	5.6 months [45]	

Figure 6 illustrates the best-case scenario which assumes the same process steps as discussed in the section "Proposed Manufacturing of Neoantigen Cancer Vaccines", and the worst-case scenario, which assumes additional costs to recover initial investments.

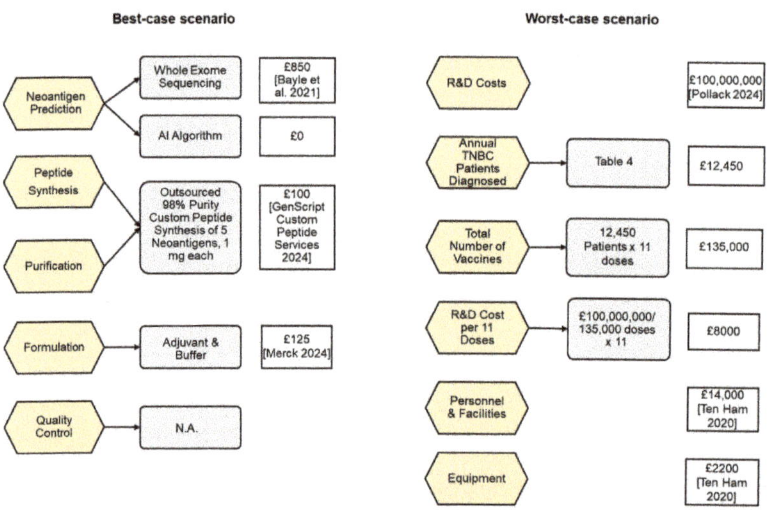

Figure 6. Cost per manufacturing step of the best-case scenario (**left**) and worst-case scenario costs (**right**). The left figure follows the manufacturing process proposed in this review [46–48].The right figure shows a calculation based on assumptions of heavy investments and mirroring costs outlined for another personalised therapy [32,49]. The value is associated with major assumptions due to the novelty of NCVs. Both costs represent the total cost per patient, as detailed in Table 7. Quality control

is not applicable for the best-case scenario based on the assumption that the neoantigens have been tested in production and this cost is included in the previous steps.

4. Results and Discussion

4.1. *Triple-Negative Breast Cancer Vaccine Clinical Trials*

Following an analysis of the different types of cancer vaccines for triple-negative breast cancer (TNBC), it was decided to prioritise peptide-based neoantigen cancer vaccines (NCVs). The data presented in Appendix A, summarised in the accompanying Figure 7, support this decision, highlighting the prevalence of ongoing clinical trials investigating peptide-based vaccines in the context of TNBC. Furthermore, TNBC tumours compared to other cancer types have a high mutational burden, resulting in large proportions of individual mutations (neoantigens). Therefore, the focus of this paper is on neoantigen formulations rather than tumour-associated cancer vaccines [50,51].

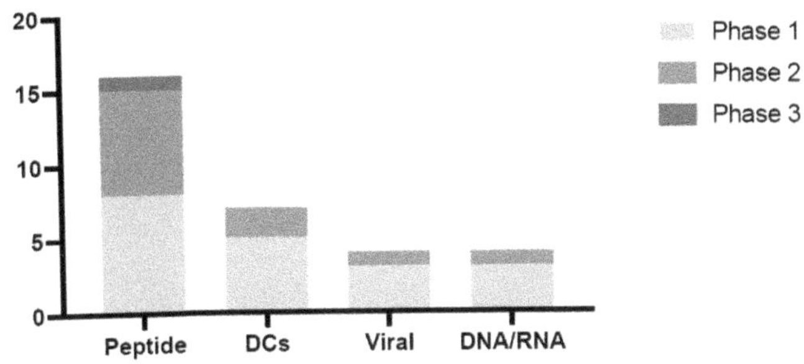

Figure 7. Breakdown of TNBC cancer vaccine platforms. The analysis demonstrates the significant industry interest in peptide-based cancer vaccines. The data are detailed in Table A1. Created from clinicaltrials.gov.

4.2. *Immunogenicity of Neoantigens*

4.2.1. Physiological Properties of Neoantigens

Neoantigens are typically categorised into short and long peptides based on their structural characteristics. Short peptides, however, often fail to induce an anti-tumour effect [52]. In contrast, long peptides, ranging from 13 to 18 amino acids, trigger both cytotoxic T-cells and CD4+ immune responses. This dual activation is attributed to the internalisation of long peptides by DCs, followed by presentation via both MHC I and II molecules, thereby bypassing immune tolerance mechanisms [53]. Synthetic long peptides (SLPs) are noteworthy for their ability to induce robust immune responses, including cytokine production and direct tumour elimination by CD4+ T-cells. Research highlights the pivotal role of CD4+ T-cells in initiating neoantigen-specific T-cell responses, emphasising the importance of utilising SLPs in cancer vaccine formulations [54]. These findings underscore the importance of researching SLPs to prolong antigen cross-presentation, thereby enhancing anti-tumour immune responses.

4.2.2. Vaccine Formulation Solutions

Further immunogenicity enhancement can be achieved by incorporating immunostimulatory adjuvants. Among the most frequently utilised agents are toll-like receptor (TLR) agonists, with polyinosinic-polycytidylic acid-poly-l-lysine carboxymethylcellulose (poly-ICLC) employed in a significant number of TNBC peptide-based NCV clinical trials highlighted in Figure 7. Studies have demonstrated that poly-ICLC can evoke robust T-cell and antibody responses, while also facilitating DC maturation and enhancing the anti-tumour efficacy of cancer vaccines [55,56].

Enhancing the immunogenicity of NCVs can also be achieved by incorporating multiple neoantigens into a single vaccine. Zhang, et al. [57] demonstrated the effectiveness of this method by successfully incorporating 11 neoantigens per vaccine per patient, resulting in a durable immune response and validating the viability of this approach. Moreover, employing a multi-neoantigen strategy promotes epitope spreading, wherein additional neoantigen-specific T-cells are generated against neoantigens not contained within the vaccine [58]. This approach shows promise in addressing the poor prognosis associated with high tumour heterogeneity in TNBC, as the expanded immune landscape may facilitate overcoming this challenge [59].

These findings outline the potential neoantigen cancer vaccine (NCV) formulation, i.e., a multi-neoantigen setting with poly-ICLC adjuvant, used to project pricing scenarios later in the review.

While peptide-based NCVs are a promising approach, their limited immunogenicity poses a challenge compared to other platforms. This can be addressed by incorporating immunogenic long-peptide neoantigens with adjuvants in a multi-neoantigen setup (Figure 8). This strategy extends neoantigen presentation on DCs, stimulating robust CD8+ and CD4+ T-cell responses and enhancing overall immune activation [54]. Incorporating toll-like receptor (TLR) agonists as adjuvants is recommended to stimulate the immune response; hence, poly-ICLC (TLR agonist) will be used in projecting the following NCV pricing scenarios.

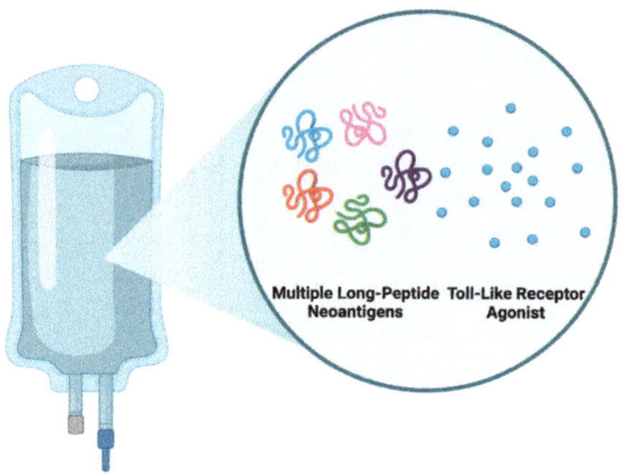

Figure 8. Recommended formulation of an NCV. To address NCVs' low immunogenicity, a formulation with multiple neoantigens and adjuvants as immunostimulators and delivery systems is proposed. Created with Biorender.

4.3. Proposed Manufacturing of Neoantigen Cancer Vaccines

Building on the findings from the previous section, an ideal TNBC NCV should feature multiple accurately identified neoantigens with high-affinity binding to HLA class II, determined through next-generation sequencing (NGS) methods. Challenges persist in identifying highly immunogenic and soluble neoantigens, necessitating further development of bioinformatic tools. Established and scalable approaches to neoantigen synthesis positively impact NCV production time. Intravenous administration of the vaccine is recommended, but further research is needed to determine optimal dosage and vaccination schedules. Quality controls (QCs) encompass safety, immunogenicity, and efficacy screening and testing, employing standard oncology endpoints and analytical assays. Overall, NCV manufacturing presents a viable aspect of launching NCVs for TNBC (illustrated in

Figure 9), yet further advancements are necessary in neoantigen prediction, formulation, and QC processes due to the early-stage R&D of NCVs.

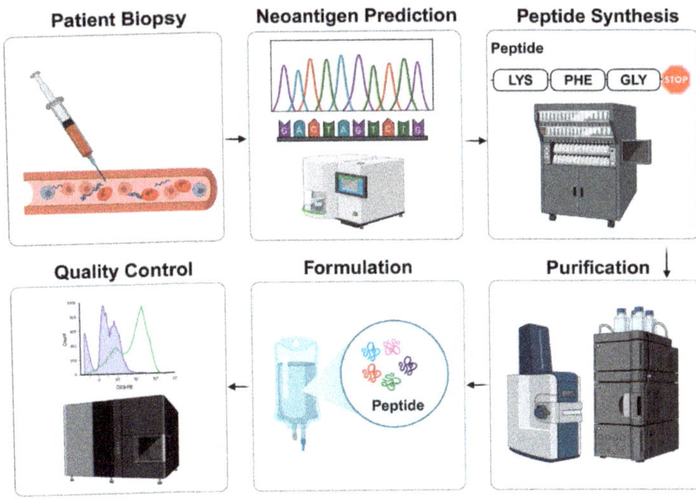

Figure 9. The proposed manufacturing process of an NCV. The process begins with obtaining a patient sample to predict immunogenic neoantigens and the arrows show the subsequent steps. The first step can utilise next-generation sequencing (NGS) tools, including whole exome sequencing, and validate the results by HLA typing, peptide processing, and peptide-MHC binding prediction. Next, the identified neoantigens synthesis will be outsourced to protein synthesising companies, significantly driving the low-cost dynamics of the process. The peptide purification will be outsourced as well, and the neoantigens will be delivered with 98% purity [47]. The proposed formulation of an NCV is an intravenous injection to stimulate a strong anti-tumour response. The quality control (QC) for an NCV will determine safety, immunogenicity, and efficacy by performing immunogenic assays and analysing adverse events and standard oncology endpoints. Created with Biorender.

4.3.1. Neoantigen Prediction

The initial phase in selecting optimal neoantigens for an NCV involves neoantigen identification, commencing with patient biopsy and tissue analysis through comparative assessment of single nucleotide variants (SNVs) between tumour and non-tumour DNA [60]. Clinical evidence shows that SNV-derived neoantigens in NCVs can induce disease regression and enhance T-cell responses [61]. Despite various genome analysis toolkits available, like whole exome sequencing, a manual review of matched tumour-normal samples is recommended due to screening tool limitations [62], potentially prolonging the turnaround time from biopsy to vaccine formulation. Research indicates multiple possible neoantigen categories, including tumour-specific fusion proteins resulting from gene translocations, which exhibit considerable genetic instability within chromosomes and can generate highly immunogenic neoantigens [63]. While research on fusion genes in TNBC is limited, the available data appear promising. Wang et al. [64] identified 22 recurring fusion proteins in TNBC patients, identifying a novel fusion biomarker. Although no other fusion proteins have been identified for TNBC, research on fusion neoantigens in other cancers has shown their ability to enhance T-cell responses and eliminate tumour cells [65]. Therefore, while additional validation of genome analysis toolkits is necessary, these findings highlight encouraging strategies for clinical application, as successfully demonstrated in the TNBC context.

Validation steps in neoantigen prediction include HLA typing, peptide processing, and peptide–MHC binding prediction. Precise HLA identification is crucial due to MHC molecule polymorphism, with over 12,000 allele modifications [66]. While next-generation sequencing (NGS) has achieved high accuracy for MHC class I, further development for class II HLA sequencing is required [67,68]. Peptide processing prediction focuses on the binding affinity between the patient's MHC molecule and the given neoantigen, with challenges, such as peptide cleavage, potentially hindering successful peptide loading onto APC [69,70]. MHC binding prediction, based on HLA typing, is considered the most selective step but results in inaccurate neoantigen predictions due to factors such as peptide immunogenicity and gaps in HLA allele datasets [68,71]. Only 20% of in silico-predicted neoantigens exhibited immunogenicity, and 55% of in vitro-predicted immunogenic neoantigens elicited an immune response after binding to HLA [72,73]. One strategy to address these challenges involves a scoring system that considers factors, including HLA mutation frequencies, neoantigen transcription abundance, and MHC binding likelihood, showing a 95% accuracy in predicting the immunogenicity of selected neoantigens [74]. Developing methods for accurately identifying the most immunogenic neoantigens is imperative, given an average of 60 neoantigen mutations per patient [73]. These findings suggest that bioinformatic tools can accurately predict neoantigens, but additional validation of the methods is needed to establish the process.

4.3.2. Peptide Synthesis

Upon completing the neoantigen identification, two primary methods are available for neoantigen production: peptide synthesis and genetic engineering. Peptide synthesis offers distinct advantages, notably in terms of cost effectiveness and production efficiency [75]. This process relies on solid-phase peptide synthesis (SPPS), which involves the sequential addition of amino acids to the growing peptide chain [76]. Various companies offer peptide synthesis at remarkably low costs, with prices typically in the region of GBP 19 per 4 mg of a peptide [47]. This affordability significantly influences the cost dynamics of NCV manufacturing. Mijalis et al. [77] demonstrated an automated SPPS approach capable of producing an amino acid residue in 40 s. Considering that neoantigens should preferably be SLPs ranging from 13 to 18 amino acids in length, the production time for a single neoantigen is approximately 12 min. Consequently, producing the required amount of a neoantigen can only take several hours. Given a concurrent neoantigen synthesis for a multi-neoantigen vaccine, the production time would not increase. Thus, peptide synthesis represents a financially feasible and scalable approach for manufacturing NCVs.

4.3.3. Purification

Once the neoantigen synthesis is completed, purification proceeds via high-performance liquid chromatography (HPLC). Mass spectrometry is commonly utilised to confirm the neoantigen structure and has demonstrated accurate sensitivity. Reversed-phase HPLC has proven effective in eliminating impurities post-neoantigen synthesis, often in combination with ion exchange or gel filtration chromatography [76,78]. However, a challenge in purifying SLPs arises from their amino acid sequence insolubility [68]. While studies have not extensively addressed this issue in neoantigens as SLPs, temporary peptide tags have demonstrated success in enhancing the solubility of other types of SLPs [79–81]. Additionally, computational tools for neoantigen prediction aim to address the purification challenges by identifying hydrophobic sequences. These tools help select the most viable neoantigen residues, serving as a decision-making tool for correct neoantigen manufacture [82]. However, neoantigens fall within the standard frame for peptide synthesis companies, which often provide peptides at 98% purity, streamlining the purification step in the manufacturing process [47]. These findings suggest that challenges related to neoantigen purification warrant further investigation; however, neoantigens as SLPs can achieve clinical-grade purity through outsourcing to peptide synthesis companies, eliminating the challenge.

4.3.4. Formulation

Although the formulation of NCVs lacks standardisation, several clinically established considerations exist. Intravenous administration of NCVs has demonstrated a stronger immune response compared to subcutaneous routes, with subcutaneous injection leading to T-cell deletion via chronic T-cell stimulation, resulting in low anti-tumour responses in clinical trials [83]. Moreover, proper stimulation timing and adjuvant selection are crucial to induce T-cell response alongside appropriate costimulation and cytokine signalling. Achieving timely APC maturation alongside neoantigen delivery is also essential for eliciting a robust anti-tumour response [75]. Another challenge in NCV manufacture is the turnaround time from biopsy to finalising the vaccine formulation, which typically takes 3–4 months [61]. This extended period may exceed the life expectancy of TNBC patients, necessitating further investigation into correct intravenous NCV formulation, along with a pressing need to shorten the vaccine production time.

4.3.5. Quality Control

Industry-standard quality controls (QCs) for NCVs include safety, immunogenicity, and efficacy (Figure 10). Both trials employ the National Cancer Institute Common Terminology Criteria for Adverse Events (NCI-CTCAE) to assess safety, while efficacy and immunogenicity are evaluated using enzyme-linked immunospot (ELISPOT) analyses, multiparametric flow cytometry, and standard oncology trial endpoints, such as the clinical response rate and overall survival [84,85]. ELISPOT assays objectively assess NCV immunogenicity by quantifying the frequency of immune cells producing specific cytokines linked to tumour-specific immune responses, validated for neoantigen-specific T-cell responses in cancer patients [86]. Multiparametric flow cytometry assesses cytokine production and the frequency of neoantigen-specific T-cells, providing a comprehensive view of the cancer vaccine efficacy [87]. The clinical response rate indicates the proportion of patients with tumour shrinkage or disappearance, reflecting vaccine efficacy, while overall survival directly reflects the vaccine's impact on patients' lives [88]. Thus, the analysis of the two NCV trials justifies current QC practices, providing authentic assessments of NCV safety, efficacy, and immunogenicity.

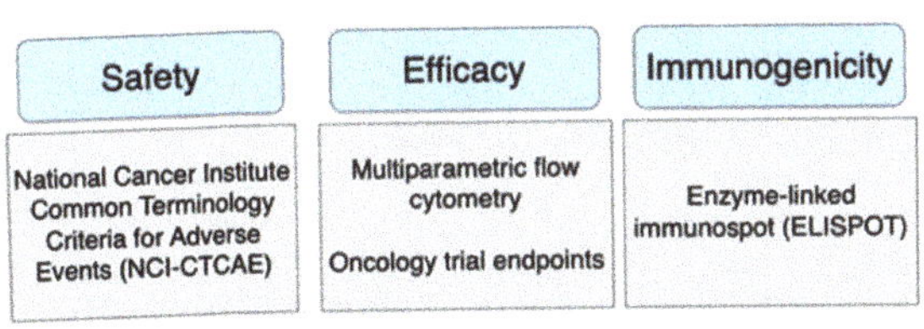

Figure 10. Quality control (QC) requirements for a safe, effective, and immunogenic NCV. These QCs were adopted from the two NCVs for TNBC trials (Section 3.1), demonstrating industry-accepted controls.

These findings suggest the overall viability of manufacturing NCVs. As a result, the following sections will focus on two main objectives: firstly, calculating the economic implications of managing TNBC in the UK using current therapies, and secondly, conducting a financial analysis of two different pricing scenarios for NCVs to assess their potential introduction to the UK market.

4.4. Financial Burden of Triple-Negative Breast Cancer

The cost of TNBC holds significant relevance due to the substantial resource utilisation associated with each TNBC stage, ranging from GBP 2200 to GBP 54,000 annually per patient, amounting to GBP 230,000,000 annually for the NHS. While attempts have been made to calculate the cost of TNBC in various countries [89], no studies have yet estimated the cost of TNBC therapies for the NHS. Although TNBC is associated with indirect costs, such as productivity losses and reduced quality of life, this review focuses solely on calculating the direct medical costs. Despite the TNBC financial burden being significant, it remains a question whether an NCV could alleviate direct costs. A potential for cost reduction at the advanced stages is in reducing the chemotherapy cycles and the regimen of immune checkpoint inhibitors.

4.4.1. Direct Medical Costs of Conventional Therapies in the United Kingdom

The calculated cost of conventional therapy ranges from GBP 2200 to GBP 22,000 per patient annually, depending on the TNBC stage, as demonstrated in Figure 11. Evaluation of these numbers against reviewed figures is challenging due to a lack of available data. The most comparable study reported a mean cumulative 15-month cost of GBP 12,595 per breast cancer patient in the UK, equivalent to GBP 14,000 as of January 2024 [90]. Notably, the study was conducted before ICIs were available for TNBC treatment, so the reported value only considered the conventional therapies. For comparison, dividing the total yearly cost by the number of patients per stage in this review yields GBP 10,400 per patient. The difference between GBP 14,000 and GBP 10,400 may be due to more costly treatment options available for other breast cancer subtypes, potentially inflating the reported mean value of the published study. Numerous limitations are inherent in estimating the financial burden of TNBC, particularly considering that therapies may extend beyond a year, which is not factored into the calculations within this review. Additionally, TNBC is more common among younger women, which might lead to higher therapy rates than those shared by NABCOP [35], as NABCOP accounted for only women over 50 years who might not be offered the TNBC treatment due to other factors (age and/or pre-existing health conditions).

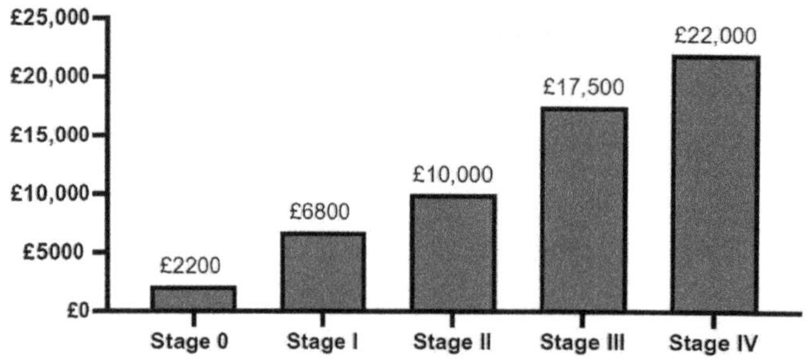

Figure 11. Annual direct medical costs of conventional therapies per patient in the United Kingdom. This figure demonstrates the cost of surgery, chemotherapy, and radiotherapy per TNBC stage, with references outlined in Table 4. These data were consolidated from various sources (shown in Table 4) due to a lack of economical appraisal of TNBC therapy costs in the United Kingdom.

The calculated costs for immune checkpoint inhibitor (ICI) therapy are shown in Figure 12. Annual pembrolizumab cost per patient was calculated to amount to GBP 21,000 and atezolizumab to GBP 32,000. The ICI therapy cost calculations are more precise due to available access to official reports, though they are likely overestimated due to discounts confidentially given to the NHS. Furthermore, as both ICI agents are available for stage III

TNBC, the more expensive treatment (atezolizumab) was assumed to project the highest possible costs.

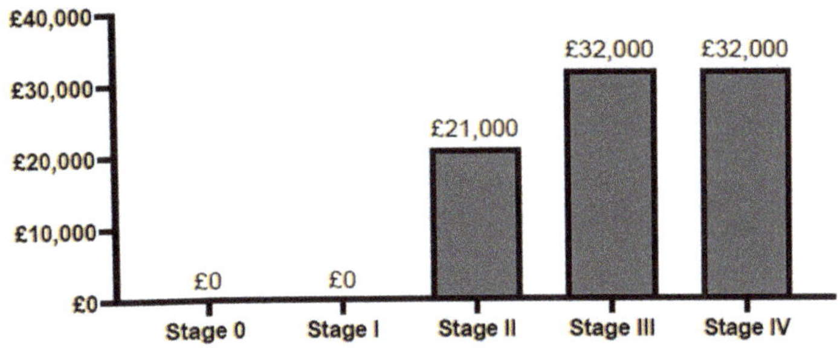

Figure 12. Annual direct medical costs of immune checkpoint inhibitor (ICI) therapies per patient in the United Kingdom. As no ICI therapy is available for stage 0 and I TNBC patients, the figure displays the annual cost of pembrolizumab per stage II TNBC patient. The stage III value represents the atezolizumab cost, although both ICI agents are available to stage III TNBC patients. Stage IV represents the atezolizumab cost.

4.4.2. Analysis of All Direct Medical Costs

The costs vary significantly across different disease progression stages, as shown in Figure 13, with notable escalations in advanced disease stages. Stage 0 and I TNBC patients typically undergo surgery, with additional chemotherapy and radiotherapy for stage I. Moreover, the shorter therapy cycles also contribute to lower associated costs [36]. Costs markedly escalate from stage II onwards due to the inclusion of ICIs, although not all patients meet the eligibility criteria for these therapies. According to the assumptions in this paper, nearly two-thirds of patients do not express PD-L1, thus receiving only conventional treatment. However, the per-patient costs shown in Figure 13 (ranging from GBP 2200 to GBP 54,000) represent the maximum potential costs per stage, including ICIs. Interestingly, costs between stages III and IV are relatively comparable (GBP 49,500 and GBP 54,000). While stage IV TNBC patients have a median survival time of 13 months, the reported overall survival time for stage III patients is 92 months [10,91]. Therefore, the substantial costs of stage IV therapy and the reduced quality of life resulting from chemotherapy may contribute to the low therapy uptake, with only 25% of stage IV patients receiving any form of treatment, as shown in Table 3 [35].

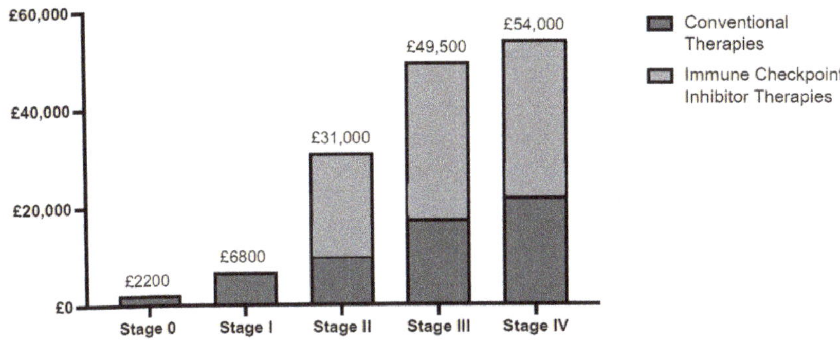

Figure 13. Yearly per-patient cost comparison per stage. Although both ICIs are available to stage III patients, the highest potential costs were assumed; therefore, atezolizumab was included (cost comparison is shown in Table 5). The cost of conventional therapies was determined from papers, aside from stage 0, which was calculated as per Figure 5. ICIs were calculated from regimen specifications from official reports (Table 5).

The annual expenditure for treating all TNBC patients in the UK is projected to reach GBP 230,000,000, with conventional therapies representing GBP 130,000,000 (Table A2), and the proportions are shown in Figure 14. The ICI therapy based on 37% patient eligibility criteria was calculated to amount to GBP 102,000,000 (Table A3), representing the minority of annual TNBC therapy costs. Another financial evaluation was performed, which considered a 50% ICI eligibility of TNBC patients. As shown in Figure 14, this leads to a significantly higher value of ICI therapy costs, estimated at GBP 138,000,000 (Table A4). In this case, the ICIs represent most of the annual expenditure of TNBC therapy, which increases to GBP 268,000,000. These data imply that it is essential to identify the correct number of eligible patients.

It can be expected that an NCV would not eliminate existing therapy options but rather serve as an additional option to control the disease more effectively. For this reason, it is advised that NCV research focuses on the introduction of NCVs to TNBC stage II onwards. This could allow for cost alleviations, e.g., by reducing the number of ICI cycles or decreasing the frequency of ICI administration. Notably, an NCV could also reduce the need for intensive chemotherapy cycles. Although the chemotherapy costs are not heavily resource intensive, it could still result in improved therapy tolerability of patients and improve their quality of life.

The upcoming section will examine the costs of conventional therapies and ICIs in comparison to two hypothetical pricing models of a TNBC NCV. The analysis will aim to assess the potential feasibility of introducing the vaccine in the UK and its potential impact on reducing TNBC treatment costs in the country.

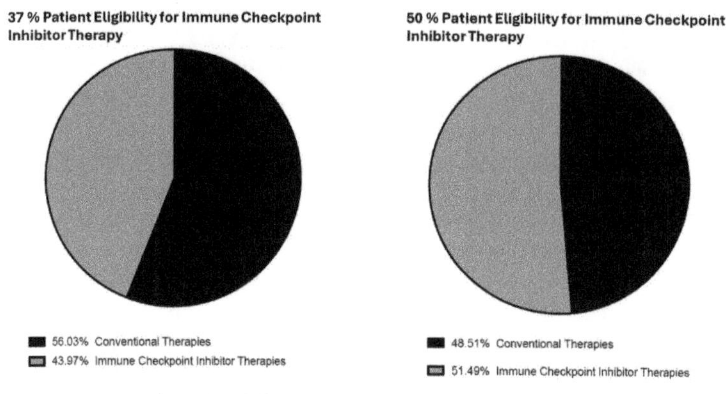

Figure 14. Annual cost breakdown of treating TNBC in the UK assuming an immune checkpoint inhibitor patient eligibility of 37% (**left**) and 50% (**right**). The left-hand graph demonstrates the total cost, which equals GBP 230,000,000 annually, with conventional therapies amounting to GBP 130,000,000 and immune checkpoint inhibitor therapies to GBP 102,000,000. The right-hand graph demonstrates the total annual cost of GBP 268,000,000. The majority of the costs are now associated with immune checkpoint inhibitor therapies (GBP 138,000,000). Data are shown in Tables A2–A4.

4.5. Pricing

4.5.1. Incremental Cost Effectiveness Ratios of Approved Therapies

The incremental cost effectiveness ratio (ICER) provides insights into the cost effectiveness of different treatments in terms of life years gained due to the medication. According to the literature, the National Institute for Health and Care Excellence (NICE) has established a willingness-to-pay therapy threshold of GBP 50,000 per life year gained [92]. Hence, the current TNBC therapies were evaluated against this upper cost limit, as shown in Table 8. All ICER calculations were found to be below the threshold, considering that ICI therapies received a discount for NICE, resulting in even lower costs than depicted in Table 8. Notably, pembrolizumab exhibited the lowest ICER, although the median progression-free survival (PFS) is not officially confirmed by the manufacturer, given the recent approval of the therapy and the confidentiality surrounding its details. Therefore, the GBP 50,000 NICE threshold offers a constructive benchmark for evaluating the two hypothetical NCV pricing scenarios.

Table 8. Incremental cost effectiveness ratio (ICER) per life year adjusted of approved TNBC therapies. Calculated cost per patient numbers are adopted from Table 5. Progression-free survival (PFS) represents the time from study initiation until tumour progression. The ICER/life year adjusted was calculated by 12 months x cost per patient/median PFS. All therapies are below the GBP 50,000 NICE threshold since the NHS received a confidential discount for atezolizumab.

	Cost per Patient	Median PFS (months)	ICER/Life Year Adjusted
Chemotherapy	GBP 17,500	5.6 [93]	GBP 38,000
Atezolizumab	GBP 32,000	7.5 [94]	GBP 52,000
Pembrolizumab	GBP 21,000	7.6 [95]	GBP 34,000

4.5.2. Pricing Scenarios Assuming a Commercialisation of a Peptide-Based Neoantigen Cancer Vaccine for Triple-Negative Breast Cancer

Should clinical trial studies indicate the usefulness of NCVs, it will be essential to have models of how these treatments could be effectively implemented by healthcare systems, such as the UK-NHS. To this end, a best-case and a worst-case scenario were proposed and analysed to assess the feasibility of a hypothetical NCV. The assumption adopted for this section is a demonstrated efficacy of the NCV in phase III trials with limited side effects that are inferior to the benefits generated from the commercialisation of the NCV. It is important to assume such a scenario due to the currently early phase but promising research about NCVs for TNBC and to allow for industry preparedness ahead of a real-life NCV launch. The proposed NCV formulation outlined in Table 7 was applied to both pricing scenarios, involving a multi-neoantigen vaccine administered in 11 doses with a PFS of 5.6 months. In the best-case scenario, treatment was assumed to be administered at cost with a decentralised approach and zero intermediary supply chain. All steps were assumed to be outsourced, following the proposed manufacturing process described in this review in Section 4.3 and shown in Figure 9. Vaccine delivery would be facilitated at existing administration locations, such as hospitals. It was further assumed that no company owned the vaccine, and no profits were generated. This approach resulted in a cost of GBP 1100 per patient, with an ICER of GBP 2400, as shown in Table 9. Conversely, the worst-case scenario assumed a privately funded NCV aimed to recover estimated initial R&D costs and the establishment of an in-house manufacturing site, albeit without any profit margin. The total cost per year amounted to GBP 25,000, resulting in an ICER of GBP 55,000, as outlined in Table 9.

Table 9 indicates that the worst-case ICER exceeds the GBP 50,000 NICE willingness-to-pay threshold. The ICER values were plotted against this threshold (Figure 15), illustrating the maximum cost of treatment per month gained. The best-case scenario analysed in this paper falls well below the NICE threshold, accounting for only 5% of the allowable cost, indicating its high feasibility. Conversely, the worst-case ICER slightly exceeds the threshold based on the assumed PFS of 5.6 months. While the characteristics of vaccine administration are based on the relevant literature, these values are approximate estimates, and the scenarios are contingent on variables that may change. Furthermore, limitations of the worst-case scenario include the assumed costs outlined in Figure 6. Given the lack of existing NCVs on the market, the assumed R&D costs amounting to GBP 100,000,000 remain a rough estimate. Similarly, uncertainties persist regarding the estimated equipment, personnel, and facility expenses, which were derived from data on the manufacturing of an autologous DC cancer vaccine due to the absence of the relevant literature on NCVs. Thus, the analysis revealed that the best-case scenario is highly feasible, whereas the worst-case scenario, associated with greater uncertainties, exceeds the NICE threshold, implying its unfeasibility.

Table 9. Costs and incremental cost effectiveness ratios (ICERs) per scenario. The total cost per regimen was calculated as outlined in Table 5; best-case costs are GBP 850 + GBP 100 + GBP 125, and worst-case costs are GBP 8000 + GBP 14,000 + 2200. The ICER/life year adjusted was calculated by 12 months x total cost per regimen/5.6 PFS. The difference in ICER values stems from the decentralised approach in the best-case scenario, contrasting with the worst-case scenario where a company aims to recover its investments. While the best-case ICER is well below the GBP 50,000 NICE threshold, the worst-case scenario exceeds it.

	Best-Case Scenario	Worst-Case Scenario
Total Cost per Regimen	GBP 1100	GBP 25,000
ICER	GBP 2400	GBP 55,000

The vaccine regimen cost is, therefore, highly sensitive to two main variables: the number of doses and the PFS. Figure 16 illustrates the cost allowances across three regimen scenarios: single-dose, five-dose, and eleven-dose administration. For instance, assuming all scenarios prolong one patient's life by 5 months, a single dose could cost up to GBP 20,833, while one dose in a five-dose regimen would be GBP 4167, and in an eleven-dose regimen, GBP 1894 per patient. Therefore, the single-dose regimen allows for the highest permissible cost per dose. This indicates that fewer doses required for the same PFS result in higher allowable costs per NCV dose. Furthermore, Figure 16 highlights the cost disparities among the regimens. Comparing the cost of doses for 5 months versus 12 months of any regimen underscores the importance of achieving a higher PFS. In the single-dose scenario, the 5-month regimen could cost GBP 20,833 per dose, while the 12-month regimen could approach the threshold of GBP 50,000. For the five-dose and eleven-dose regimens, however, the maximum allowed costs per dose would need to be considerably lower to be cost effective (Figure 16). These factors underscore the significance of minimising the number of doses and maximising each patient's life expectancy to mitigate the risk of vaccine rejection by NICE.

The main limitations in NCV pricing include the projected PFS and low immunogenicity, necessitating multiple doses to achieve an immune response. The assumed NCV PFS used in this analysis matches chemotherapy but falls short of already established ICIs, compared with Table 8. This could impact NICE approval due to perceived insufficient benefits. However, NCVs potentially offer advantages, like reduced adverse events and broader eligibility, compared to chemotherapy and ICIs. Based on current data outlined in this review, it is, however, unlikely that NCVs could be offered as a standalone treatment due to the immunogenicity challenges. For this reason, there is currently no benefit from comparing an NCV treatment directly with the existing therapies from a financial perspective. The low immunogenicity rather suggests that further research on combination therapy with existing treatments is required. Due to the lack of papers on this topic, it can only be expected that such a strategy would increase treatment costs. Our findings suggest that R&D should prioritise improving immunogenicity to reduce required doses and enhance survival outcomes to maximise the possibility of receiving NICE approval. It is highly unlikely that an NCV for TNBC would receive approval if the vaccine efficacy, i.e., immunogenicity, does not significantly improve.

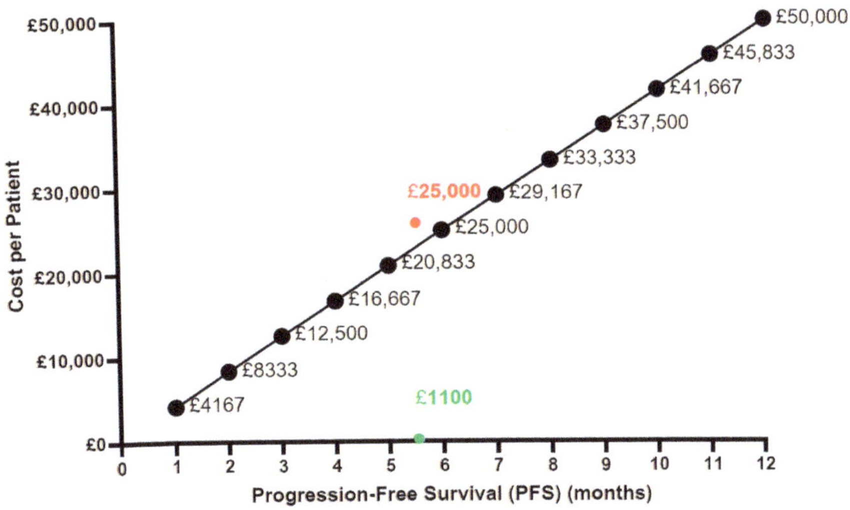

Figure 15. Cost scenarios plotted against the NICE ICER threshold in a hypothetical scenario of the commercialisation of an NCV for TNBC. This plot illustrates the maximum allowable cost per scenario based on the number of months gained by the therapy (PFS). For instance, if a therapy extends one patient's life by six months, the cost could be priced at GBP 25,000 per patient because two such regimens would prolong the life expectancy by twelve months. Therefore, extending one patient's life by 6 months would cost GBP 25,000, and extending the life by 12 months would be equal to two patients receiving such therapy, amounting to GBP 50,000 altogether. Conversely, if an NCV regimen prolonged one patient's life by just one month, the maximum allowable cost per patient would be GBP 4167 to stay within the NICE threshold for twelve months.

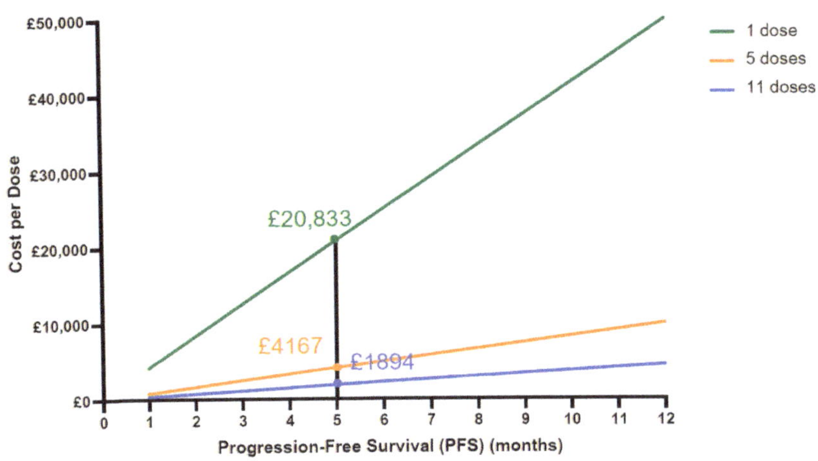

Figure 16. Maximum allowed cost per dose, dependent on PFS. This plot indicates that the fewer doses per regimen required, and the greater number of months gained by the regimen, the higher the potential price of a single dose can be. The black line shows the intersection between each regimen at 5 months PFS, demonstrating the maximum allowed cost per dose per scenario, respectively. The lower the number of doses per regimen, i.e., 1 dose, the greater the possibility of the cost per dose. Contrarily, the higher the number of doses per regimen, i.e., 11 doses, the smaller the value of cost per dose.

5. Conclusions

Neoantigen cancer vaccines (NCVs) offer a promising approach towards targeted cancer immunotherapy for triple-negative breast cancer (TNBC) treatment. The main prospect of NCVs is their feasible manufacturing process allowing for notable cost savings. However, the limited immunogenicity of NCVs is a significant challenge, and from this review, we conclude that a multi-neoantigen formulation with a toll-like receptor agonist should be further explored. The current TNBC therapy costs range between GBP 2200 and GBP 54,000, depending on the cancer stage. An opportunity for decreasing the current costs would be most impactful from stage II onwards, though it is contingent upon immune checkpoint inhibitor eligibility. It remains a question whether an NCV could alleviate some of these costs or act as an additional agent, further increasing the TNBC therapy costs. The financial feasibility of NCVs also depends on the operational setting. Calculations revealed that if the government were to manage the vaccine at cost, approval would likely be feasible. However, in a worst-case scenario where the therapy is privately owned, the cost per regimen to extend the patients' lives exceeds the GBP 50,000 NICE approval threshold. Crucial variables influencing cost include the number of doses and progression-free survival (PFS). Analyses reveal that fewer doses and higher PFS allow for higher approved costs per dose. Therefore, clinical evaluation of dosage and PFS will be critical for further refining economic appraisal.

Further research is essential to improve immunogenicity as the main hurdle of NCVs for TNBC; recommendations in this review include exploring a multi-neoantigen setting and a combination therapy with existing treatments with the aim to enhance the currently low vaccine efficacy. Obtaining the latest country-specific data on TNBC patients and therapies is required to draw accurate conclusions about the current state of the art and to provide a reliable base for further financial evaluations ahead of the commercialisation of NCVs.

In conclusion, developing an NCV for TNBC is under current circumstances unfeasible, primarily due to immunogenicity challenges, hindering the successful development. However, the NCV cost effectiveness as a standalone factor implies that the commercialisation of the therapy is possible, and the focus should be on maximising the life prolongation factor while minimising the number of doses required per patient.

Author Contributions: Conceptualisation, A.N., L.V., S.F., and S.A.M.; methodology, A.N.; formal analysis, A.N., L.V., S.F., and S.A.M.; data curation, A.N.; writing—original draft preparation, A.N.; writing—review and editing, S.F., S.A.M., and L.V.; visualisation, A.N.; supervision, S.F., S.A.M., and L.V.; project administration, S.F. All authors have read and agreed to the published version of the manuscript.

Funding: S.F. and L.V. acknowledge support from the UK Engineering and Physical Sciences Research Council (EPSRC) for the Manufacturing Research Hub for a Sustainable Future (VaxHub Sustainable) (EP/X038181/1), whereas S.A.M. acknowledges support by the Department of Health and Social Care (DHSC)/EPSRC funded by the VaxHub Global project (EP/Y530542/1).

Institutional Review Board Statement: Not applicable.

Informed Consent Statement: Not applicable.

Data Availability Statement: The original contributions presented in this study are included in the article/Appendix A. Further inquiries can be directed to the corresponding author(s).

Conflicts of Interest: The authors declare no conflicts of interest. The funders had no role in the design of the study; in the collection, analyses, or interpretation of data; in the writing of the manuscript; or in the decision to publish the results.

Appendix A

Table A1. Overview of TNBC clinical trials. NA means the therapy mode was not defined in the clinical trial description. Data were accessed from clinicaltrials.gov on 22 February 2024.

NCT Number	Status	TNBC Stage	Therapy Mode	Phase	Platform
NCT03387085	Active	All stages	Immunotherapy + chemotherapy	1b/2	Viral
NCT02316457	Completed	All stages	Immunotherapy + chemotherapy	1	RNA
NCT05504707	Recruiting	Early stage	Chemotherapy	1	DCs
NCT03199040	Terminated	Advanced	Immunotherapy	1	DNA
NCT03562637	Recruiting	Early stage	Chemotherapy	3	Peptide
NCT04674306	Recruiting	Early stage	Immunotherapy	1	Peptide
NCT04634747	Not yet recruiting	Advanced	Immunotherapy + chemotherapy	2	Peptide
NCT02938442	Completed	Early stage	Chemotherapy	1/2	Peptide
NCT03362060	Active	Metastatic	Immunotherapy	1b	Peptide
NCT03674827	Terminated	Metastatic	Immunotherapy + chemotherapy	1	Unknown
NCT02593227	Completed	Advanced	Chemotherapy	2	Peptide
NCT04348747	Recruiting	All stages	Immunotherapy	2a	DCs
NCT04024800	Active	Advanced	Immunotherapy	2	Peptide
NCT02427581	Withdrawn	Advanced and metastatic	Chemotherapy	1	Peptide
NCT02348320	Completed	All stages	Chemotherapy	1	DNA
NCT04105582	Completed		Chemotherapy	1	DCs
NCT00986609	Completed	Early stage	NA	1	Peptide
NCT02826434	Active	Early stage	Immunotherapy	1	Peptide
NCT05455658	Recruiting	Early stage	NA	2	DNA
NCT04296942	Terminated	Metastatic	Immunotherapy	1	Viral
NCT02018458	Completed	Locally advanced	Chemotherapy	1/2	DCs
NCT03012100	Active	Early stage and advanced	Chemotherapy	2	Peptide
NCT00640861	Completed	Early stage	NA	1	Peptide
NCT03606967	Recruiting	Metastatic	Chemotherapy + immunotherapy	2	peptide
NCT04879888	Completed	All stages	Chemotherapy	1	DCs
NCT05329532	Recruiting	Advanced	Immunotherapy	1/2	Peptide

Table A2. Conventional therapy costs per TNBC stage. The patient count was calculated from NABCOP [35], and per-patient costs were derived from research papers. The cost per stage increases with more advanced stages, resulting in a GBP 130,000,000 annual cost for conventional TNBC therapy in the UK.

	Stage 0	Stage I	Stage II	Stage III	Stage IV
Number of Patients	1387	3637	3637	3637	152
Cost per Patient	GBP 2200	GBP 6800	GBP 10,000	GBP 17,500	GBP 22,000
Total Yearly Cost per Stage	GBP 3,100,000	GBP 25,000,000	GBP 37,000,000	GBP 64,000,000	GBP 3,400,000

Table A3. Adjusted total annual costs of atezolizumab and pembrolizumab for TNBC. Atezolizumab is for stage III and IV TNBC, while pembrolizumab is for stage II and III TNBC. A 37% eligibility assumption due to genetic predisposition was made.

Immune Checkpoint Inhibitor	Eligible Patients (37%)	Cost per Patient	Total Cost
Atezolizumab	1402	GBP 32,000	**GBP 45,000,000**
Pembrolizumab	2692	GBP 21,000	**GBP 57,000,000**

Table A4. Adjusted number of patients eligible for immune checkpoint inhibitor (ICI) therapy. If 50% of TNBC patients exhibited the required genetic predisposition, the costs per ICI would rise significantly in the UK.

Immune Checkpoint Inhibitor	Number of Patients	Eligible Patients (50%)	Cost per Patient	Adjusted Total Cost
Atezolizumab	3789	1895	GBP 32,000	GBP 61,000,000
Pembrolizumab	7274	3637	GBP 21,000	GBP 77,000,000

References

1. Pearce, A.; Haas, M.; Viney, R.; Pearson, S.A.; Haywood, P.; Brown, C.; Ward, R. Incidence and severity of self-reported chemotherapy side effects in routine care: A prospective cohort study. *PLoS ONE* **2017**, *12*, e0184360. [CrossRef] [PubMed]
2. Barzaman, K.; Karami, J.; Zarei, Z.; Hosseinzadeh, A.; Kazemi, M.H.; Moradi-Kalbolandi, S.; Safari, E.; Farahmand, L. Breast cancer: Biology, biomarkers, and treatments. *Int. Immunopharmacol.* **2020**, *84*, 106535. [CrossRef]
3. Hsu, J.Y.; Chang, C.J.; Cheng, J.S. Survival, treatment regimens and medical costs of women newly diagnosed with metastatic triple-negative breast cancer. *Sci. Rep.* **2022**, *12*, 729. [CrossRef] [PubMed]
4. Sharma, D.; Singh, G. An institutional analysis of clinicopathological features of triple negative breast cancer. *Indian J. Cancer* **2016**, *53*, 566–568. [CrossRef] [PubMed]
5. Dieci, M.V.; Tsvetkova, V.; Orvieto, E.; Piacentini, F.; Ficarra, G.; Griguolo, G.; Miglietta, F.; Giarratano, T.; Omarini, C.; Bonaguro, S.; et al. Immune characterization of breast cancer metastases: Prognostic implications. *Breast Cancer Res.* **2018**, *20*, 62. [CrossRef]
6. Loi, S.; Michiels, S.; Salgado, R.; Sirtaine, N.; Jose, V.; Fumagalli, D.; Kellokumpu-Lehtinen, P.L.; Bono, P.; Kataja, V.; Desmedt, C.; et al. Tumor infiltrating lymphocytes are prognostic in triple negative breast cancer and predictive for trastuzumab benefit in early breast cancer: Results from the FinHER trial. *Ann. Oncol.* **2014**, *25*, 1544–1550. [CrossRef]
7. Sanchez, K.; Page, D.; McArthur, H.L. Immunotherapy in breast cancer: An overview of modern checkpoint blockade strategies and vaccines. *Curr. Probl. Cancer* **2016**, *40*, 151–162. [CrossRef]
8. Abdou, Y.; Goudarzi, A.; Yu, J.X.; Upadhaya, S.; Vincent, B.; Carey, L.A. Immunotherapy in triple negative breast cancer: Beyond checkpoint inhibitors. *npj Breast Cancer* **2022**, *8*, 121. [CrossRef]
9. Aly, H.A. Cancer therapy and vaccination. *J. Immunol. Methods* **2012**, *382*, 1–23. [CrossRef]
10. Kassam, F.; Enright, K.; Dent, R.; Dranitsaris, G.; Myers, J.; Flynn, C.; Fralick, M.; Kumar, R.; Clemons, M. Survival outcomes for patients with metastatic triple-negative breast cancer: Implications for clinical practice and trial design. *Clin. Breast Cancer* **2009**, *9*, 29–33. [CrossRef] [PubMed]
11. Srimuninnimit, V.; Pornpraserthsuk, P.; Chaiwerawattana, A.; Kongdan, Y.; Namkanisorn, T.; Somwangprasert, A.; Jatuparisuthi, C.; Puttawibul, P.; Vongsaisuwan, M.; Thongthieang, L.; et al. Real-life clinical pattern, management, and survival in Thai patients with early-stage or metastatic triple-negative breast cancer. *PLoS ONE* **2018**, *13*, e0209040. [CrossRef]
12. Pogoda, K.; Niwińska, A.; Murawska, M.; Pieńkowski, T. Analysis of pattern, time and risk factors influencing recurrence in triple-negative breast cancer patients. *Med. Oncol.* **2013**, *30*, 388. [CrossRef]
13. Gatalica, Z.; Snyder, C.; Maney, T.; Ghazalpour, A.; Holterman, D.A.; Xiao, N.; Overberg, P.; Rose, I.; Basu, G.D.; Vranic, S.; et al. Programmed cell death 1 (PD-1) and its ligand (PD-L1) in common cancers and their correlation with molecular cancer type. *Cancer Epidemiol. Biomark. Prev.* **2014**, *23*, 2965–2970. [CrossRef]
14. Pandey, A.; Shrivastava, A.; Solanki, A. Study of atherogenic lipid profile, high sensitive C-reactive protein neurological deficit and short-term outcome in stroke subtypes. *Iran. J. Neurol.* **2016**, *15*, 146–152. [PubMed]
15. Park, J.H.; Lee, H.J.; Lee, S.B.; Ahn, J.H.; Kim, J.E.; Jung, K.H.; Gong, G.; Son, B.H.; Ahn, S.H.; Kim, S.B. Intrinsic Prognostic Impact of Tumor-infiltrating Lymphocytes in Systemically Untreated Patients With Early-stage Triple-negative Breast Cancer. *Anticancer. Res.* **2019**, *39*, 3111–3119. [CrossRef] [PubMed]

16. Chu, J.; Yeo, M.K.; Lee, S.H.; Lee, M.Y.; Chae, S.W.; Kim, H.S.; Do, S.I. Clinicopathological and Prognostic Significance of Programmed Death Ligand-1 SP142 Expression in 132 Patients with Triple-negative Breast Cancer. *In Vivo* **2022**, *36*, 2890–2898. [CrossRef]
17. Yeong, J.; Lim, J.C.T.; Lee, B.; Li, H.; Ong, C.C.H.; Thike, A.A.; Yeap, W.H.; Yang, Y.; Lim, A.Y.H.; Tay, T.K.Y.; et al. Prognostic value of CD8 + PD-1+ immune infiltrates and PDCD1 gene expression in triple negative breast cancer. *J. Immunother. Cancer* **2019**, *7*, 34. [CrossRef] [PubMed]
18. Karn, T.; Denkert, C.; Weber, K.E.; Holtrich, U.; Hanusch, C.; Sinn, B.V.; Higgs, B.W.; Jank, P.; Sinn, H.P.; Huober, J.; et al. Tumor mutational burden and immune infiltration as independent predictors of response to neoadjuvant immune checkpoint inhibition in early TNBC in GeparNuevo. *Ann. Oncol.* **2020**, *31*, 1216–1222. [CrossRef]
19. Schmid, P.; Adams, S.; Rugo, H.S.; Schneeweiss, A.; Barrios, C.H.; Iwata, H.; Diéras, V.; Hegg, R.; Im, S.A.; Shaw Wright, G.; et al. Atezolizumab and Nab-Paclitaxel in Advanced Triple-Negative Breast Cancer. *N. Engl. J. Med.* **2018**, *379*, 2108–2121. [CrossRef]
20. Keenan, T.E.; Tolaney, S.M. Role of Immunotherapy in Triple-Negative Breast Cancer. *J. Natl. Compr. Canc Netw.* **2020**, *18*, 479–489. [CrossRef]
21. Taylor, E. Pembrolizumab with Carboplatin/Paclitaxel and EC Neoadjuvant Breast Cancer Regimen followed by Adjuvant Pembrolizumab. 2024. Available online: https://www.uhs.nhs.uk/Media/UHS-website-2019/Docs/Chemotherapy-SOPs1/Breastcancer/Carboplatin-Paclitaxel-EC-Pembrolizumab-Neoadjuvant.pdf (accessed on 30 October 2024).
22. NHS. *Atezolizumab/Paclitaxel Albumin (Abraxane) Triple Negative Breast Cancer, PDL1 Positive*; NICE: Manchester, UK, 2020.
23. Gajaria, P.K.; Gupta, M.R.; Patil, A.; Desai, S.B.; Shet, T.M. Programmed cell death ligand-1 expression in triple negative breast carcinoma and its prognostic significance in Indian population. *Indian J. Pathol. Microbiol.* **2021**, *64*, 664–670. [CrossRef]
24. Kim, H.S.; Do, S.I.; Kim, D.H.; Apple, S. Clinicopathological and Prognostic Significance of Programmed Death Ligand 1 Expression in Korean Patients With Triple-negative Breast Carcinoma. *Anticancer. Res.* **2020**, *40*, 1487–1494. [CrossRef]
25. Spurrell, E.L.; Lockley, M. Adaptive immunity in cancer immunology and therapeutics. *Ecancermedicalscience* **2014**, *8*, 441. [CrossRef] [PubMed]
26. Liu, J.; Fu, M.; Wang, M.; Wan, D.; Wei, Y.; Wei, X. Cancer vaccines as promising immuno-therapeutics: Platforms and current progress. *J. Hematol. Oncol.* **2022**, *15*, 28. [CrossRef] [PubMed]
27. Schneble, E.; Clifton, G.T.; Hale, D.F.; Peoples, G.E. Peptide-Based Cancer Vaccine Strategies and Clinical Results. *Methods Mol. Biol.* **2016**, *1403*, 797–817. [CrossRef] [PubMed]
28. Slingluff, C.L., Jr. The present and future of peptide vaccines for cancer: Single or multiple, long or short, alone or in combination? *Cancer J.* **2011**, *17*, 343–350. [CrossRef]
29. Ge, C.; Li, R.; Song, H.; Geng, T.; Yang, J.; Tan, Q.; Song, L.; Wang, Y.; Xue, Y.; Li, Z.; et al. Phase I clinical trial of a novel autologous modified-DC vaccine in patients with resected NSCLC. *BMC Cancer* **2017**, *17*, 884. [CrossRef]
30. Kaufman, H.L.; Kohlhapp, F.J.; Zloza, A. Oncolytic viruses: A new class of immunotherapy drugs. *Nat. Rev. Drug Discov.* **2015**, *14*, 642–662. [CrossRef]
31. Qin, F.; Xia, F.; Chen, H.; Cui, B.; Feng, Y.; Zhang, P.; Chen, J.; Luo, M. A Guide to Nucleic Acid Vaccines in the Prevention and Treatment of Infectious Diseases and Cancers: From Basic Principles to Current Applications. *Front. Cell Dev. Biol.* **2021**, *9*, 633776. [CrossRef]
32. Ten Ham, R.M.T.; Hövels, A.M.; Hoekman, J.; Frederix, G.W.J.; Leufkens, H.G.M.; Klungel, O.H.; Jedema, I.; Veld, S.A.J.; Nikolic, T.; Van Pel, M.; et al. What does cell therapy manufacturing cost? A framework and methodology to facilitate academic and other small-scale cell therapy manufacturing costings. *Cytotherapy* **2020**, *22*, 388–397. [CrossRef] [PubMed]
33. Larocca, C.; Schlom, J. Viral vector-based therapeutic cancer vaccines. *Cancer J.* **2011**, *17*, 359–371. [CrossRef] [PubMed]
34. Orrantia-Borunda, E.; Anchondo-Nuñez, P.; Acuña-Aguilar, L.E.; Gómez-Valles, F.O.; Ramírez-Valdespino, C.A. Subtypes of Breast Cancer. In *Breast Cancer*; Mayrovitz, H.N., Ed.; Exon Publications: Brisbane, Australia, 2022.
35. NABCOP. *National Audit of Breast Cancer in Older Patients*; NABCOP: London, UK, 2022; p. 94.
36. Sun, L.; Cromwell, D.; Dodwell, D.; Horgan, K.; Gannon, M.R.; Medina, J.; Pennington, M.; Legood, R.; Dos-Santos-Silva, I.; Sadique, Z. Costs of Early Invasive Breast Cancer in England Using National Patient-Level Data. *Value Health* **2020**, *23*, 1316–1323. [CrossRef]
37. Liu, M.; MacKenna, B.; Feldman, W.B.; Walker, A.J.; Avorn, J.; Kesselheim, A.S.; Goldacre, B. Projected spending for brand-name drugs in English primary care given US prices: A cross-sectional study. *J. R. Soc. Med.* **2020**, *113*, 350–359. [CrossRef]
38. Ward, M.C.; Vicini, F.; Al-Hilli, Z.; Chadha, M.; Abraham, A.; Recht, A.; Hayman, J.; Thaker, N.; Khan, A.J.; Keisch, M.; et al. Cost-Effectiveness Analysis of No Adjuvant Therapy Versus Partial Breast Irradiation Alone Versus Combined Treatment for Treatment of Low-Risk DCIS: A Microsimulation. *JCO Oncol. Pract.* **2021**, *17*, e1055–e1074. [CrossRef] [PubMed]
39. Remák, E.; Brazil, L. Cost of managing women presenting with stage IV breast cancer in the United Kingdom. *Br. J. Cancer* **2004**, *91*, 77–83. [CrossRef] [PubMed]

40. Braybrooke, J. Carboplatin & Weekly Paclitaxel / EC (Epirubicin & Cyclophosphamide) with Pembrolizumab (Breast). Somerset, Wiltshire, Avon and Gloucestershire Cancer Alliance. 2022. Available online: https://www.swagcanceralliance.nhs.uk/wp-content/uploads/2022/10/Pembro-Carbo-Wkly-Taxol-EC-v1.pdf (accessed on 30 March 2024).
41. NICE. Final appraisal document—Atezolizumab with nab-paclitaxel for treating PD-L1-positive, triple-negative, advanced breast cancer. 2020. Available online: https://www.nice.org.uk/guidance/ta639/documents/final-appraisal-determination-document (accessed on 30 March 2024).
42. Mørk, S.K.; Kadivar, M.; Bol, K.F.; Draghi, A.; Westergaard, M.C.W.; Skadborg, S.K.; Overgaard, N.; Sørensen, A.B.; Rasmussen, I.S.; Andreasen, L.V.; et al. Personalized therapy with peptide-based neoantigen vaccine (EVX-01) including a novel adjuvant, CAF®09b, in patients with metastatic melanoma. *Oncoimmunology* **2022**, *11*, 2023255. [CrossRef] [PubMed]
43. Biswas, N.; Chakrabarti, S.; Padul, V.; Jones, L.D.; Ashili, S. Designing neoantigen cancer vaccines, trials, and outcomes. *Front. Immunol.* **2023**, *14*, 1105420. [CrossRef] [PubMed]
44. Rugo, H. Study of Adagloxad Simolenin (OBI-822)/OBI-821 in the Adjuvant Treatment of Patients with Globo H Positive TNBC. 2018. Available online: https://clinicaltrials.gov/study/NCT03562637 (accessed on 20 December 2024).
45. Blass, E.; Ott, P.A. Advances in the development of personalized neoantigen-based therapeutic cancer vaccines. *Nat. Rev. Clin. Oncol.* **2021**, *18*, 215–229. [CrossRef]
46. Bayle, A.; Droin, N.; Besse, B.; Zou, Z.; Boursin, Y.; Rissel, S.; Solary, E.; Lacroix, L.; Rouleau, E.; Borget, I.; et al. Whole exome sequencing in molecular diagnostics of cancer decreases over time: Evidence from a cost analysis in the French setting. *Eur. J. Health Econ.* **2021**, *22*, 855–864. [CrossRef] [PubMed]
47. GenScript. Custom Peptide Services. 2024. Available online: https://www.genscript.com/peptide.html#resources (accessed on 2 February 2024). The original source has been removed from the website by GenScript between data anlysis and publishing. The relevant information can be requested by contacting GenScript.
48. Merck. Polyinosinic–Polycytidylic Acid Potassium Salt. 2024. Available online: https://www.sigmaaldrich.com/GB/en/product/sigma/p9582?srsltid=AfmBOopeWScrbVvYOTkA3PBPW1vxG1J7-I71wU2t4nPLJsFz9t8YE6HY (accessed on 4 February 2024).
49. Pollack, A.F.D.A. Approves 'Vaccine' to Fight Prostate Cancer. 2010. Available online: https://www.nytimes.com/2010/04/30/health/30drug.html (accessed on 2 February 2024).
50. Jiang, T.; Shi, T.; Zhang, H.; Hu, J.; Song, Y.; Wei, J.; Ren, S.; Zhou, C. Tumor neoantigens: From basic research to clinical applications. *J. Hematol. Oncol.* **2019**, *12*, 93. [CrossRef] [PubMed]
51. Brito Baleeiro, R.; Liu, P.; Chard Dunmall, L.S.; Di Gioia, C.; Nagano, A.; Cutmore, L.; Wang, J.; Chelala, C.; Nyambura, L.W.; Walden, P.; et al. Personalized neoantigen viro-immunotherapy platform for triple-negative breast cancer. *J. Immunother. Cancer* **2023**, *11*. [CrossRef] [PubMed]
52. Melief, C.J.M.; van der Burg, S.H. Immunotherapy of established (pre)malignant disease by synthetic long peptide vaccines. *Nat. Rev. Cancer* **2008**, *8*, 351–360. [CrossRef] [PubMed]
53. Chen, X.; Yang, J.; Wang, L.; Liu, B. Personalized neoantigen vaccination with synthetic long peptides: Recent advances and future perspectives. *Theranostics* **2020**, *10*, 6011–6023. [CrossRef] [PubMed]
54. Kreiter, S.; Vormehr, M.; van de Roemer, N.; Diken, M.; Löwer, M.; Diekmann, J.; Boegel, S.; Schrörs, B.; Vascotto, F.; Castle, J.C.; et al. Mutant MHC class II epitopes drive therapeutic immune responses to cancer. *Nature* **2015**, *520*, 692–696. [CrossRef] [PubMed]
55. Takeoka, T.; Nagase, H.; Kurose, K.; Ohue, Y.; Yamasaki, M.; Takiguchi, S.; Sato, E.; Isobe, M.; Kanazawa, T.; Matsumoto, M.; et al. NY-ESO-1 Protein Cancer Vaccine With Poly-ICLC and OK-432: Rapid and Strong Induction of NY-ESO-1-specific Immune Responses by Poly-ICLC. *J. Immunother.* **2017**, *40*, 140–147. [CrossRef]
56. Wang, C.; Zhuang, Y.; Zhang, Y.; Luo, Z.; Gao, N.; Li, P.; Pan, H.; Cai, L.; Ma, Y. Toll-like receptor 3 agonist complexed with cationic liposome augments vaccine-elicited antitumor immunity by enhancing TLR3-IRF3 signaling and type I interferons in dendritic cells. *Vaccine* **2012**, *30*, 4790–4799. [CrossRef]
57. Zhang, X.; Goedegebuure, S.P.; Myers, N.B.; Vickery, T.; McLellan, M.D.; Gao, F.; Sturmoski, M.A.; Chen, M.Y.; Kim, S.W.; Chen, I.; et al. Neoantigen DNA vaccines are safe, feasible, and capable of inducing neoantigen-specific immune responses in patients with triple negative breast cancer. *medRxiv* **2024**, *16*, 131. [CrossRef]
58. Zaidi, N. Can Personalized Neoantigens Raise the T Cell Bar? *Cell* **2020**, *183*, 301–302. [CrossRef] [PubMed]
59. Yadav, M.; Jhunjhunwala, S.; Phung, Q.T.; Lupardus, P.; Tanguay, J.; Bumbaca, S.; Franci, C.; Cheung, T.K.; Fritsche, J.; Weinschenk, T.; et al. Predicting immunogenic tumour mutations by combining mass spectrometry and exome sequencing. *Nature* **2014**, *515*, 572–576. [CrossRef] [PubMed]
60. Xu, C. A review of somatic single nucleotide variant calling algorithms for next-generation sequencing data. *Comput. Struct. Biotechnol. J.* **2018**, *16*, 15–24. [CrossRef] [PubMed]
61. Ott, P.A.; Hu, Z.; Keskin, D.B.; Shukla, S.A.; Sun, J.; Bozym, D.J.; Zhang, W.; Luoma, A.; Giobbie-Hurder, A.; Peter, L.; et al. An immunogenic personal neoantigen vaccine for patients with melanoma. *Nature* **2017**, *547*, 217–221. [CrossRef]

62. Barnell, E.K.; Ronning, P.; Campbell, K.M.; Krysiak, K.; Ainscough, B.J.; Sheta, L.M.; Pema, S.P.; Schmidt, A.D.; Richters, M.; Cotto, K.C.; et al. Standard operating procedure for somatic variant refinement of sequencing data with paired tumor and normal samples. *Genet. Med.* **2019**, *21*, 972–981. [CrossRef]
63. Mansfield, A.S.; Peikert, T.; Smadbeck, J.B.; Udell, J.B.M.; Garcia-Rivera, E.; Elsbernd, L.; Erskine, C.L.; Van Keulen, V.P.; Kosari, F.; Murphy, S.J.; et al. Neoantigenic Potential of Complex Chromosomal Rearrangements in Mesothelioma. *J. Thorac. Oncol.* **2019**, *14*, 276–287. [CrossRef] [PubMed]
64. Wang, M.Y.; Huang, M.; Wang, C.Y.; Tang, X.Y.; Wang, J.G.; Yang, Y.D.; Xiong, X.; Gao, C.W. Transcriptome Analysis Reveals MFGE8-HAPLN3 Fusion as a Novel Biomarker in Triple-Negative Breast Cancer. *Front. Oncol.* **2021**, *11*, 682021. [CrossRef] [PubMed]
65. Biernacki, M.A.; Foster, K.A.; Woodward, K.B.; Coon, M.E.; Cummings, C.; Cunningham, T.M.; Dossa, R.G.; Brault, M.; Stokke, J.; Olsen, T.M.; et al. CBFB-MYH11 fusion neoantigen enables T cell recognition and killing of acute myeloid leukemia. *J. Clin. Investig.* **2020**, *130*, 5127–5141. [CrossRef] [PubMed]
66. Robinson, J.; Halliwell, J.A.; Hayhurst, J.D.; Flicek, P.; Parham, P.; Marsh, S.G. The IPD and IMGT/HLA database: Allele variant databases. *Nucleic Acids Res.* **2015**, *43*, D423–D431. [CrossRef]
67. Kiyotani, K.; Mai, T.H.; Nakamura, Y. Comparison of exome-based HLA class I genotyping tools: Identification of platform-specific genotyping errors. *J. Hum. Genet.* **2017**, *62*, 397–405. [CrossRef] [PubMed]
68. Richters, M.M.; Xia, H.; Campbell, K.M.; Gillanders, W.E.; Griffith, O.L.; Griffith, M. Best practices for bioinformatic characterization of neoantigens for clinical utility. *Genome Med.* **2019**, *11*, 56. [CrossRef] [PubMed]
69. Jurtz, V.; Paul, S.; Andreatta, M.; Marcatili, P.; Peters, B.; Nielsen, M. NetMHCpan-4.0: Improved Peptide-MHC Class I Interaction Predictions Integrating Eluted Ligand and Peptide Binding Affinity Data. *J. Immunol.* **2017**, *199*, 3360–3368. [CrossRef]
70. Calis, J.J.; Reinink, P.; Keller, C.; Kloetzel, P.M.; Keşmir, C. Role of peptide processing predictions in T cell epitope identification: Contribution of different prediction programs. *Immunogenetics* **2015**, *67*, 85–93. [CrossRef]
71. Calis, J.J.; Maybeno, M.; Greenbaum, J.A.; Weiskopf, D.; De Silva, A.D.; Sette, A.; Keşmir, C.; Peters, B. Properties of MHC class I presented peptides that enhance immunogenicity. *PLoS Comput. Biol.* **2013**, *9*, e1003266. [CrossRef] [PubMed]
72. Castle, J.C.; Kreiter, S.; Diekmann, J.; Löwer, M.; van de Roemer, N.; de Graaf, J.; Selmi, A.; Diken, M.; Boegel, S.; Paret, C.; et al. Exploiting the mutanome for tumor vaccination. *Cancer Res.* **2012**, *72*, 1081–1091. [CrossRef] [PubMed]
73. Aparicio, B.; Repáraz, D.; Ruiz, M.; Llopiz, D.; Silva, L.; Vercher, E.; Theunissen, P.; Tamayo, I.; Smerdou, C.; Igea, A.; et al. Identification of HLA class I-restricted immunogenic neoantigens in triple negative breast cancer. *Front. Immunol.* **2022**, *13*, 985886. [CrossRef] [PubMed]
74. Leoni, G.; D'Alise, A.M.; Tucci, F.G.; Micarelli, E.; Garzia, I.; De Lucia, M.; Langone, F.; Nocchi, L.; Cotugno, G.; Bartolomeo, R.; et al. VENUS, a Novel Selection Approach to Improve the Accuracy of Neoantigens' Prediction. *Vaccines* **2021**, *9*, 880. [CrossRef]
75. Kumai, T.; Kobayashi, H.; Harabuchi, Y.; Celis, E. Peptide vaccines in cancer-old concept revisited. *Curr. Opin. Immunol.* **2017**, *45*, 1–7. [CrossRef] [PubMed]
76. Corradin, G.; Kajava, A.V.; Verdini, A. Long Synthetic Peptides for the Production of Vaccines and Drugs: A Technological Platform Coming of Age. *Sci. Transl. Med.* **2010**, *2*, 50rv3. [CrossRef] [PubMed]
77. Mijalis, A.J.; Thomas, D.A., III; Simon, M.D.; Adamo, A.; Beaumont, R.; Jensen, K.F.; Pentelute, B.L. A fully automated flow-based approach for accelerated peptide synthesis. *Nat. Chem. Biol.* **2017**, *13*, 464–466. [CrossRef]
78. Demine, R.; Sherev, T.; Walden, P. Biochemical determination of natural tumor-associated T-cell epitopes. *Mol. Biotechnol.* **2003**, *25*, 71–78. [CrossRef] [PubMed]
79. Hara, T.; Tainosho, A.; Nakamura, K.; Sato, T.; Kawakami, T.; Aimoto, S. Peptide purification by affinity chromatography based on alpha-ketoacyl group chemistry. *J. Pept. Sci.* **2009**, *15*, 369–376. [CrossRef] [PubMed]
80. Hossain, M.A.; Belgi, A.; Lin, F.; Zhang, S.; Shabanpoor, F.; Chan, L.; Belyea, C.; Truong, H.T.; Blair, A.R.; Andrikopoulos, S.; et al. Use of a temporary "solubilizing" peptide tag for the Fmoc solid-phase synthesis of human insulin glargine via use of regioselective disulfide bond formation. *Bioconjug Chem.* **2009**, *20*, 1390–1396. [CrossRef] [PubMed]
81. Villain, M.; Vizzavona, J.; Rose, K. Covalent capture: A new tool for the purification of synthetic and recombinant polypeptides. *Chem. Biol.* **2001**, *8*, 673–679. [CrossRef] [PubMed]
82. Rubinsteyn, A.; Hodes, I.; Kodysh, J.; Hammerbacher, J. Vaxrank: A computational tool for designing personalized cancer vaccines. *bioRxiv* **2017**. [CrossRef]
83. Hailemichael, Y.; Dai, Z.; Jaffarzad, N.; Ye, Y.; Medina, M.A.; Huang, X.F.; Dorta-Estremera, S.M.; Greeley, N.R.; Nitti, G.; Peng, W.; et al. Persistent antigen at vaccination sites induces tumor-specific $CD8^+$ T cell sequestration, dysfunction and deletion. *Nat. Med.* **2013**, *19*, 465–472. [CrossRef] [PubMed]
84. ClinicalTrials.gov. Safety and Immunogenicity of a Personalized Synthetic Long Peptide Breast Cancer Vaccine Strategy in Patients with Persistent Triple-Negative Breast Cancer Following Neoadjuvant Chemotherapy. Available online: https://clinicaltrials.gov/study/NCT02427581?cond=TNBC,%20Triple%20Negative%20Breast%20Cancer&term=cancer%20vaccine&limit=100&page=1&rank=18 (accessed on 20 February 2024).

85. ClinicalTrials.gov. Testing the Addition of an Individualized Vaccine to Nab-Paclitaxel, Durvalumab and Tremelimumab and Chemotherapy in Patients with Metastatic Triple Negative Breast Cancer. Available online: https://clinicaltrials.gov/study/NCT03606967?cond=TNBC,%20Triple%20Negative%20Breast%20Cancer&term=cancer%20vaccine&limit=100&page=1&rank=31 (accessed on 20 February 2024).
86. Nemunaitis, J.; Senzer, N.; Olivares, J.; Kumar, P.; Barve, M.; Kuhn, J.; Nemunaitis, T.; Magee, M.; Yu, Y.; Wallraven, G.; et al. Immune response and survival of refractory cancer patients who received TGF-β2 antisense/GM-CSF gene modified autologous tumor cell (TAG) vaccine. *Gene Ther.* **2013**, *20*, 875–879. [CrossRef]
87. Whiteside, T.L. Methods to monitor immune response and quality control. *Dev. Biol.* **2004**, *116*, 219–228; discussion 229–236.
88. Shahnazari, M.; Samadi, P.; Pourjafar, M.; Jalali, A. Therapeutic vaccines for colorectal cancer: The progress and future prospect. *Int. Immunopharmacol.* **2020**, *88*, 106944. [CrossRef]
89. Huang, M.; Haiderali, A.; Fox, G.E.; Frederickson, A.; Cortes, J.; Fasching, P.A.; O'Shaughnessy, J. Economic and Humanistic Burden of Triple-Negative Breast Cancer: A Systematic Literature Review. *Pharmacoeconomics* **2022**, *40*, 519–558. [CrossRef]
90. Hall, P.S.; Hamilton, P.; Hulme, C.T.; Meads, D.M.; Jones, H.; Newsham, A.; Marti, J.; Smith, A.F.; Mason, H.; Velikova, G.; et al. Costs of cancer care for use in economic evaluation: A UK analysis of patient-level routine health system data. *Br. J. Cancer* **2015**, *112*, 948–956. [CrossRef] [PubMed]
91. Bajpai, J.; Kashyap, L.; Vallathol, D.H.; Das, A.; Singh, M.; Pathak, R.; Rath, S.; Sekar, A.; Mohanta, S.; Reddy, A.; et al. Outcomes of non-metastatic triple negative breast cancers: Real-world data from a large Indian cohort. *Breast* **2022**, *63*, 77–84. [CrossRef]
92. Njoroge, M.W.; Walton, M.; Hodgson, R. Understanding the National Institute for Health and Care Excellence Severity Premium: Exploring Its Implementation and the Implications for Decision Making and Patient Access. *Value Health* **2024**, *27*, 730–736. [CrossRef] [PubMed]
93. Cortes, J.; Rugo, H.S.; Cescon, D.W.; Im, S.A.; Yusof, M.M.; Gallardo, C.; Lipatov, O.; Barrios, C.H.; Perez-Garcia, J.; Iwata, H.; et al. Pembrolizumab plus Chemotherapy in Advanced Triple-Negative Breast Cancer. *N. Engl. J. Med.* **2022**, *387*, 217–226. [CrossRef]
94. NICE. Atezolizumab with Nabpaclitaxel for Untreated PD-L1-positive, Locally Advanced or Metastatic, Triple-Negative Breast Cancer. 2020. Available online: https://www.nice.org.uk/guidance/ta639 (accessed on 30 March 2024).
95. Cortes, J.; Cescon, D.W.; Rugo, H.S.; Nowecki, Z.; Im, S.A.; Yusof, M.M.; Gallardo, C.; Lipatov, O.; Barrios, C.H.; Holgado, E.; et al. Pembrolizumab plus chemotherapy versus placebo plus chemotherapy for previously untreated locally recurrent inoperable or metastatic triple-negative breast cancer (KEYNOTE-355): A randomised, placebo-controlled, double-blind, phase 3 clinical trial. *Lancet* **2020**, *396*, 1817–1828. [CrossRef] [PubMed]

vaccines

MDPI

Article

Development of a Recombinant Fusion Vaccine Candidate Against Lethal *Clostridium botulinum* Neurotoxin Types A and B

Eun-Sun Choi [1], Seong-Wook Pyo [1], So-Hyeon Kim [1], Jun-Ho Jeon [2], Gi-Eun Rhie [3], Mi-Ran Yun [4], Hwajung Yi [1] and Yoon-Seok Chung [1,*]

1 Division of High-Risk Pathogens, Department of Laboratory Diagnosis and Analysis, Korea Disease Control and Prevention Agency, KDCA, Cheongju 28159, Republic of Korea; pearlces86@korea.kr (E.-S.C.); swde29@korea.kr (S.-W.P.); ssonaki82@korea.kr (S.-H.K.); pobee@korea.kr (H.Y.)

2 Division of Infectious Disease Diagnosis, Chungcheong Regional Center for Disease Control and Prevention, Korea Disease Control and Prevention Agency, KDCA, Cheongju 28159, Republic of Korea; jhjeon78@korea.kr

3 Director General, Center for Vaccine Research, National Institute of Health, Korea Disease Control and Prevention Agency, KDCA, Cheongju 28159, Republic of Korea

4 Division of Infectious Disease Vaccine Research, Center for Vaccine Research, National Institute of Health, Korea Disease Control and Prevention Agency, KDCA, Cheongju 28159, Republic of Korea; ivareve125@korea.kr

* Correspondence: rollstone93@korea.kr; Tel.: +82-43-719-8270

Abstract: Background: Botulinum neurotoxins (BoNTs), produced by *Clostridium botulinum*, are potent protein toxins that can cause botulism, which leads to death or neuroparalysis in humans by targeting the nervous system. BoNTs comprise three functional domains: a light-chain enzymatic domain (LC), a heavy-chain translocation domain (HC_N), and a heavy-chain receptor-binding domain (HC_C). The HC_C domain is critical for binding to neuronal cell membrane receptors and facilitating BoNT internalization via endocytosis. Accordingly, it may serve as a vaccine candidate, inducing anti-BoNT-neutralizing antibodies in animals. Here, we aimed to develop a vaccine capable of simultaneously defending against both BoNT/A and B. Methods: We combined the HC_C domains of botulinum neurotoxin type A (BoNT/A) and botulinum neurotoxin type B (BoNT/B) in *Escherichia coli* to produce a recombinant protein (rHC_CB-L-HC_CArHCcB) that offers dual protection against both toxins by inhibiting their receptor binding. To evaluate the efficacy of the vaccine, mice were immunized intramuscularly with rHC_CB-L-HC_CA plus alum thrice at 2-week intervals, followed by the assessment of immunogenicity and protective efficacy. Results: The antibody titer in mice immunized with rHC_CB-L-HC_CA was significantly higher than that in mice immunized with alum alone, protecting them from the lethal challenges of BoNT/A (10^5 50% lethal dose, LD_{50}) and B (10^3 LD_{50}). Conclusion: These findings suggest that rHC_CB-L-HC_CA may simultaneously be an effective vaccine candidate against BoNT/A and B.

Keywords: *Clostridium botulinum*; botulism; neurotoxin; fusion vaccine; receptor binding domain

1. Introduction

Botulinum neurotoxins (BoNTs), produced by the bacterium *Clostridium botulinum*, are the primary agents responsible for botulism and rank among the most lethal substances known. These toxins are classified into eight serotypes (A–H), each with a similar structure but distinct antigenic properties [1–3]. BoNTs are initially synthesized as single polypeptide chains, which are then post-translationally cleaved into dichains consisting of a 100 kDa

https://doi.org/10.3390/vaccines13010039

heavy chain (HC) and a 50 kDa light chain (LC) connected by a disulfide bond. The HC is further subdivided into two functionally independent domains: the N-terminal translocation domain (HC_N) and the C-terminal receptor-binding domain (HC_C) [4]. The HC_N (~50 kDa) facilitates the transport of the LC across the endosomal membrane, whereas the HC_C (~50 kDa) is essential for binding to specific receptors on cholinergic nerve cells. BoNTs achieve high affinity and specificity for neurons by binding to two receptors: gangliosides and one of the synaptic vesicle proteins, either synaptotagmin (Syt) or synaptic vesicle protein 2 (SV2). BoNT/A uses SV2 as its protein receptor, whereas BoNT/B binds to Syt, specifically the Syt-I and Syt-II isoforms [5,6]. After receptor binding, the toxin is internalized into endosomes via receptor-mediated endocytosis. LC acts as a zinc-dependent endoprotease that selectively cleaves three crucial proteins involved in the docking and fusion of acetylcholine-containing synaptic vesicles with the plasma membrane. The inactivation of a synaptosomal-associated protein of 25 kDa, synaptic vesicle-associated membrane protein, or syntaxin by BoNTs prevents acetylcholine release, leading to neuromuscular paralysis. When exposed to BoNTs, early symptoms may include ptosis, ambiopia, blurred vision, dysphonia, and a dry, sore throat. High doses of BoNT can cause respiratory muscle paralysis, leading to dyspnea, respiratory failure, and potentially death [7–9].

Botulism can occur naturally following the colonization of the gastrointestinal tract by neurotoxigenic clostridia (infant or intestinal botulism), consumption of contaminated food (foodborne botulism), or anaerobic wound infections (wound botulism) [10]. The Centers for Disease Control and Prevention (CDC) has reported an average of 208 cases annually between 2015 and 2019 [11]. While botulism is rare in South Korea, the Korea Disease Control and Prevention Agency (KDCA) conducts annual diagnostic tests to detect and confirm cases of the disease. From 2003 to 2024, eleven cases of botulism were reported. Of these, eight cases were foodborne botulism, one case was infant botulism, and two cases occurred through an unknown route. Among the eleven patients, serotypes A (three cases) and B (four cases) were the most common, although these cases occurred in 2003 and 2004, respectively [12]. Since 2019, one case of each serotype Ab, Bf, and E has been reported. In the first case of infant botulism, we described the genome of *C. botulinum* type Ab, which contains two different toxin genes [13]. In the USA, where bivalent toxins have been continuously monitored since their discovery in 1976 [14], cases caused by the bivalent strains Ab, Ba, and Bf account for only 2% (30/1514) of all infant botulism cases [15]. However, three-quarters of patients with bivalent strain-induced botulism experienced respiratory failure during hospitalization, suggesting that patients with bivalent toxin may require more urgent treatment.

Pentavalent botulinum toxoid (PBT) is used as an investigational drug by the CDC for military and research personnel exposed to the toxin. However, PBT has not received FDA approval because of numerous shortcomings in its existing form. The development of new-generation recombinant vaccines may alleviate many such problems associated with toxoids [16]. Due to their extreme toxicity, botulinum toxins have been considered prime candidates for bioweapons, prompting the KDCA to research vaccines and treatments for over a decade to prepare for its potential use in terrorism. The threat is increasing worldwide, and South Korea faces heightened risks as a divided nation. Therefore, developing and stockpiling vaccines for military personnel, researchers, and other frontline personnel to prepare them against bioterrorism scenarios as well as natural occurrences is essential. Therefore, this study aimed to develop a vaccine capable of providing simultaneous protection against both BoNT/A and BoNT/B, addressing the critical need for effective countermeasures against bioterrorism and natural outbreaks.

2. Materials and Methods

2.1. Construction of Synthetic Genes and Cloning

Genes encoding the HCc fragments of BoNT/A (*hccA*, strain 19397; GenBank accession number NC_009697) and BoNT/B (*hccB*, strain Okra; GenBank accession number NC_010516), as well as the fused HCc of BoNT/B and A (hccB-linker-*hccA*), were synthesized by Bioneer Co. (Daejeon, South Korea). A (Gly)3 linker was introduced between the two HCc fragments to facilitate proper folding. After digestion with the restriction enzymes *Nde*I and *Bam*HI, the gene fragments were cloned into the pET19b vector for expression in *E. coli*. The gene sequences and their predicted structures are shown in Figure 1. Gene synthesis was conducted in compliance with the national regulations governing experiments involving genetically modified organisms. All the experimental procedures were performed in a biosafety laboratory and certified by the appropriate authority [17].

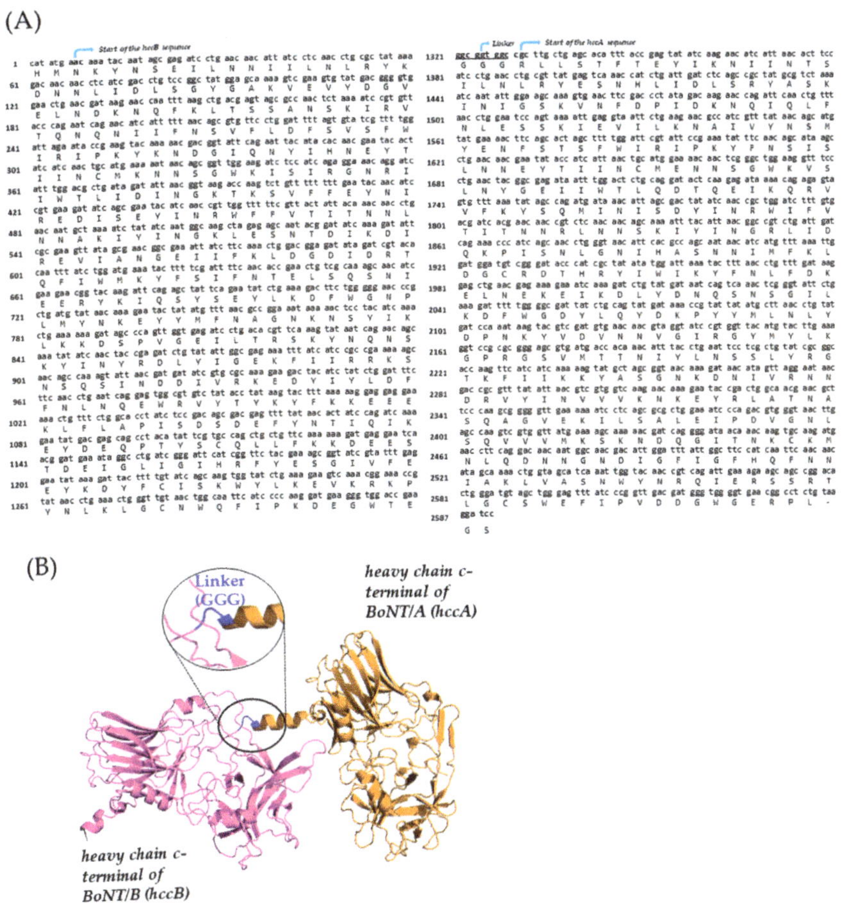

Figure 1. Gene sequence and predicted protein structure of rHCcB-L-HCcA. (**A**) The synthetic gene for rHCcB-L-HCcA expression in *Escherichia coli* is shown with its translated amino acid sequence below the nucleotide sequence. The initial codons of each subunit and the (Gly)3 linker codons are written in bold and marked with arrows. (**B**) Visualization of the three-dimensional structure of the rHCcB-L-HCcA construct, comprising rHCcB (violet), (Gly)3 linker (blue), and rHCcA (orange), predicted using the AlphaFold2 program.

2.2. Expression and Purification of Recombinant Antigens

Plasmids (pET19b-*hccA*, pET19b-*hccB*, and pET19b-*hccB-L-hccA*) were transformed into different *E. coli* strains to optimize expression: pET19b-*hccA* was transformed into *E. coli* BL21(DE3) RIPL Codon Plus cells, pET19b-*hccB* into *E. coli* BL21(DE3) pLysS cells, and pET19b-*hccB-L-hccA* into *E. coli* BL21(DE3) SoluBL21 cells. The cultures (400 mL for each strain) were grown in Terrific Broth, induced with 0.5 mM isopropyl-β-D-thiogalactopyranoside at an OD_{600} of 0.6 ± 0.1, and incubated at 16 °C for 96 h. The incubated *E. coli* were harvested by centrifugation and resuspended in lysis buffer (50 mM Tris-HCl, 1.5 M NaCl, 1 mM PMSF, 50 µg/mL lysozyme, and 0.1% Triton X100, pH 8.0). The lysed cells were centrifuged to remove the precipitate and filtered through a 0.45 µm disposable filter. The clear supernatant with rHCcA, rHCcB, and rHCcB-L-HCcA antigens was loaded onto a 20 mL column of Ni-NTA superflow (Qiagen, Hilden, Germany), which was equilibrated with 50 mM of Tris-HCl and 1.5 M of NaCl containing 5 mM of imidazole with pH 8.0. The column was washed with washing buffer of different concentrations (50 mM of Tris-HCl and 1.5 M of NaCl containing 60 or 80 mM of imidazole with pH 8.0). Bound rHCcA and rHCcB were eluted from the column using imidazole (50 mM of Tris-HCl and 1.5 M of NaCl containing 100, 200, or 400 mM imidazole with pH 8.0). The bound rHCcB-L-HCcA protein was similarly eluted (50 mM of Tris-HCl and 1.5 M of NaCl containing 250 or 500 mM of imidazole with pH 8.0). Each 5 µL protein sample collected during the purification process was mixed with a loading buffer and loaded onto an SDS-PAGE gel to assess the samples at each step of purification. The eluted proteins were subjected to a final purification step using a fast protein liquid chromatography system (FPLC, Bioneer, Daejeon, South Korea) equipped with a Superdex 200 size-exclusion column (Sigma, Darmstadt, Germany). A 1 mL volume of each eluted protein was loaded onto the column, and fractions containing proteins with a final concentration exceeding 0.5 mg/mL were collected. The eluted rHCcA, rHCcB, and rHCcB-L-HCcA proteins were subsequently dialyzed in 50 mM of sodium citrate buffer (pH 5.5) using a Slide-A-Lyzer Dialysis Cassette (Thermo Scientific, Waltham, MA, USA). The purified proteins were stored at −80 °C until further use.

2.3. Identification of Antigens

The BiolineTM Bioterror Pathogens and Toxins Test Kit (Abbott, Seoul, South Korea) was used to verify the identity of the purified antigens. This lateral flow assay, designed for the rapid detection of bioterrorism agents, was adapted to confirm the presence of the BoNT/A and B antigens. The strips were coated with antibodies specific for BoNT/A and B and designed to allow differential detection of the two toxin types on a single strip. Purified rHCcA, rHCcB, and rHCcB-L-HCcA antigens were mixed with the sample diluent, added to the cassette wells, and absorbed. The results were documented after a 30 min incubation.

2.4. Preparation of Toxins

BoNT/A was harvested from *C. botulinum* strain ATCC19397 following a 6-day anaerobic culture as described previously [18,19]. BoNT/B complex was purchased from List Bio Laboratory Inc. (Campbell, CA, USA). The potencies of the toxins were determined using standard mouse bioassays with established LD_{50} values for BoNT/A and B. The LD_{50} values of BoNT/A and B in mice were confirmed to be 0.1 ng and 0.18 ng, respectively.

2.5. Vaccination and Challenge of Mice

BALB/c mice (female, 5–6 weeks old, KOATECH, South Korea) were immunized with the purified antigens adsorbed onto 0.2% aluminum hydroxide ($Al(OH)_3$). A group of five mice was vaccinated intramuscularly at 0, 2, and 4 weeks with 1 μg of rHCcA, rHCcB, rHCcB-L-HCcA, or an antigen mixture, which combined 1 μg of rHCcA and 1 μg of rHCcB, all mixed with alum (25 μg) in a total volume of 0.2 mL. Mice injected with PBS or alum were used as negative controls. Two weeks after the last vaccination, mice were challenged with a 10^5 LD_{50} dose of BoNT/A or 10^3 LD_{50} dose of BoNT/B by intraperitoneal injection and observed for 14 days. All animal procedures were approved by the Institutional Animal Care and Use Committee of KDCA (KDCA-IACUC-046-17-2A, 2017).

2.6. Measurement of Serum Antibody Titers

Serum samples collected at specified time points were analyzed for antigen-specific antibodies using indirect ELISA. Briefly, ELISA plates (Corning Incorporated, Corning, NY, USA) were coated with an optimal concentration of purified rHCcA or rHCcB (1 μg/mL in bicarbonate, 100 μL/well) overnight at 4 °C. Plates were washed with PBS containing 0.05% Tween 20 (PBST) using a Plate Washer (BioTek, Agilent, CA, USA). The plates were blocked for 1 h with 5% skimmed milk at 37 °C, then washed as described above. Serum samples were initially diluted 1:50, followed by five-fold serial dilutions (1:50–1:3,906,250), and incubated for 2 h at 37 °C. After washing with PBST, a 1:5000 dilution of anti-mouse IgG-HRP (Jackson ImmunoResearch Inc., West Grove, PA, USA) was incubated for 1 h at 37 °C. After washing with PBST, TMB substrate was added to each well and incubated for 10 min at room temperature (25 °C). The colorimetric reaction was stopped with 2 N sulfuric acid, and absorbance at 450 nm was determined using a microplate reader (Molecular Devices, San Jose, CA, USA).

2.7. Statistical Analysis

Statistical significance across groups was assessed using one-way analysis of variance (ANOVA), followed by the Kruskal–Wallis test and then Dunn's multiple comparison test to identify specific group differences. All analyses were conducted using GraphPad Prism 5 (GraphPad, La Jolla, CA, USA). The Kruskal–Wallis test was selected to evaluate differences among groups due to its suitability for non-parametric data. Post-hoc tests, specifically Dunn's multiple comparison tests, were applied to control for type 1 error in multiple comparisons. Statistical significance was defined as $p < 0.05$. Asterisks (*) in the figures indicate p-values less than 0.05, and double asterisks (**) indicate *p*-values less than 0.01, denoting significant differences between groups. Data are presented as mean ± standard deviation (SD) unless otherwise noted.

3. Results

3.1. Protein Expression and Verification

Codon optimization was employed to facilitate the high-level expression of recombinant BoNT/A HC_C (rHCcA), BoNT/B HCc (rHCcB), and rHCcB-L-HCcA. Synthetic genes for *hccA*, *hccB*, and *hccB-L-hccA* were engineered to target the C-terminal fragment of the heavy chain in BoNT/A and B, as illustrated in Figure 1A. To ensure proper folding of each HCc domain, a three-glycine linker was incorporated between the *hccB* and *hccA* segments. The recombinant proteins (rHCcA, HcB, and rHCcB-L-HCcA) were purified from 1 L of the culture using a Ni^{2+} affinity chromatography column. Each purified protein fraction was verified using SDS-PAGE. The results confirmed that the rHCcA and rHCcB proteins were approximately 50 kDa (Figure 2A,B), whereas the rHCcB-L-HCcA fusion protein was approximately 100 kDa (Figure 2C). Thus, the rHCcB-L-HCcA fusion protein exhibited a higher molecular weight owing to the synthesis of rHCcA and rHCcB. To further enhance protein purity, the eluted fractions were subjected to additional purification steps using an FPLC system with Superdex200 column, and the proteins were analyzed by SDS-PAGE

(Figure 2D). The results showed that all three proteins collected from the elution buffer possessed a molecular size similar to the 50 kDa of rHCcA and rHCcB proteins and 100 kDa of rHCcB-L-HCcA fusion protein, with high purity. The next experiment was conducted to verify the specific binding of each purified protein antigen with its respective antibody, using a Bioline™ Bioterror Pathogens and Toxins Test Kit developed in previous research to prepare for biological terrorism scenarios. This rapid antigen detection kit features membrane strips coated with specific polyclonal antibodies against BoNT/A and B, enabling the simultaneous detection of these antigens. The assay results revealed that rHCcA and rHCcB were specifically bound to anti-BoNT/A and B antibodies, respectively, which manifested as purple bands. Remarkably, the rHCcB-L-HCcA fusion protein bound to both antibody sets and displayed two distinct purple bands (Figure 2E). These results confirmed that rHCcA, rHCcB, and rHCcB-L-HCcA were specifically bound to their respective antibodies, demonstrating that each protein exhibited high specificity for its intended target.

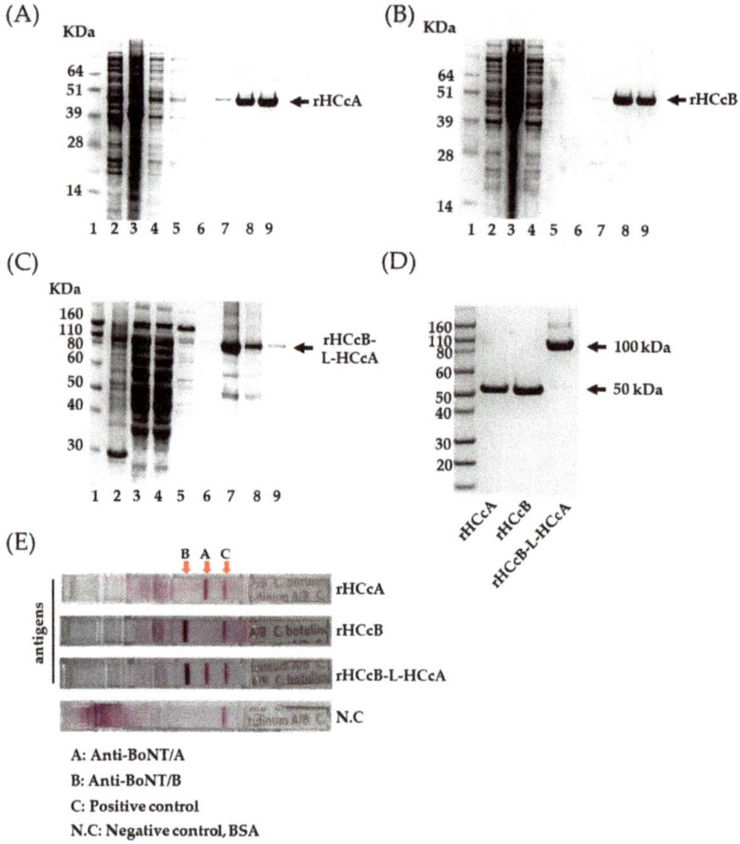

Figure 2. Purification and verification of protein from *E. coli* BL21(DE3) with pET19b-*hccA*, pET19b-*hcB*, and pET19b-*hccB-L-hccA*. (**A–C**) SDS-PAGE analysis of samples from the purification process, showing molecular mass markers (Lane 1), soluble cell fraction (Lane 2), insoluble cell fraction (Lane 3), flow-through from the soluble cell fraction in the Ni^{2+} column (Lane 4), wash fractions (Lanes 5–6), and eluted protein (Lanes 7–9). (**D**) SDS-PAGE analysis of purified proteins rHCcA, rHCcB, and rHCcB-L-HCcA, showing expected molecular weights of ~50 kDa and ~100 kDa. (**E**) Verification of purified proteins using an Antigen Rapid Detection Test Kit (Abbott) based on a lateral flow assay.

3.2. Immunogenicity and Protective Efficacy

In the next experiment, we evaluated the immunogenicity induced by the purified antigens (rHCcA, rHCcB, and rHCcB-L-HCcA) and an antigen mixture (rHCcA and rHCcB). BALB/c mice (n = 5/group) were immunized with each antigen mixed with alum (25 μg) thrice at 2-week intervals, as depicted in Figure 3A. One week after the third immunization, blood was collected from the facial veins of mice and separated into serum samples. Serum was then used to determine the binding antibody titers for each antigen via ELISA using plates coated with rHCcA and rHCcB antigens. The experimental results showed that anti-BoNT/A-specific titers in mice immunized with rHCcA, rHCcB-L-HCcA, and antigen mixture were significantly higher than those in the negative controls (mice immunized with alum alone), with all three antigens showing statistical significance ($p < 0.05$; Figure 3B). The results shown in Figure 3C indicate that the anti-BoNT/B-specific titers in mice immunized with rHCcB-L-HCcA were significantly higher ($p < 0.05$) than those in the negative control group. While the rHCcB and antigen mixture groups did not demonstrate statistical significance, it is noteworthy that three out of five mice in the rHCcB group exhibited antibody titers comparable to or exceeding those observed antibody titers comparable to or exceeding those observed in the rHCcB-L-HCcA group (Figure 3C). These results suggest that rHCcA and rHCcB-L-HCcA antigens have the potential to act as vaccines to protect against BoNT/A, with a strong immunogenic response. While the rHCcB antigen exhibited variability among mice, leading to statistically non-significant outcomes, this may be attributed to the small sample size used in the experiment, which could have limited the detection of significant differences. Notably, rHCcB-L-HCcA displayed consistent and robust immunogenicity, indicating its potential to serve as a vaccine candidate for simultaneous protection against both BoNT/A and BoNT/B.

In subsequent experiments, to evaluate the protective efficacy of each antigen, 10^5 50% lethal dose (LD_{50}) of BoNT/A (equivalent to 10 μg per mouse) and 10^3 LD_{50} of BoNT/B (equivalent to 0.18 μg per mouse) were injected intraperitoneally into the immunized mice, which were then observed for 2 weeks. As shown in Table 1, the groups immunized with rHCcA, rHCcB-L-HCcA, and antigen mixture exhibited 100% survival against 10^5 LD_{50} of BoNT/A. Similarly, groups immunized with rHCcB, rHCcB-L-HCcA, and antigen mixture showed 100% survival against 10^3 LD_{50} of BoNT/B. Conversely, the groups immunized with single antigens rHCcA or rHCcB did not survive when challenged with BoNT/B or BoNT/A, respectively. Through this experiment, we confirmed that there were no significant differences in the ability of single antigens, fusion antigens, and antigen mixtures to protect against BoNTs.

Table 1. Survival rate of mice immunized [1] with antigen following challenge with BoNT/A or BoNT/B.

Antigens	Dose	BoNT/A (10^5 LD_{50})	BoNT/B (10^3 LD_{50})
		% (Number of Survivors/Total)	
Alum	25 μg	0 (0/5)	0 (0/5)
rHCcA	1 μg	100 (5/5)	0 (0/5)
rHCcB	1 μg	0 (0/5)	100 (5/5)
rHCcB-L-HCcA	1 μg	100 (5/5)	100 (5/5)
rHCcA + rHCcB	1 μg + 1 μg	100 (5/5)	100 (5/5)

[1] Mice were immunized thrice at weeks 0, 2, and 4 with 1 μg of rHCcA, rHCcB, or rHCcB-L-HCcA, each mixed with alum as an adjuvant to enhance the immune response. The antigen mixture (rHCcA + rHCcB) was prepared in the same manner as other antigens by combining 1 μg of rHCcA and 1 μg of rHCcB, then mixing with alum before administration to mice. Four weeks after the final booster immunization, mice were challenged with 10^5 LD_{50} of BoNT/A and 10^3 LD_{50} of BoNT/B. Challenge numbers indicate the survival rate as the number of surviving mice out of the total number of mice in each group.

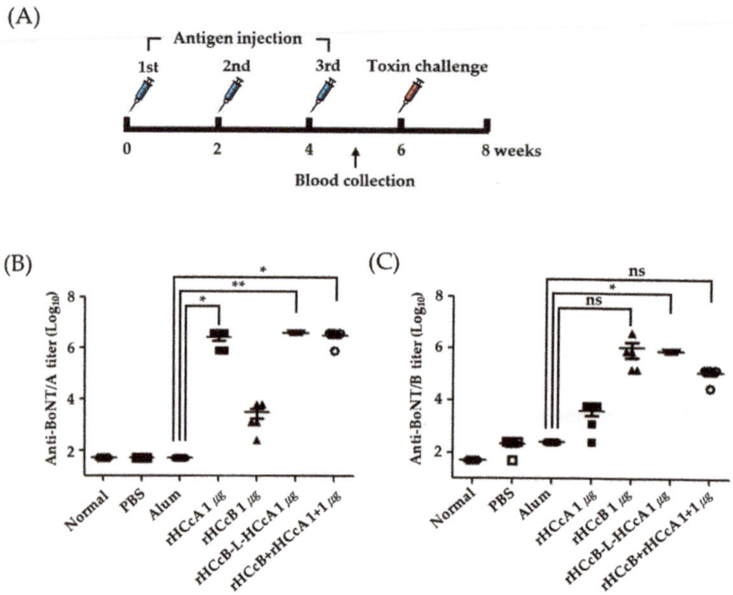

Figure 3. Antibody responses in mice after vaccination with rHCcA, rHCcB, rHCcB-L-HCcA, or a mixture of rHCcB and rHCcA antigens. (**A**) Outline of the immunization study to assess antibody responses post-vaccination in BALB/c mice. (**B**,**C**) Evaluation of antibody response in mice injected with PBS, alum, rHCcA, rHCcB, rHCcB-L-HCcA, or antigen mixture, tested individually using ELISA. The median values for each group are depicted with a bar. Significance levels are indicated as * $p < 0.05$, ** $p < 0.01$; ns indicates no significant difference. Each point on the graph represents an individual mouse.

We conducted additional studies to evaluate the protective efficacy when mice were simultaneously challenged with BoNT/A and B. Four mice were immunized with either the rHCcB-L-HCcA antigen or a mixture of rHCcA and rHCcB, with each mouse receiving a 5 μg dose mixed with alum (25 μg) and administered intramuscularly at 2-week intervals for a total of three doses. Two weeks after the final immunization, the mice were challenged intraperitoneally with a mixture of 10^3 LD_{50} of BoNT/A and 10^3 LD_{50} of BoNT/B, as well as a mixture of 10^4 LD_{50} of BoNT/A and 10^4 LD_{50} of BoNT/B, and were observed for two weeks. The results showed that the group immunized with the rHCcB-L-HCcA antigen had a 100% survival rate when challenged with 10^3 LD_{50} of BoNT/A + BoNT/B, whereas, in the mixture group, one out of four mice died, resulting in a 75% survival rate. However, both groups succumbed to the challenge with 10^4 LD_{50} of BoNT/A + BoNT/B (Table 2). These experimental results highlight the unique advantage of the rHCcB-L-HCcA antigen, which demonstrates protective efficacy comparable to single antigens. Additionally, the ability of rHCcB-L-HCcA to protect against both BoNT/A and B simultaneously at lower doses than the antigen mixture suggests a significant advantage as a potential vaccine candidate.

Table 2. Protective efficacy of rHCcB-L-HCcA and antigen mixture against combined BoNT/A and B exposure in mice [1].

Antigens	Dose	BoNT/A (10^3 LD_{50}) + BoNT/B (10^3 LD_{50})	BoNT/A (10^4 LD_{50}) + BoNT/B (10^4 LD_{50})
		% (Number of Survivors/Total)	
Alum	25 μg	0 (0/4)	0 (0/4)
rHCcB-L-HCcA	5 μg	100 (4/4)	0 (0/4)
rHCcA + rHCcB	5 μg + 5 μg	75 (3/4)	0 (0/4)

[1] Mice were immunized with three intramuscular injections of 5 μg of the rHCcB-L-HCcA or antigen mixture, prepared by combining 5 μg of rHCcA and 5 μg of rHCcB per injection, administered at 2-week intervals. Following immunization, mice were challenged intraperitoneally with a mixture of BoNT/A and BoNT/B at doses of 10^3 LD_{50} and 10^4 LD_{50}.

4. Discussion

Botulism is a rare disease worldwide; however, in South Korea—a divided nation with potential bioterrorism risks—the development of a vaccine as part of preparedness measures is crucial. Given the potential use of botulinum toxins in bioterrorism and the absence of licensed vaccines, developing an effective dual-protection vaccine remains a pressing global priority. Vaccination was previously recommended only for high-risk groups, including healthcare providers, researchers, first responders, and military personnel at risk of exposure to BoNTs. In 2011, however, the CDC discontinued the investigational PBT (ABCDE) vaccine due to its limited efficacy. As a result, no licensed vaccine is currently available to prevent intoxication caused by the botulinum serotypes most commonly associated with human diseases, namely serotypes A, B, E, and F [20,21]. While post-exposure administration of antitoxins can effectively treat rare cases of life-threatening botulism, these therapies are insufficient for protecting large populations during a potential bioterrorism event involving the dissemination of BoNTs [22]. Thus, there is an urgent need for the proactive development of new therapies and vaccination strategies to mitigate the risk of botulinum neurotoxin intoxication.

The objective of this study was to develop a fusion vaccine capable of simultaneously protecting against botulinum toxin serotypes A and B, with the aim of establishing independent domestic vaccine production. To achieve this, we designed a recombinant fusion protein antigen by combining the heavy chain C-terminal domains of BoNT/A and B. The fusion protein, named rHCcB-L-HCcA, incorporates a glycine linker ((Gly)3) to optimize protein folding, enhance production yield, and improve antibody accessibility (Figure 1). This design aims to overcome common challenges in protein misfolding and low production efficiency often encountered in vaccine development [23–25]. The synthetic genes *hccB*, *hccA*, and *hccB-L-hccA* were cloned into the pET19b expression vector, and each plasmid was transformed into *E. coli* BL21(DE3) RIPL Codon Plus, pLysS, and SoluBL21, respectively. Following protein expression, the rHCcA, rHCcB, and rHCcB-L-HCcA antigens were purified using a Ni^{2+} column. We attempted to express a synthetic gene with *hccA* placed upstream, *hccA-L-hccB*, by cloning the pET19b-*hccA-L-hccB* plasmid into *E. coli* BL21(DE3) SoluBL21; however, a pure protein was not obtained. Therefore, we selected the rHCcB-L-HCcA fusion protein as a vaccine candidate against BoNT/A and B and evaluated its efficacy.

The final purified proteins were obtained in sufficient quantities (0.5–1 mg) for experimental use. SDS-PAGE analysis confirmed the purity of each protein, revealing single antigen bands at the expected molecular weights: 50 kDa for the individual proteins and 100 kDa for the fusion protein (Figure 2A–D). The purified proteins (rHCcA, rHCcB, and rHCcB-L-HCcA) were further tested for their reactivity using the BiolineTM Bioterror Pathogens and Toxin Test Kit, enabling the detection of immune reactions with anti-

BoNT/A or anti-BoNT/B antibodies coated in the kit. The results confirmed that the rHCcA, rHCcB, and rHCcB-L-HCcA proteins specifically bound to anti-BoNT/A, anti-BoNT/B, and both anti-BoNT/A and anti-BoNT/B simultaneously, respectively (Figure 2E). These results not only demonstrate the successful purification of the antigens but also suggest the potential for generating antibodies specifically targeting each single antigen.

The purified protein antigens (rHCcA, rHCcB, and rHCcB-L-HCcA), each at a dose of 1 μg, along with a mixed antigen containing 1 μg each of rHCcB and rHCcA, were administered intramuscularly with 25 μg of alum to groups of five mice. Immunizations were performed three times at 2-week intervals. As a negative control, phosphate-buffered saline (PBS) as the antigen diluent, combined with 25 μg of alum, was administered under the same conditions as the antigens (Figure 3A). To assess the immunogenicity of the antigen–antibody response, blood samples were collected from the mice one week after the final immunization. The serum was analyzed using ELISA, and the antibody titers for each antigen were logarithmically transformed and statistically evaluated using GraphPad Prism 5. The results shown in Figure 3B indicate that the antigens rHCcA, rHCcB-L-HCcA, and the antigen mixture elicited significantly higher antibody titers when bound to coated rHCcA compared to alum alone. This finding suggests a strong potential for protection against BoNT/A. Among these, the fusion protein rHCcB-L-HCcA demonstrated the highest significance, further emphasizing its promise as a viable vaccine candidate.

Figure 3C shows that both the rHCcB and rHCcB-L-HCcA fusion protein antigens elicited high antibody titers. However, the antigens rHCcB and the antigen mixture did not show statistically significant differences compared to alum. The antibody titer results revealed considerable variability among the five mice in the rHCcB-immunized group, leading to a large standard deviation. One study reported that a small amount of antibodies targeting the HN domain of BoNT/A could block critical active sites of the toxin [26]. This suggests that the protective efficacy observed in certain antigen groups, despite low immunogenicity, may result from functional mechanisms independent of antibody titers. It emphasizes that the structural or functional properties of antigens play a significant role in determining protective efficacy. Furthermore, even with low titers, existing antibodies may act as neutralizing antibodies, effectively targeting and neutralizing the toxin's active sites [27]. The slightly elevated antibody titer observed in the alum group may have contributed to the lack of statistically significant differences when compared to rHCcB. Another consideration is the heterogeneity often observed among mice in immunization experiments. Small group sizes, such as five mice, can lead to considerable variability in results. To mitigate this issue, future experiments will increase the group size to at least ten mice per group, ensuring more robust statistical reliability.

Despite these challenges, the rHCcB-L-HCcA-immunized group showed statistically significant differences compared to the alum group. These findings strongly suggest that the rHCcB-L-HCcA antigen has dual protective potential against both BoNT/A and BoNT/B, further reinforcing its promise as an effective vaccine candidate.

In the protection assays, mice immunized with each antigen were intraperitoneally challenged with 10^5 LD50 (10 μg) of BoNT/A and 10^3 LD50 (0.18 μg) of BoNT/B. The results showed that all mice in the negative control groups (PBS and Alum) succumbed to the toxin challenge. In contrast, mice immunized with rHCcA, rHCcB-L-HCcA, and the antigen mixture demonstrated 100% survival, as expected due to their strong protective efficacy against BoNT/A. Furthermore, mice immunized with rHCcB, rHCcB-L-HCcA, and the antigen mixture also achieved 100% survival against BoNT/B despite exhibiting low antibody titers. As previously mentioned, the results suggest that rHCcB or the antigen mixture, despite having low antibody titers, may effectively block critical active sites of BoNT/B. It is also possible that the antigens directly bind to the toxin, thereby neutralizing its activity. These findings from the protection assays support the potential of the rHCcB-L-HCcA antigen as a promising vaccine candidate capable of providing strong protective efficacy against both BoNT/A and BoNT/B. Furthermore, they highlight the importance of the functional properties of antigens in determining protective efficacy. To investigate whether increasing the antigen dose could enhance antibody titers and protective efficacy, the concentrations of rHCcB, rHCcB-L-HCcA, and the antigen mixture were increased to 5 μg and 10 μg. These antigens were mixed with 25 μg of Alum and administered intramuscularly to mice at 2-week intervals for three immunizations. After the final immunization, blood samples were collected to assess antibody titers and protective efficacy. The experimental results showed that increasing the antigen dose to 10 μg resulted in significant differences in antibody titers for the rHCcB and rHCcB-L-HCcA groups compared to the Alum group (Figure S1). However, despite the increased dose and significant differences in antibody titers, mice in all antigen groups succumbed to a higher toxin challenge of 10^4 LD50 BoNT/B (1.8 μg) (Table S1). These findings suggest that increasing the antigen dose alone is insufficient to achieve protective efficacy against BoNT/B. The literature also suggests that the lack of protective efficacy, despite high immunogenicity in some antigen groups, can be attributed to glycosylation [28]. Glycosylated forms of BoNT/B(HC) and TeNT(HC) failed to induce protective immunity, while their protective capabilities were restored after undergoing deglycosylation. This indicates that glycosylation can alter the immunogenicity of protein antigens. In this study, we plan to investigate the immunogenicity and protective efficacy of rHCcB after subjecting it to deglycosylation to further assess its potential.

Finally, the protective efficacy of the rHCcB-L-HCcA antigen and the antigen mixture was evaluated against simultaneous challenges with BoNT/A and BoNT/B. The results showed that mice immunized with the rHCcB-L-HCcA antigen survived a mixture of 10^3 LD50 of BoNT/A and BoNT/B but succumbed to a higher dose of 10^4 LD50 of the same toxins. In contrast, mice immunized with the antigen mixture exhibited a 75% survival rate against 10^3 LD50 of BoNT/A and BoNT/B but did not survive the higher toxin dose (Table 2). According to the Supplementary Data, both the rHCcB-L-HCcA antigen and the antigen mixture elicited high antibody titers (Figure S1). However, despite the elevated antibody titers, both groups were only able to protect mice against up to 10^3 LD50 of BoNT/A and BoNT/B. The exact cause of this limitation remains unclear, but as previously mentioned, the structural or functional properties of the antigens may play a crucial role in determining protective efficacy. It is necessary to analyze antigen-antibody interactions, increase the size of the mouse groups, and evaluate immune responses under various conditions to improve the reliability of the results and clarify the defense mechanisms against BoNT/B. Nonetheless, the rHCcB-L-HCcA antigen is confirmed to be a strong and promising vaccine candidate capable of protecting against 10^5 LD50 of BoNT/A and 10^3 LD50 of BoNT/B. These findings not only highlight the potential of the rHCcB-L-HCcA antigen but also provide a foundation for further investigations to optimize its protective efficacy and broaden its application as a dual-protection vaccine against botulinum neurotoxins.

5. Conclusions

This study demonstrated that the rHCcB-L-HCcA fusion protein is a promising vaccine candidate capable of providing dual protection against BoNT/A and BoNT/B. The antigen showed strong immunogenicity and protective efficacy against BoNT/A, while the protective efficacy against BoNT/B was achieved despite low antibody titers, highlighting the potential role of functional mechanisms beyond antibody titers. However, the limited protection observed at higher toxin concentrations suggests the need for further optimization. Future research should focus on improving the protective efficacy against BoNT/B through antigen modifications and investigating glycosylation effects and antigen-antibody interactions. These findings provide valuable insights for the development of effective vaccines against botulinum neurotoxins.

Supplementary Materials: The following supporting information can be downloaded at https://www.mdpi.com/article/10.3390/vaccines13010039/s1. Table S1: Protective efficacy of rHCcB and rHCcB-L-HCcA antigens against high-concentration BoNT/B exposure in mice. Figure S1: Evaluation of antibody response in mice injected with PBS, alum, rHCcB, rHCcB-L-HCcA, or antigen mixture, tested individually using ELISA.

Author Contributions: Conceptualization, J.-H.J. and G.-E.R.; methodology, J.-H.J.; software, E.-S.C. and M.-R.Y.; validation, S.-W.P. and S.-H.K.; formal analysis, E.-S.C. and J.-H.J.; investigation, E.-S.C. and S.-W.P. writing—original draft preparation, E.-S.C.; writing—review and editing, G.-E.R., S.-H.K., H.Y. and Y.-S.C.; visualization, E.-S.C. and M.-R.Y.; supervision, Y.-S.C.; project administration, E.-S.C. and J.-H.J. All authors have read and agreed to the published version of the manuscript.

Funding: This research was funded by the Korea Disease Control and Prevention Agency, grant number 4845-300-210-13.

Institutional Review Board Statement: The animal study protocol was approved by the Institutional Animal Care and Use Committee of the Korea Disease Control and Prevention Agency (KDCA-IACUC-046-17-2A; 2017).

Informed Consent Statement: Not applicable.

Data Availability Statement: Data are contained within the article.

Conflicts of Interest: The authors declare no conflicts of interest.

References

1. Maslanka, S.E.; Lúquez, C.; Dykes, J.K.; Tepp, W.H.; Pier, C.L.; Pellett, S.; Raphael, B.H.; Kalb, S.R.; Barr, J.R.; Rao, A.; et al. A novel botulinum neurotoxin, previously reported as Serotype H, has a hybrid-like structure with regions of similarity to the structures of Serotypes A and F and is neutralized with Serotype A antitoxin. *J. Infect. Dis.* **2016**, *213*, 379–385. [CrossRef]
2. Zhang, S.; Masuyer, G.; Zhang, J.; Shen, Y.; Lundin, D.; Henriksson, L.; Miyashita, S.-I.; Martínez-Carranza, M.; Dong, M.; Stenmark, P. Identification and characterization of a novel botulinum neurotoxin. *Nat. Commun.* **2017**, *8*, 14130. [CrossRef] [PubMed]
3. Arnon, S.S.; Schechter, R.; Inglesby, T.V.; Henderson, D.A.; Bartlett, J.G.; Ascher, M.S.; Eitzen, E.; Fine, A.D.; Hauer, J.; Layton, M.; et al. Botulinum toxin as a biological weapon: Medical and public health management. *JAMA* **2001**, *285*, 1059–1070. [CrossRef] [PubMed]
4. Pirazzini, M.; Rossetto, O.; Eleopra, R.; Montecucco, C. Botulinum neurotoxins: Biology, pharmacology, and toxicology. *Pharmacol. Rev.* **2017**, *69*, 200–235. [CrossRef]
5. Chai, Q.; Arndt, J.W.; Dong, M.; Tepp, W.H.; Johnson, E.A.; Chapman, E.R.; Stevens, R.C. Structural basis of cell surface receptor recognition by botulinum neurotoxin B. *Nature* **2006**, *444*, 1096–1100. [CrossRef] [PubMed]
6. Ben David, A.; Diamant, E.; Barnea, A.; Rosen, O.; Torgeman, A.; Zichel, R. The receptor binding domain of botulinum neurotoxin serotype A (BoNT/A) inhibits BoNT/A and BoNT/E intoxications in vivo. *Clin. Vaccine Immunol.* **2013**, *20*, 1266–1273. [CrossRef] [PubMed]
7. Rusnak, J.M.; Smith, L.A. Botulinum neurotoxin vaccines: Past history and recent developments. *Hum. Vaccines* **2009**, *5*, 794–805. [CrossRef]
8. Montal, M. Botulinum neurotoxin: A marvel of protein design. *Annu. Rev. Biochem.* **2010**, *79*, 591–617. [CrossRef] [PubMed]
9. Brunger, A.T.; Breidenbach, M.A.; Jin, R.; Fischer, A.; Santos, J.S.; Montal, M. Botulinum neurotoxin heavy chain belt as an intramolecular chaperone for the light chain. *PLoS Pathog.* **2007**, *3*, 1191–1194. [CrossRef]
10. Centers for Disease Control and Prevention. *Botulism in the United States, 1899–1998. Handbook for Epidemiologists, Clinicians, and Laboratory Workers*; Public Health Service, United States Department of Health and Human Services: Atlanta, GA, USA, 1998.
11. National Botulism Surveillance. Available online: https://www.cdc.gov/botulism/php/national-botulism-surveillance/index.html (accessed on 29 November 2024).
12. Infectious Disease Portal. Available online: https://dportal.kdca.go.kr/pot/is/inftnsdsEDW.do (accessed on 25 November 2024).

13. Jeon, J.H.; Choi, C.H.; Kim, J.H.; Hyun, J.; Choi, E.S.; Choi, S.Y.; Shin, Y.W.; Pyo, S.W.; Kim, D.W.; Kang, B.H.; et al. Genetic characterization of Clostridium botulinum isolated from the first case of infant botulism in Korea. *Ann. Lab. Med.* **2021**, *41*, 489–492. [CrossRef] [PubMed]
14. Edmond, B.J.; Guerra, F.A.; Blake, J.; Hempler, S. Case of infant botulism in Texas. *Tex. Med.* **1977**, *73*, 85–88. [CrossRef]
15. Panditrao, M.V.; Chung, C.H.; Khouri, J.M.; Barash, J.R.; Motter, R.N.; Dover, N.; Arnon, S.S. Dual-toxin ('bivalent') infant botulism in California, 1976–2020: Epidemiologic, clinical, and laboratory aspects. *J. Pediatr.* **2023**, *253*, 8–13. [CrossRef] [PubMed]
16. Webb, R.P.; Smith, L.A. What next for botulism vaccine development? *Expert Rev. Vaccines* **2013**, *12*, 481–492. [CrossRef] [PubMed]
17. Sun, D.; Wu, L.; Fan, G. Laboratory information management system for biosafety laboratory: Safety and efficiency. *J. Biosaf. Biosecur.* **2021**, *3*, 28–34. [CrossRef]
18. Malizio, C.J.; Goodnough, M.C.; Johnson, E.A. Purification of *Clostridium botulinum* type A neurotoxin. *Methods Mol. Biol.* **2000**, *145*, 27–39. [CrossRef]
19. Choi, E.S.; Jeon, J.H.; Kim, Y.R.; Cha, K.; Rhie, G. Enhancement of antibody-mediated botulinum toxin A neutralization by conjugating annexin V to the antibody in the mouse model. *Korea J Microbiol.* **2021**, *57*, 169–173.
20. Smith, L.A.; Rusnak, J.M. Botulinum neurotoxin vaccines: Past, present, and future. *Crit. Rev. Immunol.* **2007**, *27*, 303–318. [CrossRef] [PubMed]
21. Centers for Disease Control and Prevention (CDC). Notice of CDC's discontinuation of investigational pentavalent (ABCDE) botulinum toxoid vaccine for workers at risk for occupational exposure to botulinum toxins. *MMWR Morb. Mortal. Wkly Rep.* **2011**, *60*, 1454–1455.
22. Scott, V.L.; Villarreal, D.O.; Hutnick, N.A.; Walters, J.N.; Ragwan, E.; Bdeir, K.; Yan, J.; Sardesai, N.Y.; Finnefrock, A.C.; Casimiro, D.R.; et al. DNA vaccines targeting heavy chain C-terminal fragments of *Clostridium botulinum* neurotoxin serotypes A, B, and E induce potent humoral and cellular immunity and provide protection from lethal toxin challenge. *Hum. Vaccines Immunother.* **2015**, *11*, 1961–1971. [CrossRef] [PubMed]
23. Chen, X.; Zaro, J.L.; Shen, W.C. Fusion protein linkers: Property, design and functionality. *Adv. Drug Deliv. Rev.* **2013**, *65*, 1357–1369. [CrossRef]
24. Zhao, H.L.; Yao, X.Q.; Xue, C.; Wang, Y.; Xiong, X.H.; Liu, Z.M. Increasing the homogeneity, stability and activity of human serum albumin and interferon-alpha2b fusion protein by linker engineering. *Protein Expr. Purif.* **2008**, *61*, 73–77. [CrossRef]
25. Amet, N.; Lee, H.F.; Shen, W.C. Insertion of the designed helical linker led to increased expression of Tf-based fusion proteins. *Pharm. Res.* **2009**, *26*, 523–528. [CrossRef] [PubMed]
26. Ayyar, B.V.; Tajhya, R.B.; Beeton, C.; Atassi, Z. Antigenic sites on the HN domain of botulinum neurotoxin A stimulate protective antibody responses against active toxin. *Sci. Rep.* **2015**, *5*, 15776. [CrossRef]
27. Cheng, L.W.; Stanker, L.H.; Henderson II, T.D.; Lou, J.; Marks, J.D. Antibody protection against botulinum neurotoxin intoxication in mice. *Infect. Immun.* **2009**, *77*, 4305–4313. [CrossRef] [PubMed]
28. Smith, L.A. Development of recombinant vaccines for botulinum neurotoxin. *Toxicon* **1998**, *36*, 1539–1648. [CrossRef]

vaccines

MDPI

Review

Oncolytic Viruses: An Inventory of Shedding Data from Clinical Trials and Elements for the Environmental Risk Assessment

Sheela Onnockx *, Aline Baldo and Katia Pauwels

Sciensano, Service Biosafety and Biotechnology, Rue Juliette Wytsmanstraat 14, B-1050 Brussels, Belgium; aline.baldo@sciensano.be (A.B.); katia.pauwels@sciensano.be (K.P.)

* Correspondence: sheela.onnockx@sciensano.be; Tel.: +32-2-642-58-12

Abstract: Attenuated and/or genetically modified oncolytic viruses (OV) gain increasing interest as a promising approach for cancer therapy. Beside the assessment of subject safety, quality and efficacy aspects of medicinal products for human use, genetically modified viruses are also governed by EU regulatory frameworks requiring an environmental risk assessment (ERA). An important element to be assessed as part of the ERA is the incidence of exposure to OV of individuals, other than the trial subjects, and the environment. The evidence-based evaluation of shedding data is considered to be decisive in that context, as it may impact the OV capacity to be transmitted. This is particularly true for OV still able to (conditionally) replicate as opposed to replication-defective viral vectors commonly used in gene therapy or vaccination. To our knowledge, this article presents the most extensive and up-to-date review of shedding data reported with OV employed in clinics. Besides the identification of a topical need for improving the collection of shedding data, this article aims at providing an aid to the design of an appropriate shedding study, thereby relying on and further complementing principles described in existing guidelines issued by European and international institutions.

Keywords: oncolytic virus; shedding; environmental risk assessment; biosafety; clinical trials; cancer

1. Introduction

Oncolytic viruses (OV) are (conditionally) replication competent viruses (with low pathogenicity) that are designed to be able to selectively replicate in tumor cells, leading to their destruction by the direct lysis of host tumor cells, while sparing normal cells. Accumulating evidence in oncovirotherapy demonstrates that OV infection can also trigger specific antitumor immune effects. Cellular proteins released from OV-lysed tumor cells elicit an interaction with the innate immune system through the activation of dendritic cells, which in turn stimulate adaptive immunity (Figure 1).

OV can be naturally occurring viruses that have natural tropism to neoplastic cells, such as Reoviruses [1], Newcastle disease virus (NDV) [2] and Vesicular stomatitis virus (VSV) [3]. OV can also be laboratory-adapted attenuated virus strains, such as attenuated Measles viruses, which acquired the ability to use, for viral entry, receptors that are overexpressed on the surface of malignant cells [4]. Some OV have also been genetically modified (GM) to enhance their antitumor specificity, safety and immunogenicity, for example by delivering immuno-stimulatory agents or therapeutic agents or by triggering novel cancer-specific acquired immune responses against tumor antigens. As reported by Madeco et al., in 2020, approximately two-thirds of the studies involving OV use GM viruses [5]. The growing list of virus platforms applied as oncolytic virotherapy or even as oncolytic immunotherapy illustrates the increasing clinical interest in OV as effective cancer therapeutics, either as a single-agent therapeutics or in combination with chemotherapy, radiation treatment or immune-based therapeutic regimens. OV under clinical investigation include Adenovirus (Ad) (48), Herpesvirus (39), Reovirus (24) and Poxvirus (vacciniavirus 21/22; fowlpox virus 1/22), along with other candidate viruses, such as Measles virus, Gamma-Herpes virus, Parvovirus, Retrovirus and VSV that have been reported in single or a limited number of clinical trials (Figure 2). Characteristics of the most widely used OV such as their structure, virion size and receptor usage, as well as some of the main advantages and disadvantages, have been reviewed elsewhere [6].

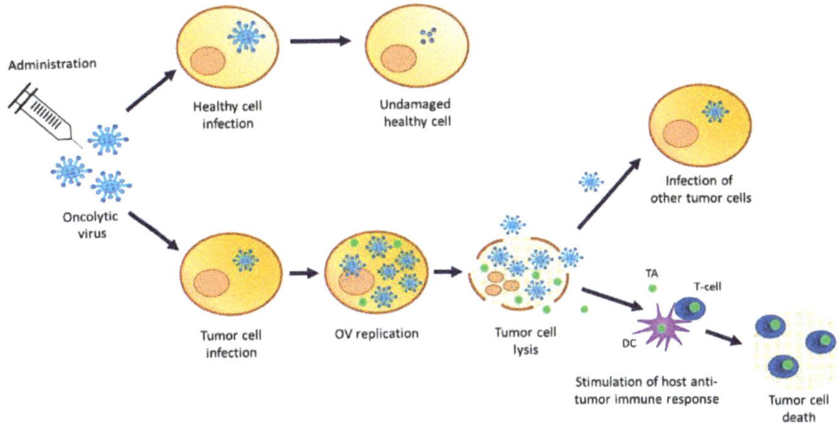

Figure 1. Mechanism of action of oncolytic viruses. OV infect healthy cells but cannot replicate. High infection of cancer cells where OV replicate and package for the production of new viral particles. A high viral load inside the cell causes tumor cell lysis releasing viral particles and tumor antigens in the cancer microenvironment. The viral particles' progeny can infect other tumor cells while the released tumor antigens stimulate the host anti-tumor immune response. TA = tumor antigen; DC = dendritic cell.

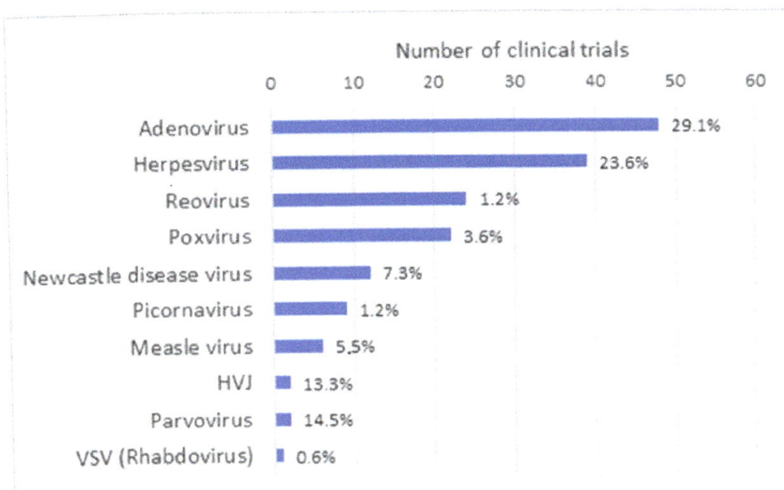

Figure 2. Type of oncolytic viruses used in oncolytic virus clinical trials. Based on the results obtained in the Supplementary Table S1 of this article, a graph representing the number of clinical trials that have been performed by type of oncolytic virus all over the world has been generated. Taken together, the number of clinical trials with Adenovirus and Herpesvirus represents slightly more than half of all clinical trials with OV.

While the approval in the US and Europe in 2015 [7–9] (and later also elsewhere) of Imlygic®® (also known as talimogene laherparepvec, T-VEC and OncoVex), an oncolytic Herpes Simplex Virus (HSV), for the treatment of advanced melanoma can be considered as a milestone in the development of OV therapy, it should be noticed that three other OV have been approved for commercialization. A wild-type Enteric Cytopathogenic Human Orphan type 7 (ECHO-7) Picornavirus, with trade name Rigvir®®, was first approved in 2004 in Latvia for the treatment of melanoma [10]. Earlier in 2019, the distribution of this medicinal product was stopped due to manufacturing issues and finally suspended for marketing authorization in mid-2019 [11]. A GM Adenovirus called Oncorine (H101) was approved in 2005 in China for subjects with head and neck cancer [12]. More recently, in June 2021, a GM HSV known as Teserpaturev/G47Δ (Delytact®®) received conditional approval in Japan for the treatment of glioblastoma [13]. Meanwhile, a number of OV have also reached an advanced stage of clinical development and are used in phase III clinical trials, such as a Newcastle disease virus to treat colorectal cancer [14,15], a vaccinia virus called Pexa-Vec (formerly JX-594) for the treatment of hepatocellular cancer [16], a Reovirus, Reolysin, as part of a combination therapy for the treatment of squamous cell carcinoma of the head and neck [17], and CG0070 Adenovirus for the treatment of non-muscle-invasive bladder cancer [18].

The clinical development of investigational products is subject to strict regulatory requirements concerning, in particular, quality, efficacy and safety aspects. In the case of GM viruses, these requirements not only pertain to the safety of the subject itself, but also to the safety of human health at large and the environment. The identification and evaluation of potential adverse effects on human health and the environment when directly exposed to the GM viruses are performed within a dedicated environmental risk assessment (ERA) as part of the regulatory application for clinical trials or marketing applications of medicinal products containing genetically modified organisms (GMO).

The evaluation of exposure pathways through which GM viruses and viral vectors with their inserted DNA sequence may interact with humans (other than subjects receiving treatment with the viral vector), or the environment, is of major importance in the ERA. Pathways of exposure include leakage upon administration (spreading) of the investigational product, accidental release during its administration, and shedding of the product by the trial subject. Shedding corresponds to the dissemination of viral (vector) particles in any form into the environment via excreta (feces, secreta (e.g., urine, sweat, saliva, nasopharyngeal fluids, lacrimal fluid, semen)), skin (wounds, pustules, sores) and blood from the treated subject [19]. Unlike gene therapy with recombinant viruses or viral vectors that are rendered replication-defective, oncovirotherapy is based on the (conditional) replication competency of the OV. As a consequence, the shedding of OV may be compared to replication-deficient viral vectors. Collecting information on whether and how OV may be released into the environment from subjects is therefore a critical step in the ERA. In addition, the likelihood of the exposure of personnel handling the vaccine or involved in clinical care (occupational exposure), close contacts of the subjects (living under the same roof or caregiver at the subject's home) and the environment (including animals, plants and micro-organisms) necessitates an evaluation of several aspects, including the environmental stability of the OV, the person-to-person or person-to-animal transmissibility of the OV, and their capacity to exchange genetic information with circulating viruses.

While several guidelines are recommending to examine shedding as early as possible in the clinical development (see hereunder), in practice, rather limited attention is given to shedding data compared to the relatively extensive collection and assessment of data supporting the safety, quality and efficacy assessment of the OV.

This paper presents a review of shedding data collected during the clinical development of OV and aims at providing an aid in the design of an appropriate shedding study.

2. Materials and Methods

Literature Review

Based on general reviews on OV recently published in PubMed [5,20], a first list of manuscripts containing results of clinical trial data using an OV was created. This list was completed by a literature review in the PubMed database on 8 June 2023. The search for the keywords "oncolytic virus therapy" was filtered for "clinical trials" and "randomized controlled trials". In this second list, only manuscripts written in English and containing reports of clinical trial data using an OV were kept. Reports of preclinical data, clinical protocols without data, review manuscripts and retrospective studies were rejected from the list. Both lists were put together and different manuscripts related to the same clinical trial were combined as a single entry in a final list.

This final list counts 165 manuscripts representing 165 different clinical trials and each trial was evaluated for multiple variables. Variables assessed included the phase of the clinical trial, the number of subjects treated, the type of virus used, the nature of the viral backbone (i.e., native virus, modified or recombinant virus), the transgene, the type of cancer treated, the use of single-agent or combination regimens and viral genome shedding data. With respect to the viral genome shedding, the authors assessed for each of the studies whether viral genome shedding was assessed and reported, and more particularly, which body tissues and/or fluids were assessed for viral particles, which detection test was used, whether viral particles were detected and for how long, and whether shed particles contained infectious viral particles. This final list of 165 manuscripts can be found in online Supplementary Table S1.

3. Environmental Risk Assessment

In addition to the regulatory requirements common to all (investigational) medicinal products, the use of GM viruses for pre-clinical investigation, clinical trials as well as their marketing as medicinal product is covered by the legislation regulating the use of GMO, which encompasses an ERA.

The ERA relies on a well-defined methodology and should be conducted on a case-by-case basis. It starts with the identification and characterization of potential hazards associated with the GMO on human health, with focus on individuals other than subjects or those vaccinated, and on the environment at large, including animals, plants and microorganisms. Concurrently and as part of a second risk component, the probability of occurrence of potential hazards under the conditions of use is assessed. Both components led to an estimation of the risk to human health and the environment posed by each identified hazard of the GMO by combining the probability of its occurrence and the magnitude of its consequences. An overall risk is then determined by combining all of the individual risks [21,22]. The ERA is based on a weight of evidence methodology encompassing both qualitative and quantitative considerations, and is described using qualitative terms ranging from high to moderate, low and negligible [23]. After overall risk determination, it is examined whether risk management measures need to be implemented in order to minimize the likelihood of adverse effects occurring. If no risks are identified that require management, no risk management strategy need be defined.

Numerous viruses have been used to design and develop OV therapy. The identification of potential hazards, the first step in the ERA, should take into account the characteristics of the OV and the properties of the inserted gene sequences and the gene products. This implies that due consideration of aspects such as the extent of attenuation, the replication capacity, tropism, biodistribution, genetic stability and the capacity to recombine with other wild-type viruses should be evaluated on a case-by-case basis. The properties of the parental viruses from which OV are derived may provide valuable starting information, taking into account that, in general, OV developed for therapeutic application are less virulent or infectious.

The development of different oncolytic viral systems for cancer therapeutic applications relies to a major extent on the genetic modification of viruses. Several strategies to enhance the therapeutic effect of oncolytic virotherapy involve the genetic "arming" of replicating viruses with transgenes, such as tumor suppressor genes, immune regulatory genes, apoptosis inducing genes, angiogenesis inhibitory genes and genes coding for prodrug converting enzymes or heat shock proteins. Besides the insertion of transgenes with an inherent therapeutic effect, other sequences can be inserted or deleted that are involved in the targeting of OV [24].

Inserted gene sequences and their gene products should be considered for their potential impact on the viral life cycle alterations (e.g., viral tropism, entry, transcription/translation, replication, transmission), on the capacity of recombination of the virus or on the host (e.g., immune modulation, pathogenesis). All of these elements may alter biodistribution and persistence in the subjects and may impact shedding following administration of the OV.

In the next section, we will focus on elements that may have an impact on the shedding properties of OV, based on examples in the clinical field, and elaborate on the assessment of shedding data as one of the key aspects in the outcome of the ERA of OV.

4. Shedding Analysis

4.1. Definition

As mentioned above, shedding corresponds to the dissemination of viral (vector) particles in any form into the environment via the excreta or secreta, skin and blood from the treated subject [19]. While indirectly related, the evaluation of the shedding pattern of OV addresses issues that are distinct from biodistribution, because the latter focuses on dissemination and persistence within the host tissues, thereby mainly impacting the subject, while shedding can be considered as one of the main pathways through which GM OV may come into contact with individuals other than the treated subject. Another consideration to be made for the purpose of this article is that blood and related products, like peripheral blood mononuclear cells, serum or plasma, are not considered as biological fluids that can spontaneously be shed into the environment. However, blood and related products could be a source of exposure for personnel in clinical settings (e.g., during intravenous administration of the product, etc.) or for close contacts of the trial subjects (e.g., direct contact with open wounds). Addressing the release of OV through secretions and/or excreta of the subject is a key element to be performed during the ERA of the clinical use of OV and should be examined as early as possible in the clinical process.

4.2. Detection

From our review of the literature (see Supplementary Table S1), it is observed that the results of shedding analysis are available in about half of the early phases of the OV development. Shedding analysis and results were reported in 70 clinical trials (42.4%) (all phases confounded), while it was not specified whether shedding analysis was conducted in 95 clinical trials (57.6%) (Figure 3).

The test method used to assess the shedding potential of oncolytic viruses should be sufficiently sensitive [25–27]. Polymerase chain reaction (PCR) and infectivity are mainly used for the detection of shed virus/vector. A quantitative PCR assay to detect viral genetic material is recommended to quantify viral genetic material. Unless full-length complete genome amplification is demonstrated after a nuclease treatment, it should be emphasized that the detection of viral genomic material by qPCR or RT-PCR is not suitable to confirm the presence of infectious viral particles. This is because qPCR or RT-PCR can detect a fragment of the viral genome even in situations where no complete genomes and/or infectious viral material are present. To have a better insight into the potential for transmission, it is recommended to perform infectivity assays involving the in vitro culturing of shed material with a permissive cell line or growth tests (e.g., plaque assay) if qPCR results reach a level above the limit of detection (LOD) [25–27]. qPCR or RT-PCR results should be accompanied with the determination of the LOD and limit of quantification (LOQ) to enable an evaluation of the sensitivity and the reliability of the assay. Also, the inclusion of suitable controls (e.g., spiking with a reference standard or an internal positive control) should be considered to account for possible effects that could lead to an underestimation of the level of shedding, for example due to the nature of the matrix of the biological sample.

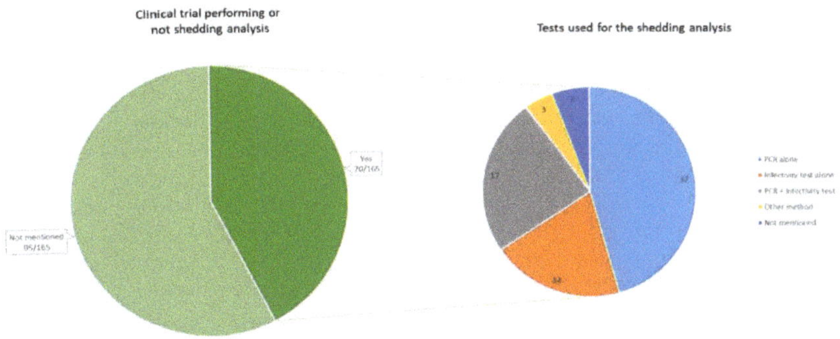

Figure 3. On the left, the number of clinical trials that reported information on viral genome shedding ($n = 70$). On the right, the method of detection used during the shedding analyses, reported within the 70 clinical trials. The method "PCR" includes all types of PCR (quantitative PCR, real-time PCR, reverse transcription PCR, etc.). The infectivity test includes cell culture and plaque assays. Other methods include viruria and direct fluorescence hexon protein assay.

Our review of the literature shows that many studies limit the collection of shedding data by conducting quantitative real-time PCR (qRT-PCR) analyses. Of the 70 clinical trials mentioning shedding analysis, 4 did not mention the method. In 32 of the clinical trials, only a PCR test was performed, while 14 of the studies did only perform an infectivity test such as a cell culture or a plaque assay test. In 17 of the trials, both a PCR and a cell culture or plaque assay were performed.

In most of the clinical trials that performed infectivity tests alone or in combination with a PCR, no infectious particles were observed in the various shedding samples analyzed. However, in a few trials (6/32), the presence of infectious particles was shown by cell culture or plaque assay in some shedding samples. This was the case for some saliva samples from metastatic prostate cancer subjects treated with a high dose of the oncolytic Adenovirus CG7870 [28], and for three subjects with solid tumors repeatedly treated intratumorally with the oncolytic Adenovirus ONCOS-102 and presenting infectious viral particles in buccal samples and, for one subject, also in the urine [29]. The presence of shed infectious particles in samples was also observed with other OV such as the Herpesvirus Imlygic®®, for which swabs from the surface of injected lesions from subjects with unresectable recurrent melanoma tested positive for infectivity [30], as well as the Parvovirus H-1, which was injected in subjects with metastatic pancreatic ductal adenocarcinoma (PDAC) and for which infectious particles were detected in feces swabs of five of the seven subjects [31]. We also observed the naturally Picornavirus Seneca Valley Virus (SVV-001), showing infectious virus in nasal secretions, sputum, blood, urine, and stool in all dose cohorts during the first weeks after injection [32], and the Vaccinia Virus (GL-ONC1), for which skin rash swabs were found positive for a virus in 2 out of 19 subjects with locoregionally advanced head and neck carcinoma [33]. All these examples illustrate that even if the shedding of infectious viral particles seems to be a rare event, it cannot be excluded.

4.3. *Aspects of the ERA Impacting Shedding*

A proper ERA of OV addresses several aspects that may impact the release of the viral particles by the host. This includes among others an examination of the genetic stability, the conditions under which replication is occurring, replication competence and the route of administration of the OV. Characteristics from the wild-type virus from which the OV has been derived, such as the pathogenicity, the tropism, the host range, the natural route of transmission and the shedding pattern, may provide valuable information to perform the ERA of OV. Furthermore, each of these aspects may be altered by the overall design and the genetic modification proper to a given OV [24,34].

With regard to the type of virus from which OV is derived, the detection of a viral DNA/RNA genome was observed at least once for all virus families (Figure 4). A rather clear picture is depicted for Adenovirus vectors, as the detection of the viral genome during shedding analysis was observed in 89% of the clinical trials with subjects treated with an adenoviral vector. It remains difficult to retrieve a general consideration for the other OV. As observed in Table 1, for oncolytic Herpesvirus vectors, the detection of the viral genome within shedding samples varies depending on the vector. Shedding has been observed only with the Herpesvirus Imlygic®® [30] and OrienX010 [35]. No shedding has been observed with the Herpesvirus OH2 [36], G207 [37–39], G47Δ [40], HF10 [41] or HSV176 [42,43]. Imlygic®® and OrienX010 both express the transgene GM-CSF used to boost the anti-tumor immune response by promoting dendritic cell recruitment and activation following tumor antigens' liberation from lysing tumor cells. Although OH2 also expresses the transgene GM-CSF, no shedding of viral particles has been observed [36].

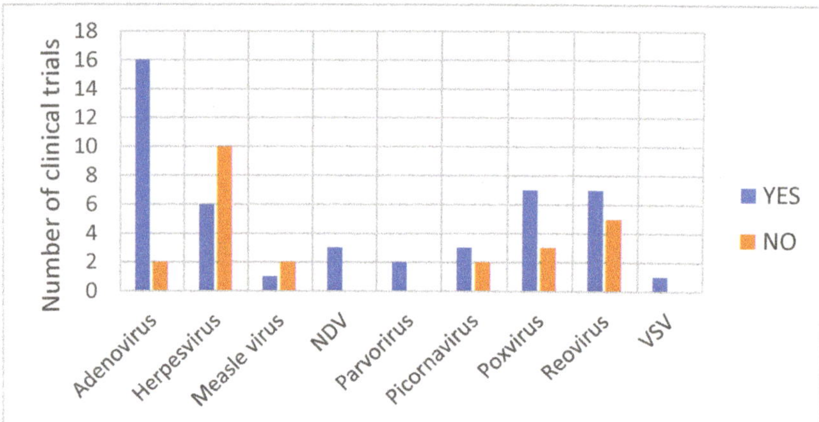

Figure 4. The number of clinical trials (by type of viral vector) for which the detection of viral genome was observed or was not observed in shedding samples.

Table 1. Overview of different oncolytic Herpesvirus vectors for which shedding analyses have been performed and the shedding observation.

Herpesvirus Vectors	Genetic Modifications [44]	Administration Route	Viral Genome Shedding	References
Imlygic®®	Armed recombinant HSV [1] with GM-CSF [2] transgen	IT [3]	Yes	[30]
OrienX010	Armed recombinant HSV with GM-CSF transgen	IT	Yes	[35]
OH2	Armed recombinant HSV with GM-CSF transgen	IT	No	[36]
G207	Conditionally replicating HSV with multiple mutations	IT	No	[37–39]
G47Δ	Conditionally replicating HSV with multiple mutations	IT	No	[40]
HF10	Conditionally replicating HSV with multiple mutations	IT	No	[41]

Table 1. *Cont.*

Herpesvirus Vectors	Genetic Modifications [44]	Administration Route	Viral Genome Shedding	References
HSV1716	Conditionally replicating HSV with multiple mutations	IT	No	[42,43]
NV1020	Conditionally replicating HSV with multiple mutations	Hepatic arterial injection	Yes and No	[45,46]

[1] HSV: Herpes Simplex Virus; [2] GM-CSF: Granulocyte-macrophage colony-stimulating factor; [3] IT: intratumoral injection.

Differences in shedding pattern have also been observed within the Picornaviruses class. Shedding of the viral particles from subjects treated with the naturally occurring replication-competent Picornavirus, Coxsackievirus [47] or Seneca Valley virus [32,48] has been observed, whereas no shedding has been observed from subjects treated with the recombinant Poliovirus PVS-RIPO [49,50]. For other types of OV, an analysis of the shedding pattern does not reveal any general trends, partly due to the relatively low number of studies reporting shedding analysis results.

In addition to the intrinsic properties of the OV and irrespective of the type of virus, due account should be given to the interaction of the OV with the host, which may have an effect on this interaction and hence on the shedding pattern. One should therefore remain cautious with extrapolating pre-clinical data to human beings. For example, the results of quantitative real-time PCR (qRT-PCR) indicate that VSV-IFNβ-NIS RNA was detectable in some early nasal, oral, and rectal swabs of inoculated pigs [51], or in some buccal swabs, urine or fecal samples of inoculated cancer dogs with detectable VSV-N gene copies close to or below the limit of detection (LOD) [52], with no infectious virus detected in any collected samples. These data are consistent with shedding results obtained during a clinical trial with subjects with hematologic malignancies intravenously injected with VSV-IFNβ-NIS. Quantitative RT-PCR at day 2 revealed a low level of viral genome in the saliva with no infectious virus detected [53]. Although, in non-clinical studies in non-human primates, presenting many similarities with humans, qRT-PCR analysis revealed no detection of viral genome in shedding buccal swab samples from these animals treated with the oncolytic virus VSV-IFNβ [54].

The route of administration used during clinical application usually differs from the natural portal of entry of the wild-type virus from which the OV are derived, and may also impact shedding pattern (Figure 5A,B). Intraperitoneal, intratumoral, intravenous or hepatic arterial injections are all routes of administration that may change the biodistribution and the shedding properties of the OV. In a phase I study with subjects with advanced solid tumors, treated with the replicating Adenovirus ONCOS-102, quantifiable levels of viral genomes were found in urine and buccal swabs after treatment, among which three subjects were found positive for infective virus 3 days after the first intravenous administration with 20% of the dose. However, all samples were found negative when the entire dose of ONCOS-102 was given intratumorally [29]. In another study investigating the safety and tolerability of an oncolytic H-1 Parvovirus, subjects were assigned to two arms differing in the route of administration of the initial virus application consisting either of a single intratumoral injection or five intravenous virus infusions on days 1 to 5. While in the intratumorally injected subjects, the viral genome was only detected in fecal samples at the highest dose, feces samples of all but one of the intravenously injected subjects were found positive at the lower doses [55]. No shedding of Measles virus MeV-NIS was observed when administrated intraperitoneally in subjects with ovarian cancer [56], whereas shedding was observed when administrated intravenously to subjects with recurrent or refractory multiple myeloma [57].

The same observation can be made with two oncolytic Poxvirus GL-ONC1 and Pexa-Vec. Shedding was observed when GL-ONC1 was delivered intravenously to subjects with advanced head and neck carcinoma [33], whereas no shedding was observed with the intraperitoneal injection of GL-ONC1 [58]. In a phase I clinical trial with intratumoral injection of the modified poxvirus Pexa-Vec/JX-594 into subjects with refractory primary or metastatic liver cancer, no evidence of viral genome shedding was observed by plaque assay analyses of urine and throat swab samples [59]. However, in a phase IIb clinical trial with Pexa-Vec given as a single IV infusion followed by up to five IT injections in subjects with advanced hepatocellular carcinoma, Pexa-Vec was recovered from throat swabs at day 8 post-IV (and before IT injection) in 36% (9/25) of the subjects, but not thereafter. All urine samples were tested negative at all timepoints [60]. Hence, it is important to consider that the location of the cancer and the concomitant choice of delivery of the investigated OV may affect subsequent shedding.

For oncovirotherapy, direct intratumoral injection is a preferred route of administration for brain tumors (18/23), despite the fact that it may pose significant challenges. Intratumoral injection of the OV is also mainly used for easily injectable tumors, such as melanoma (16/22), or head and neck cancers (6/8) (Figure 5C).

OV are also often administered intravenously in subjects with metastatic tumors. In this case, OV encounter many physiological barriers before reaching cancer lesions and repeated doses may be necessary, thereby triggering the recognition and attack by the immune system and clearance of the OV by neutralizing antibodies. While the latter is a concern for efficacy reasons, elicitation of a strong immune response may also result in a shorter duration of shedding.

As has been observed by Dunn et al. [61] and Weil et al. [62], the immune status of the subject could also have an effect on viral replication and subsequent viral genome shedding. Therefore, another aspect that could influence the viral vector shedding pattern is the use of concomitant drugs or treatments (e.g., radiotherapy, chemotherapy). Given the heterogeneity of cancer types, OV are likely to be administrated as part of combination regimens involving the modulation of immuno-inhibitory pathways and the T lymphocyte activation. Roulstone et al. reported that the shedding of RT3D RNA was more frequent when Reovirus was administrated together with cyclophosphamide than with Reovirus alone, or with combination regimens of RT3D and conventional chemotherapy [63].

Finally, the reactivation of latent OV, influenced by the immune status of the subject, could possibly lead to a shedding pattern that is different from what could have been predicted from former clinical experiences. For oncolytic viruses with the potential for latency reactivation, the collection of additional samples for shedding analysis when subjects show signs of infection due to reactivation could be planned.

4.4. Shedding Study Design

Each of the above-mentioned elements contributes to a risk-based approach in the design and the extent of shedding studies. It may provide insights into the choice of biological samples to be analyzed, as well as the frequency and the duration of monitoring.

Samples most commonly collected include urine and oral swabs. Other sample types such as feces, nasal swabs and injection site samples are also collected, but less commonly (see Figure 6).

The collection of data should also take into account the occurrence of metastasis. For example, secondary tumors may also be located in the oral cavity, larynx, pharynx or esophagus, justifying the collection of saliva samples.

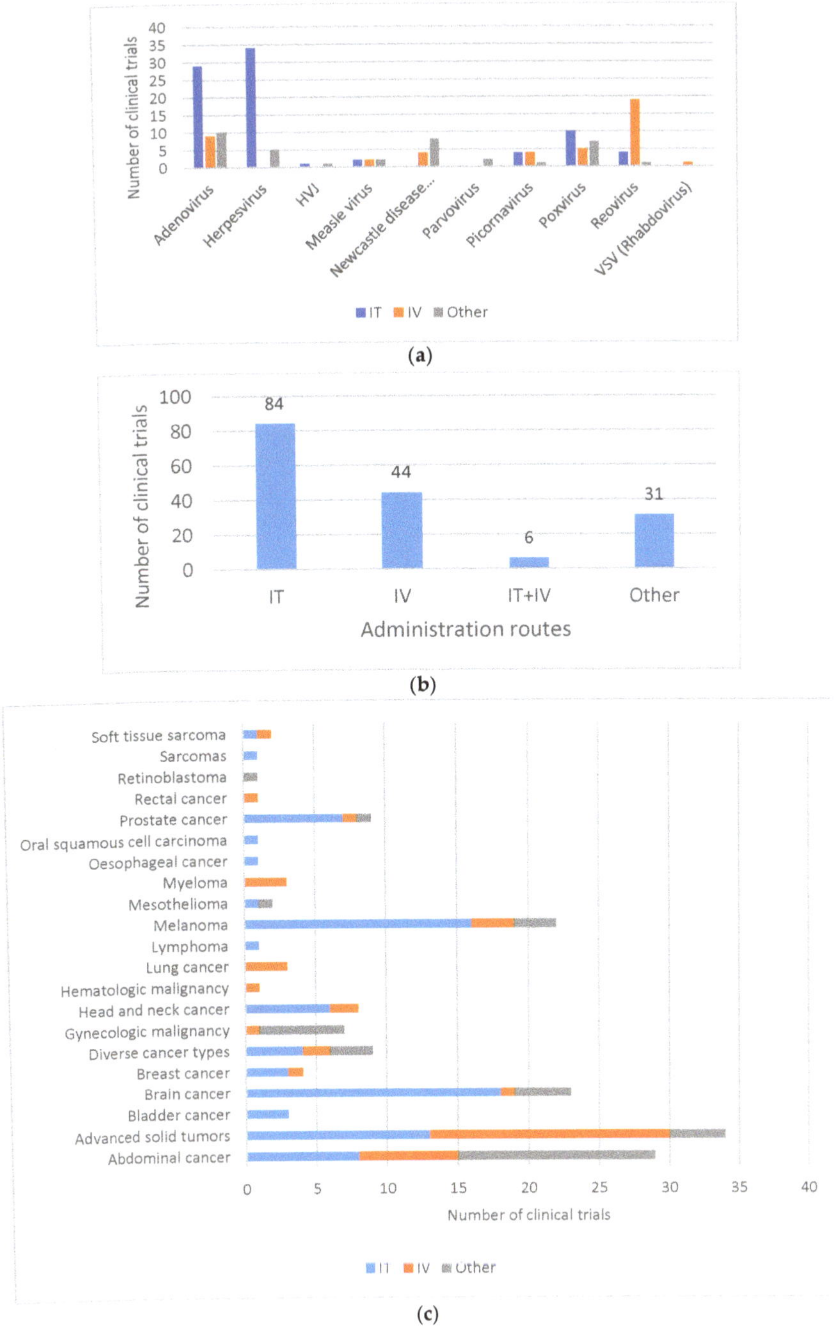

Figure 5. Routes of administration for oncolytic viruses in clinical trials. (**a**) Route of administration by type of oncolytic vectors. (**b**) Most commonly used administration routes in clinical trials. Most virus deliveries were performed by intratumoral route (n = 84). Other routes include, among others,

intradermal injection (8/165), intramuscular injection (1/165) and hepatic arterial injection (4/165). (**c**) Route of administration by type of cancer. IT = intratumoral; IV = intravenous. Sarcomas also include soft-tissue sarcoma. Brain cancers include central nervous system (CNS) cancer, glioma and glioblastoma. Gynecologic malignancies include ovarian cancer, tubal cancer, endometrial cancer or peritoneal cancer. Abdominal cancers include liver cancer, colorectal cancer, pancreatic cancer, kidney cancer (renal cell cancer) and stomach cancer (gastric cancer).

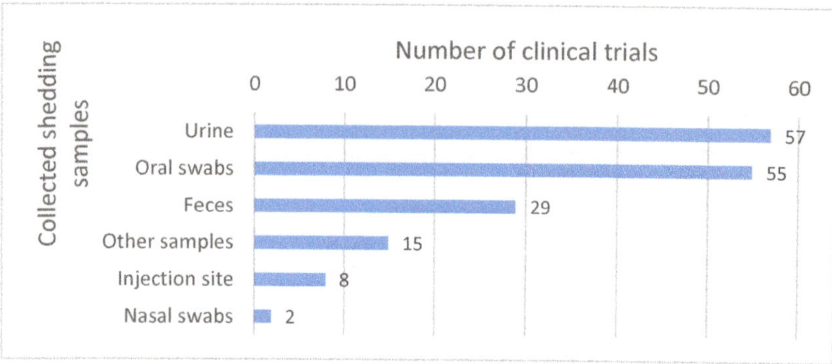

Figure 6. Body fluids collected for the shedding analysis. The numbers reported in the graph correspond to the number of clinical trials in which the corresponding samples were collected. Other samples include, among others, dressing swabs, lesion swabs, rash swabs, pustules swabs, etc.

When OV are administrated by the intradermal route, there is a possibility of transmission of the OV through skin contact. Therefore, the collection of skin swabs at the site of injection, in addition to samples routinely assessed for shedding, should be recommended in order to determine whether an appropriate occlusive dressing is required as a precautionary measure. According to our analysis, none of the trials performing intradermal injection reported shedding results. On the other hand, eight trials where the OV were administrated intratumorally included swabs from the injection site in their shedding analysis. From these eight trials, shed viral DNA at the injection site was observed in five trials. Of these five clinical trials, four trials were performed with Imlygic®® [30,64–66] and one with the Adenovirus Ad.hIFN-beta [67]. Detectable Imlygic®® DNA was observed on the surface of injected lesions for all treated subjects, and it was still detected for 14% of subjects during the safety follow-up period. Of the 740 swabs from the surface of injected lesions, 8 tested positive for infectivity [30]. The Adenovirus Ad.hIFN-beta DNA was detected and remained in the injection site area for at least 8 days [67].

The duration and frequency of sample collection should be decided on a case-by-case basis, taking into account the characteristics of the parental virus, the conditionally replicative competence of the OV and the immune status of the subject. As most of the OV are still replication-competent, the duration of sample collection should also take into account the possible appearance of a secondary peak of shedding. As one of the numerous examples of viral replication, it was shown that in subjects treated with the intratumorally injected HSP70, a telomerase-specific replication-competent oncolytic Adenovirus (telomelysin), viral DNA was detectable in plasma or sputum at days 7 and 14 post-treatment, despite being below detectable levels at 24 h post-treatment [68].

4.5. Risk Management Measures

The identification and characterization of potential adverse effects associated with the use of a given OV and the assessment of their likelihood of occurrence may lead to the identification of potential risks. It is also possible that the case-specific assessment reveals remaining uncertainties, precluding any conclusion on the risks for human health and the environment. In the first case, the set-up and implementation of risk management measures aim at minimizing identified risks, while in the second case, these could serve as precautionary measures.

In cases wherein data support the low likelihood of shedding or where no risk related to the shedding is identified for human health or the environment, good working practices involving proper hand hygiene, personal protective equipment (PPE) and proper decontamination and waste procedures at the clinical setting will be effective to limit the inadvertent exposure of personnel and the possible dissemination of the OV into the environment (Table 2). The correct implementation of these measures necessitates personnel trained and experience in handling infectious material.

Table 2. Examples of good working practices for personnel manipulating oncolytic vectors to prevent or manage risks for human health and/or the environment.

Preventing Measures	PPE	- Always use a lab coat and gloves to avoid any skin contamination during OV preparation and administration - Workers should wear a mask that conforms with the norm NBN EN 529, a FFP2 type (EN149:2001) with a P2 filter (EN 143:2000)
	Needle preparation	- The needle preparation of vials containing the oncolytic vector may generate aerosols. The preparation of the OV for administration is recommended to be conducted in a class II Biosafety Cabinet. Otherwise, the use of goggles and masks should be mandatory during the puncture of the vial and needle preparation - Removal of the syringe should occur by means of hands-free operation (i.e., hands do not touch the needle) into a closed container
	Spill kits	- Spill kits containing materials for spill clean-up should be on hand (or must be easily accessible to personnel) before handling the OV - The spill kit should contain liquid disinfectant, personal protective equipment (i.e., gloves, safety glasses, laboratory coat, shoe covers, mask), absorptive paper towels, tongs or forceps, a sharp container and biohazard waste bags
Risk Management Measures	Skin contact	- Skin contamination through spills should be handled by first placing an absorbent tissue on the affected area to adsorb all viral particles. An effective disinfectant should then be applied to the tissue. After removing the tissue, the skin should be washed with soap and water thoroughly and the tissue should be disposed of as a biohazard material
	Mucus membrane or eye contact	- In the case of accidental contact with open mouth or eye, rinse mouth or eye thoroughly over a closing basin. The collected washing liquid should be decontaminated with appropriate disinfectant before disposal - In the case of accidental ingestion, do not induce vomiting
	Accidental spill	In the case of accidental spills or breakage of a vial containing the GMO: - People in the area of the spill should be alerted and asked to leave the area - All personnel involved with the spill should remove contaminated clothes before leaving the area - The area should be closed to allow aerosols to be carried away and heavier particles to settle and a message "DO NOT ENTER" should be posted - After 30 min, the area can be entered again by wearing a clean lab coat, disposable gloves, glasses, disposable shoe covers and a mask - The spill should be covered with towels or other absorbent material starting from the edge toward the center. Appropriate disinfectant should be poured over the absorbent material starting from the edge to the center. Sufficient contact time should be allowed so as to ensure inactivation of the GMO by the disinfectant - After that, the paper towels and broken vials should be removed with tongs or forceps and discarded in a biohazard waste bag. The PPE should be discarded in the biohazard bag. The lab coat should be decontaminated before disposal - The medical staff should report the incident to the responsible member on the site

When shedding by the treated subject cannot be excluded and potential risks for human health and the environment have been identified, risk management measures should also focus on minimizing the exposure of third parties outside the clinical setting, thereby giving particular attention to immunosuppressed or any vulnerable people (e.g., pregnant women, newborns, infants, elderly people). A list of possible measures that may be considered, taking into account the considerations made as part of a case-specific risk assessment, is provided in a guidance document endorsed by several national competent authorities involved in the risk assessment GMOs [27] and has been further adapted in Figure 7.

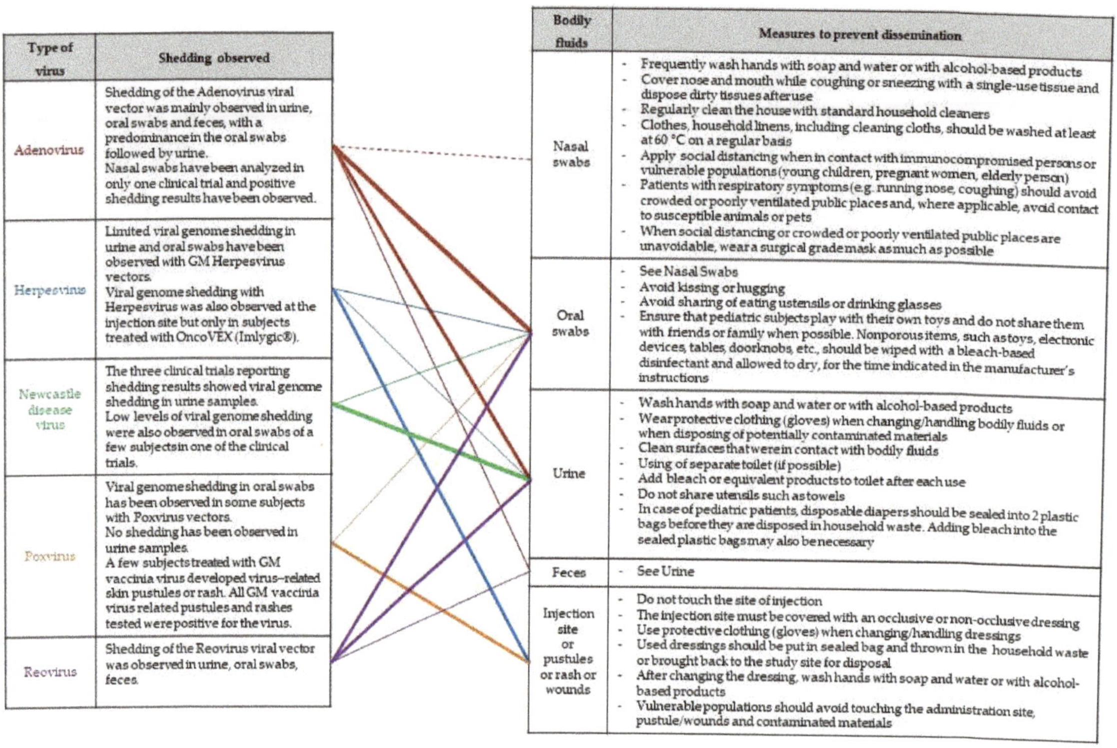

Figure 7. Possible risk-mitigation measures. The lines indicate observed trends in shedding results obtained from clinical trials involving OV. The thickness of the lines is proportional to shedding results per OV type.

Geletneky et al. indicated in their article that glioblastoma subjects treated with the oncolytic Parvovirus H-1 were obliged to stay isolated in the study center until shed viral genomes were no longer detected in feces, urine or saliva, or until the first occurrence of H-1-specific antibodies [55].

It could be hypothesized that OV applications that have entered the market and that have successfully gone through the several stages of clinical development would rely on shedding data to determine risk management measures, if deemed relevant according to a proper risk assessment, and that data on the occurrence of transmission to close contacts would allow further refinement of risk management measures. In this ideal scenario, evidence-based data would contribute to a set of management measures that are as proportionate as possible to the environmental risk. However, the occurrence of secondary infections is barely addressed during clinical development. Given that these viral vectors are often derived from infectious viruses, any studies that contribute to the assessment of possible secondary infection would further contribute to the ERA of the medicinal product.

During a phase II clinical trial with modified Herpesvirus Imlygic®®, Andtbacka et al. reported that some mucosal or skin lesions were observed in close contact, and investigators all tested negative for T-VEC. However, none of the lesions were tested for wild-type HSV-1 or HSV-2, leaving an uncertainty as to the origin of the lesion [30].

The precautionary measures that were implemented for the subject during this phase II study with Imlygic®® are also found in the current subject brochure for Imlygic®®, which stipulates measures to be taken by the subject to avoid the direct contact of thirds with the subjects' bodily fluids or injection sites, such as covering injection sites with airtight and watertight dressings, implementing a proper disposal of used dressings and cleaning material to prevent household contacts from directly touching them [69].

An ongoing post-marketing study of melanoma subjects treated with Imlygic®®, started in 2017, is among others counting the numbers of herpetic infections, with the detection of T-DNA among close contacts and healthcare providers as a secondary outcome [70]. This exemplifies that efforts to collect information on the effective transmission of Imlygic®® are being pursued.

Finally, if animals may be infected, appropriate measures to limit exposure to susceptible pets or other animals in the immediate surroundings of the treated subject should be considered. Newcastle disease virus (NDV), for example, is a naturally occurring oncolytic virus that causes severe illness in birds and poultry, and could therefore pose an environmental risk even if it is non-pathogenic in humans. In three clinical trials with intravenously injected NDV-PV701 in subjects with advanced solid cancer [71–73], low levels of viral genome shedding in urine have been observed up to 3 weeks after injection. Pecora et al. [73] also observed low and transient levels of viral genome shedding in sputum. Although, Pecora et al. suggested that the levels of shed PV701 are orders of magnitude below the standard avian vaccine dose required for an antibody response, appropriate biosafety measures to prevent environmental spread of the virus should be considered when administrating high-dose oncolytic NDV. Subjects working with birds and poultry or subjects having a pet bird or poultry at home could be asked to avoid contact with these NDV host species for a certain time after injection of the IMP, in order to reduce the potential environmental impact of viral shedding on the most susceptible host species.

Another example of clinical trials where measures to avoid contact with animals have been proposed involved the use of a recombinant chimeric Vesicular stomatitis virus, in which the VSV glycoprotein was replaced to abrogate neurotoxicity and pathogenicity [74]. As the OV were derived from a vector-borne virus causing significant disease in pigs, cattle and horses, instructions for avoiding contact with livestock for seven days following administration of the OV have been proposed [75].

5. Discussion and Recommendations

The inventory presented in this paper provides a state-of-the-art of the shedding analysis of OV in clinical practice, and raises the question: to what extent it is possible to build upon the experience gained so far with shedding data to draw conclusions for each of the different types of OV? This may be particularly relevant in cases where historical shedding data have been obtained for well-characterized OV, of which the designs present relevant similarities with a novel investigational OV. Our literature search reveals that in 89% of the studies with Adenovirus-derived OV reporting shedding analysis, positive shedding results were obtained. However, as illustrated above by the several examples developed in this paper, the shedding patterns remain diverse and complex, as well as for Adenovirus-derived OV, thereby hindering the development of a standardized study design. Diversity in shedding patterns was observed even when using OV derived from the same type of virus. A number of elements may impact the shedding pattern, such as the specific design of the viral vector and the transgene harbored by the viral vector, the interaction of the OV with their host organisms, the immune status of the patient or the variety of the clinical protocols, such as differences in the administration route or the use of concomitant drugs.

Valuable information and insights into the toxicity, biodistribution and shedding pattern of OV could be obtained from non-clinical studies. As compared to clinical studies, animal studies are more amenable to be conducted in the early stages of the development of investigational OV. However, it should be taken into account that data are not readily extrapolable from animals to human, in particular when different routes of administration are used or no data have been collected in larger animals, such as non-human primates. Also, an animal model fails to mimic the patient-specific immune status. This means that an absence of viral shedding in animal studies does not necessarily preclude viral shedding in humans, as a different host organism may induce a different behavior of the virus (viral replication, viral clearance, viral tropism).

Because the shedding pattern strongly depends on different factors and because it can also differ between animals and humans, the collection of shedding data in the earliest phase of clinical development of investigational OV is strongly recommended regardless of the OV vector.

The FDA guidance for the design and analysis of shedding studies also recommends the collection of shedding data on OV in the earliest phase of clinical development (phase I) and anytime afterwards if the dose, the route of administration, the regimen or the indication are modified [25]. Likewise, both an EMA guideline on scientific requirements for the ERA of Gene Therapy Medicinal Products and an EC consideration document specifically addressing the evaluation of shedding with OV recommend addressing shedding analysis as early as possible in the clinical development, and more particularly during a phase I study [23,26]. Whilst the time point of sample collection for shedding has not been further specified in the EC consideration document, the FDA guidance recommends sampling on days 1, 3, 7 and 10, and then weekly, until the shedding analysis reveals three consecutive results below the LOD of the assay. Notably, all guidance emphasizes the need of a case-by-case approach taking into account the properties of the OV (replication competence, known persistence or possibility of latency reactivation of the parental virus from which the OV are derived) and the interaction with the host (immune status of the patient and thirds, single versus multiple round of administration and effect on clearance by the immune system) [21,23,25,26]. For example, in the case of subsequent rounds of dose administration, the time point of sampling can be adapted when justified by a proper shedding analysis obtained with a single-dose administration.

A possible concern, for which we could not find experimental data, is the likelihood of an in vivo recombination between the OV and endogenous viruses circulating in the trial participants. This assessment should not be neglected because recombination events could lead to the formation of uncharacterized variants that could be more virulent and that could affect the shedding pattern and the potential for transmission. These newly generated viruses could therefore compromise the environmental safety. In general, the likelihood of the recombination between viruses significantly increases with the prevalence of co-circulating viruses in the population, and with their genetic homology. High viral loads, often a relevant feature of replication-competent OV, increase the chance of exchanging strands, explaining why, in many cases, recombination is often replication-dependent [76]. Moreover, Buijs et al. [77] mentioned the relevance of assessing the recombination of these OV with wild-type viruses given the ongoing strategies to use more virulent conditionally replicating viruses. A possible explanation for the fact that the likelihood of the recombination of OV has been barely examined is that, unless there is scientific evidence pointing to recombination, such as in in vitro experiments demonstrating the generation of novel and uncharacterized recombinants, developers could be hesitant to pursue this research due to the anticipated low occurrence and the technical hurdles of the lower limit of detection and quantification associated with the monitoring of viral particles.

Whilst the collection of shedding data undoubtedly supports an evidence-based ERA, it is important to be aware that the shedding of OV or any other viral vector or virus does not necessarily involve a risk. Potential adverse effects for close contacts or the environment that could arise following shedding do not only result from the presence of viral particles in the shedding samples, but also depend on the stability of the shed viral particles under environmental conditions outside the host, the route of transmission (e.g., spreading through aerosols, fecal–oral route of transmission via direct contact or contaminated fluids, vector-borne transmission, through parenteral exposure), the capacity of the shed particles to infect cells of other persons or animals, and, as a last element in the chain of events for environmental risk to occur, the capacity of the OV to cause adverse effects in the novel host organism. To possibly alleviate remaining uncertainties in secondary transmission, it is therefore important to answer the questions of whether the observed shed particles are only vector DNA/RNA or a remnant thereof, and whether these shed particles are still infectious. These observations will contribute to a proportionate risk management by allowing the determination of appropriate precautionary measures.

Indeed, a fundamental question when uncertainties remain regarding the actual risk associated to the shedding of OV is what level of risk management measures should be taken, or what level of uncertainty would warrant precautionary measures. If it remains unclear whether shedding may occur and what risks it may entail for human health and the environment, a drastic and conservative scenario would be to eliminate any possibility of release of OV into the environment by keeping patients for several weeks/months in the hospital setting. However, the implementation of stringent measures may carry drawbacks, as it may increase costs and time not only for the appropriate training of personnel, the set-up and follow-up of waste disposal procedures and logistics, but also for the recruitment of subjects requiring their informed consent and the training of close contacts if the trial participant is discharged. Ideally, risk management measures should be as proportionate as possible to the actual risk posed so as not to hinder the development of research and innovation and to safeguard patient access to innovative treatments, while ensuring the proper protection of human health at large and the environment. A way to contribute to proportionate risk management is to continue to gathering data-based evidence by including within the shedding analysis the determination of the fraction of infectious particles in early phases of the clinical development of OV.

6. Concluding Recommendations

With the diversity of OV that entered the clinical research and development landscape, this work demonstrates the current gaps in data-based evidence on shedding and the challenge of defining risk management measures that are proportionate to the actual risk posed for human health and the environment. In accordance with GMO legislation requiring a case-specific and risk-proportionate approach, this paper aims at encouraging the collection of shedding data as early as possible in the developmental plan in the rapidly growing area of OV. The demonstration of the shedding of infectious particles may warrant assessments of the potential of secondary transmission. The collection of real-world transmission data is expected to provide a better understanding of transmissibility, which is key to characterizing the risk for the human population and the environment. It will also benefit future clinical trials developers in establishing a clinical protocol based on evidence-based risk assessment.

Supplementary Materials: The following supporting information can be downloaded at: https://www.mdpi.com/article/10.3390/vaccines11091448/s1, Table S1: Final list of 165 manuscripts.

Author Contributions: Conceptualization, writing—original draft preparation, writing—review and editing: S.O., A.B. and K.P. All authors have read and agreed to the published version of the manuscript.

Funding: This work received support from the Brussels-Capital Region, the Flemish Region, Wallonia and the Federal Agency for Medicines and Health Products (FAMHP).

Institutional Review Board Statement: Not applicable.

Informed Consent Statement: Not applicable.

Data Availability Statement: Data sharing not applicable.

Acknowledgments: The authors thank Didier Breyer, Amaya Leunda, Emilie Descamps and Fanny Coppens (Sciensano) for their critical reading of a late phase of the manuscript.

Conflicts of Interest: The authors declare no conflict of interest.

References

1. Müller, L.; Berkeley, R.; Barr, T.; Ilett, E.; Errington-Mais, F. Past, Present and Future of Oncolytic Reovirus. *Cancers* **2020**, *12*, 3219. [CrossRef]
2. Schirrmacher, V.; van Gool, S.; Stuecker, W. Breaking Therapy Resistance: An Update on Oncolytic Newcastle Disease Virus for Improvements of Cancer Therapy. *Biomedicines* **2019**, *7*, 66. [CrossRef] [PubMed]
3. Zhang, Y.; Nagalo, B.M. Immunovirotherapy Based on Recombinant Vesicular Stomatitis Virus: Where Are We? *Front. Immunol.* **2022**, *13*, 898631. [CrossRef] [PubMed]
4. Msaouel, P.; Opyrchal, M.; Domingo Musibay, E.; Galanis, E. Oncolytic Measles Virus Strains as Novel Anticancer Agents. *Expert Opin. Biol. Ther.* **2013**, *13*, 483–502. [CrossRef] [PubMed]
5. Macedo, N.; Miller, D.M.; Haq, R.; Kaufman, H.L. Clinical Landscape of Oncolytic Virus Research in 2020. *J. Immunother. Cancer* **2020**, *8*, e001486. [CrossRef] [PubMed]
6. Watanabe, N.; McKenna, M.K.; Rosewell Shaw, A.; Suzuki, M. Clinical CAR-T Cell and Oncolytic Virotherapy for Cancer Treatment. *Mol. Ther.* **2021**, *29*, 505–520. [CrossRef] [PubMed]
7. FDA: U.S. Food & Drug Administration: Imlygic. STN: 125518. Available online: https://www.fda.gov/vaccines-blood-biologics/cellular-gene-therapy-products/imlygic (accessed on 11 July 2023).
8. European Medicines Agency: Imlygic (Talimogene Laherparepvec). EMEA/H/C/002771. Available online: https://www.ema.europa.eu/en/medicines/human/EPAR/imlygic (accessed on 11 July 2023).
9. European Commission: Public Health—Union Register of Medicinal Products—Imlygic: EU/1/15/1064. Active Substance: Talimogene Laherparepvec. Available online: https://ec.europa.eu/health/documents/community-register/html/h1064.htm (accessed on 11 July 2023).
10. Alberts, P.; Tilgase, A.; Rasa, A.; Bandere, K.; Venskus, D. The Advent of Oncolytic Virotherapy in Oncology: The Rigvir®® Story. *Eur. J. Pharmacol.* **2018**, *837*, 117–126. [CrossRef] [PubMed]
11. State Agency of Medicines Republic of Latvia: Rigvir Marketing Authorisation Suspended; Information for Current Patients. 3 July 2019. Available online: https://www.zva.gov.lv/en/news-and-publications/news/rigvir-marketing-authorisation-suspended-information-current-patients (accessed on 11 July 2023).
12. Wei, D.; Xu, J.; Liu, X.-Y.; Chen, Z.-N.; Bian, H. Fighting Cancer with Viruses: Oncolytic Virus Therapy in China. *Hum. Gene Ther.* **2018**, *29*, 151–159. [CrossRef]
13. Report on the Deliberation Results from the Committee on Regenerative Medicine Products and Biotechnology. Brand Name: Delytact Injection. 24 May 2021. Available online: https://www.pmda.go.jp/files/000242808.pdf (accessed on 11 July 2023).
14. Schulze, T.; Kemmner, W.; Weitz, J.; Wernecke, K.-D.; Schirrmacher, V.; Schlag, P.M. Efficiency of Adjuvant Active Specific Immunization with Newcastle Disease Virus Modified Tumor Cells in Colorectal Cancer Patients Following Resection of Liver Metastases: Results of a Prospective Randomized Trial. *Cancer Immunol. Immunother.* **2009**, *58*, 61–69. [CrossRef]
15. Liang, W.; Wang, H.; Sun, T.-M.; Yao, W.-Q.; Chen, L.-L.; Jin, Y.; Li, C.-L.; Meng, F.-J. Application of Autologous Tumor Cell Vaccine and NDV Vaccine in Treatment of Tumors of Digestive Tract. *World J. Gastroenterol.* **2003**, *9*, 495–498. [CrossRef]
16. Abou-Alfa, G.K.; Galle, P.R.; Chao, Y.; Brown, K.T.; Heo, J.; Borad, M.J.; Luca, A.; Pelusio, A.; Agathon, D.; Lusky, M.; et al. PHOCUS: A Phase 3 Randomized, Open-Label Study Comparing the Oncolytic Immunotherapy Pexa-Vec Followed by Sorafenib (SOR) vs. SOR in Patients with Advanced Hepatocellular Carcinoma (HCC) without Prior Systemic Therapy. *JCO* **2016**, *34*, TPS4146. [CrossRef]
17. U.S. National Institutes of Health, ClinicalTrials.gov. Efficacy Study of REOLYSIN®® in Combination with Paclitaxel and Carboplatin in Platinum-Refractory Head and Neck Cancers. Official Title: Randomized, Double-Blind, Multicenter Two-Stage Adaptive Phase 3 Study of Intravenous Administration of REOLYSIN (Reovirus Type 3 Dearing) in Combination with Paclitaxel and Carboplatin Versus the Chemotherapy Alone in Patients with Metastatic or Recurrent Squamous Cell Carcinoma of the Head and Neck Who Have Progressed on or After Prior Platinum-Based Chemotherapy. Identifier: NCT01166542. Available online: https://clinicaltrials.gov/study/NCT01166542 (accessed on 11 July 2023).
18. U.S. National Institutes of Health, ClinicalTrials.gov. An Integrated Phase II/III, Open Label, Randomized and Controlled Study of the Safety and Efficacy of CG0070 Adenovirus 679 Vector Expressing GM-CSF in Patients With NMIBC With Carcinoma In Situ Disease Who Have Failed BCG. Identifier: NCT01438112. Available online: https://clinicaltrials.gov/study/NCT01438112 (accessed on 11 July 2023).
19. Schenk-Braat, E.A.M.; van Mierlo, M.M.K.B.; Wagemaker, G.; Bangma, C.H.; Kaptein, L.C.M. An Inventory of Shedding Data from Clinical Gene Therapy Trials. *J. Gene Med.* **2007**, *9*, 910–921. [CrossRef]

20. Cook, M.; Chauhan, A. Clinical Application of Oncolytic Viruses: A Systematic Review. *Int. J. Mol. Sci.* **2020**, *21*, 7505. [CrossRef] [PubMed]
21. EMEA 2008. Committee for the Medicinal Product for Human Use (CHMP)—Guideline on Scientific Requirements for the Environmental Risk Assessment of Gene Therapy Medicinal Products. EMEA/CHMP/GTMP/125491/2006. Available online: https://www.ema.europa.eu/en/documents/scientific-guideline/guideline-scientific-requirements-environmental-risk-assessment-gene-therapy-medicinal-products_en.pdf (accessed on 11 July 2023).
22. Baldo, A.; van den Akker, E.; Bergmans, H.E.; Lim, F.; Pauwels, K. General Considerations on the Biosafety of Virus-Derived Vectors Used in Gene Therapy and Vaccination. *Curr. Gene Ther.* **2013**, *13*, 385–394. [CrossRef]
23. EC Commission Decision 2002/623/EC of 24 July 2002 Establishing Guidance Notes Supplementing Annex II to Directive 2001/18/EC of the European Parliament and of the Council on the Deliberate Release into the Environment of Genetically Modified Organisms and Repealing Council Directive 90/220/EEC. Official Journal L 200, 30/07/2002 P. 0022-0033. Available online: http://data.europa.eu/eli/dec/2002/623/oj (accessed on 11 July 2023).
24. van den Akker, E.; van der Vlugt, C.J.B.; Bleijs, D.A.; Bergmans, H.E. Environmental Risk Assessment of Replication Competent Viral Vectors Applied in Clinical Trials: Potential Effects of Inserted Sequences. *Curr. Gene Ther.* **2013**, *13*, 395–412. [CrossRef] [PubMed]
25. FDA 2015. Design and Analysis of Shedding Studies for Virus or Bacteria-Based Gene Therapy and Oncolytic Products—Guidance for Industry. Available online: https://www.fda.gov/media/89036/download (accessed on 11 July 2023).
26. EMEA 2009. IHC Considerations: General Principles to Address Virus and Vector Shedding. EMEA/CHMP/ICH/449035/2009. Available online: https://www.ema.europa.eu/en/documents/scientific-guideline/international-conference-harmonisation-technical-requirements-registration-pharmaceuticals-human-use_en-10.pdf (accessed on 11 July 2023).
27. Oncolytic Viruses: Considerations for Evaluation of Shedding. Version 2 January 2022 European Commission. Available online: https://health.ec.europa.eu/system/files/2022-01/oncolytic_evaluation_en.pdf (accessed on 11 July 2023).
28. Small, E.J.; Carducci, M.A.; Burke, J.M.; Rodriguez, R.; Fong, L.; van Ummersen, L.; Yu, D.C.; Aimi, J.; Ando, D.; Working, P.; et al. A Phase I Trial of Intravenous CG7870, a Replication-Selective, Prostate-Specific Antigen-Targeted Oncolytic Adenovirus, for the Treatment of Hormone-Refractory, Metastatic Prostate Cancer. *Mol. Ther.* **2006**, *14*, 107–117. [CrossRef] [PubMed]
29. Ranki, T.; Pesonen, S.; Hemminki, A.; Partanen, K.; Kairemo, K.; Alanko, T.; Lundin, J.; Linder, N.; Turkki, R.; Ristimäki, A.; et al. Phase I Study with ONCOS-102 for the Treatment of Solid Tumors—An Evaluation of Clinical Response and Exploratory Analyses of Immune Markers. *J. Immunother. Cancer* **2016**, *4*, 17. [CrossRef] [PubMed]
30. Andtbacka, R.H.I.; Amatruda, T.; Nemunaitis, J.; Zager, J.S.; Walker, J.; Chesney, J.A.; Liu, K.; Hsu, C.-P.; Pickett, C.A.; Mehnert, J.M. Biodistribution, Shedding, and Transmissibility of the Oncolytic Virus Talimogene Laherparepvec in Patients with Melanoma. *EBioMedicine* **2019**, *47*, 89–97. [CrossRef]
31. Hajda, J.; Leuchs, B.; Angelova, A.L.; Frehtman, V.; Rommelaere, J.; Mertens, M.; Pilz, M.; Kieser, M.; Krebs, O.; Dahm, M.; et al. Phase 2 Trial of Oncolytic H-1 Parvovirus Therapy Shows Safety and Signs of Immune System Activation in Patients With Metastatic Pancreatic Ductal Adenocarcinoma. *Clin. Cancer Res.* **2021**, *27*, 5546–5556. [CrossRef]
32. Rudin, C.M.; Poirier, J.T.; Senzer, N.N.; Stephenson, J.; Loesch, D.; Burroughs, K.D.; Reddy, P.S.; Hann, C.L.; Hallenbeck, P.L. Phase I Clinical Study of Seneca Valley Virus (SVV-001), a Replication-Competent Picornavirus, in Advanced Solid Tumors with Neuroendocrine Features. *Clin. Cancer Res.* **2011**, *17*, 888–895. [CrossRef]
33. Mell, L.K.; Brumund, K.T.; Daniels, G.A.; Advani, S.J.; Zakeri, K.; Wright, M.E.; Onyeama, S.-J.; Weisman, R.A.; Sanghvi, P.R.; Martin, P.J.; et al. Phase I Trial of Intravenous Oncolytic Vaccinia Virus (GL-ONC1) with Cisplatin and Radiotherapy in Patients with Locoregionally Advanced Head and Neck Carcinoma. *Clin. Cancer Res.* **2017**, *23*, 5696–5702. [CrossRef] [PubMed]
34. Bergmans, H.; Logie, C.; Van Maanen, K.; Hermsen, H.; Meredyth, M.; Van Der Vlugt, C. Identification of Potentially Hazardous Human Gene Products in GMO Risk Assessment. *Environ. Biosaf. Res.* **2008**, *7*, 1–9. [CrossRef] [PubMed]
35. Cui, C.; Wang, X.; Lian, B.; Ji, Q.; Zhou, L.; Chi, Z.; Si, L.; Sheng, X.; Kong, Y.; Yu, J.; et al. OrienX010, an Oncolytic Virus, in Patients with Unresectable Stage IIIC-IV Melanoma: A Phase Ib Study. *J. Immunother. Cancer* **2022**, *10*, e004307. [CrossRef] [PubMed]
36. Zhang, B.; Huang, J.; Tang, J.; Hu, S.; Luo, S.; Luo, Z.; Zhou, F.; Tan, S.; Ying, J.; Chang, Q.; et al. Intratumoral OH2, an Oncolytic Herpes Simplex Virus 2, in Patients with Advanced Solid Tumors: A Multicenter, Phase I/II Clinical Trial. *J. Immunother. Cancer* **2021**, *9*, e002224. [CrossRef] [PubMed]
37. Friedman, G.K.; Johnston, J.M.; Bag, A.K.; Bernstock, J.D.; Li, R.; Aban, I.; Kachurak, K.; Nan, L.; Kang, K.-D.; Totsch, S.; et al. Oncolytic HSV-1 G207 Immunovirotherapy for Pediatric High-Grade Gliomas. *N. Engl. J. Med.* **2021**, *384*, 1613–1622. [CrossRef] [PubMed]
38. Markert, J.M.; Medlock, M.D.; Rabkin, S.D.; Gillespie, G.Y.; Todo, T.; Hunter, W.D.; Palmer, C.A.; Feigenbaum, F.; Tornatore, C.; Tufaro, F.; et al. Conditionally Replicating Herpes Simplex Virus Mutant, G207 for the Treatment of Malignant Glioma: Results of a Phase I Trial. *Gene Ther.* **2000**, *7*, 867–874. [CrossRef] [PubMed]
39. Markert, J.M.; Liechty, P.G.; Wang, W.; Gaston, S.; Braz, E.; Karrasch, M.; Nabors, L.B.; Markiewicz, M.; Lakeman, A.D.; Palmer, C.A.; et al. Phase Ib Trial of Mutant Herpes Simplex Virus G207 Inoculated Pre-and Post-Tumor Resection for Recurrent GBM. *Mol. Ther.* **2009**, *17*, 199–207. [CrossRef]
40. Todo, T.; Ino, Y.; Ohtsu, H.; Shibahara, J.; Tanaka, M. A Phase I/II Study of Triple-Mutated Oncolytic Herpes Virus G47Δ in Patients with Progressive Glioblastoma. *Nat. Commun.* **2022**, *13*, 4119. [CrossRef]

41. Kasuya, H.; Kodera, Y.; Nakao, A.; Yamamura, K.; Gewen, T.; Zhiwen, W.; Hotta, Y.; Yamada, S.; Fujii, T.; Fukuda, S.; et al. Phase I Dose-Escalation Clinical Trial of HF10 Oncolytic Herpes Virus in 17 Japanese Patients with Advanced Cancer. *Hepatogastroenterology* **2014**, *61*, 599–605.
42. Danson, S.J.; Conner, J.; Edwards, J.G.; Blyth, K.G.; Fisher, P.M.; Muthana, M.; Salawu, A.; Taylor, F.; Hodgkinson, E.; Joyce, P.; et al. Oncolytic Herpesvirus Therapy for Mesothelioma—A Phase I/IIa Trial of Intrapleural Administration of HSV1716. *Lung Cancer* **2020**, *150*, 145–151. [CrossRef]
43. Streby, K.A.; Geller, J.I.; Currier, M.A.; Warren, P.S.; Racadio, J.M.; Towbin, A.J.; Vaughan, M.R.; Triplet, M.; Ott-Napier, K.; Dishman, D.J.; et al. Intratumoral Injection of HSV1716, an Oncolytic Herpes Virus, Is Safe and Shows Evidence of Immune Response and Viral Replication in Young Cancer Patients. *Clin. Cancer Res.* **2017**, *23*, 3566–3574. [CrossRef] [PubMed]
44. Menotti, L.; Avitabile, E. Herpes Simplex Virus Oncolytic Immunovirotherapy: The Blossoming Branch of Multimodal Therapy. *Int. J. Mol. Sci.* **2020**, *21*, 8310. [CrossRef] [PubMed]
45. Fong, Y.; Kim, T.; Bhargava, A.; Schwartz, L.; Brown, K.; Brody, L.; Covey, A.; Karrasch, M.; Getrajdman, G.; Mescheder, A.; et al. A Herpes Oncolytic Virus Can Be Delivered via the Vasculature to Produce Biologic Changes in Human Colorectal Cancer. *Mol. Ther.* **2009**, *17*, 389–394. [CrossRef] [PubMed]
46. Geevarghese, S.K.; Geller, D.A.; de Haan, H.A.; Hörer, M.; Knoll, A.E.; Mescheder, A.; Nemunaitis, J.; Reid, T.R.; Sze, D.Y.; Tanabe, K.K.; et al. Phase I/II Study of Oncolytic Herpes Simplex Virus NV1020 in Patients with Extensively Pretreated Refractory Colorectal Cancer Metastatic to the Liver. *Hum. Gene Ther.* **2010**, *21*, 1119–1128. [CrossRef] [PubMed]
47. Annels, N.E.; Mansfield, D.; Arif, M.; Ballesteros-Merino, C.; Simpson, G.R.; Denyer, M.; Sandhu, S.S.; Melcher, A.A.; Harrington, K.J.; Davies, B.; et al. Phase I Trial of an ICAM-1-Targeted Immunotherapeutic-Coxsackievirus A21 (CVA21) as an Oncolytic Agent Against Non Muscle-Invasive Bladder Cancer. *Clin. Cancer Res.* **2019**, *25*, 5818–5831. [CrossRef]
48. Burke, M.J.; Ahern, C.; Weigel, B.J.; Poirier, J.T.; Rudin, C.M.; Chen, Y.; Cripe, T.P.; Bernhardt, M.B.; Blaney, S.M. Phase I Trial of Seneca Valley Virus (NTX-010) in Children with Relapsed/Refractory Solid Tumors: A Report of the Children's Oncology Group. *Pediatr. Blood Cancer* **2015**, *62*, 743–750. [CrossRef]
49. Desjardins, A.; Gromeier, M.; Herndon, J.E.; Beaubier, N.; Bolognesi, D.P.; Friedman, A.H.; Friedman, H.S.; McSherry, F.; Muscat, A.M.; Nair, S.; et al. Recurrent Glioblastoma Treated with Recombinant Poliovirus. *N. Engl. J. Med.* **2018**, *379*, 150–161. [CrossRef]
50. Beasley, G.M.; Nair, S.K.; Farrow, N.E.; Landa, K.; Selim, M.A.; Wiggs, C.A.; Jung, S.-H.; Bigner, D.D.; True Kelly, A.; Gromeier, M.; et al. Phase I Trial of Intratumoral PVSRIPO in Patients with Unresectable, Treatment-Refractory Melanoma. *J. Immunother. Cancer* **2021**, *9*, e002203. [CrossRef]
51. Velazquez-Salinas, L.; Naik, S.; Pauszek, S.J.; Peng, K.-W.; Russell, S.J.; Rodriguez, L.L. Oncolytic Recombinant Vesicular Stomatitis Virus (VSV) Is Nonpathogenic and Nontransmissible in Pigs, a Natural Host of VSV. *Hum. Gene Ther. Clin Dev* **2017**, *28*, 108–115. [CrossRef]
52. Naik, S.; Galyon, G.D.; Jenks, N.J.; Steele, M.B.; Miller, A.C.; Allstadt, S.D.; Suksanpaisan, L.; Peng, K.W.; Federspiel, M.J.; Russell, S.J.; et al. Comparative Oncology Evaluation of Intravenous Recombinant Oncolytic Vesicular Stomatitis Virus Therapy in Spontaneous Canine Cancer. *Mol. Cancer Ther.* **2018**, *17*, 316–326. [CrossRef]
53. Cook, J.; Peng, K.-W.; Witzig, T.E.; Broski, S.M.; Villasboas, J.C.; Paludo, J.; Patnaik, M.; Rajkumar, V.; Dispenzieri, A.; Leung, N.; et al. Clinical Activity of Single-Dose Systemic Oncolytic VSV Virotherapy in Patients with Relapsed Refractory T-Cell Lymphoma. *Blood Adv.* **2022**, *6*, 3268–3279. [CrossRef] [PubMed]
54. Jenks, N.; Myers, R.; Greiner, S.M.; Thompson, J.; Mader, E.K.; Greenslade, A.; Griesmann, G.E.; Federspiel, M.J.; Rakela, J.; Borad, M.J.; et al. Safety Studies on Intrahepatic or Intratumoral Injection of Oncolytic Vesicular Stomatitis Virus Expressing Interferon-Beta in Rodents and Nonhuman Primates. *Hum. Gene Ther.* **2010**, *21*, 451–462. [CrossRef] [PubMed]
55. Geletneky, K.; Hajda, J.; Angelova, A.L.; Leuchs, B.; Capper, D.; Bartsch, A.J.; Neumann, J.-O.; Schöning, T.; Hüsing, J.; Beelte, B.; et al. Oncolytic H-1 Parvovirus Shows Safety and Signs of Immunogenic Activity in a First Phase I/IIa Glioblastoma Trial. *Mol. Ther.* **2017**, *25*, 2620–2634. [CrossRef] [PubMed]
56. Galanis, E.; Atherton, P.J.; Maurer, M.J.; Knutson, K.L.; Dowdy, S.C.; Cliby, W.A.; Haluska, P.; Long, H.J.; Oberg, A.; Aderca, I.; et al. Oncolytic Measles Virus Expressing the Sodium Iodide Symporter to Treat Drug-Resistant Ovarian Cancer. *Cancer Res.* **2015**, *75*, 22–30. [CrossRef] [PubMed]
57. Dispenzieri, A.; Tong, C.; LaPlant, B.; Lacy, M.Q.; Laumann, K.; Dingli, D.; Zhou, Y.; Federspiel, M.J.; Gertz, M.A.; Hayman, S.; et al. Phase I Trial of Systemic Administration of Edmonston Strain of Measles Virus Genetically Engineered to Express the Sodium Iodide Symporter in Patients with Recurrent or Refractory Multiple Myeloma. *Leukemia* **2017**, *31*, 2791–2798. [CrossRef] [PubMed]
58. Lauer, U.M.; Schell, M.; Beil, J.; Berchtold, S.; Koppenhöfer, U.; Glatzle, J.; Königsrainer, A.; Möhle, R.; Nann, D.; Fend, F.; et al. Phase I Study of Oncolytic Vaccinia Virus GL-ONC1 in Patients with Peritoneal Carcinomatosis. *Clin. Cancer Res.* **2018**, *24*, 4388–4398. [CrossRef]
59. Park, B.-H.; Hwang, T.; Liu, T.-C.; Sze, D.Y.; Kim, J.-S.; Kwon, H.-C.; Oh, S.Y.; Han, S.-Y.; Yoon, J.-H.; Hong, S.-H.; et al. Use of a Targeted Oncolytic Poxvirus, JX-594, in Patients with Refractory Primary or Metastatic Liver Cancer: A Phase I Trial. *Lancet Oncol.* **2008**, *9*, 533–542. [CrossRef]
60. Moehler, M.; Heo, J.; Lee, H.C.; Tak, W.Y.; Chao, Y.; Paik, S.W.; Yim, H.J.; Byun, K.S.; Baron, A.; Ungerechts, G.; et al. Vaccinia-Based Oncolytic Immunotherapy Pexastimogene Devacirepvec in Patients with Advanced Hepatocellular Carcinoma after Sorafenib Failure: A Randomized Multicenter Phase IIb Trial (TRAVERSE). *Oncoimmunology* **2019**, *8*, 1615817. [CrossRef]

61. Dunn, G.; Klapsa, D.; Wilton, T.; Stone, L.; Minor, P.D.; Martin, J. Twenty-Eight Years of Poliovirus Replication in an Immunodeficient Individual: Impact on the Global Polio Eradication Initiative. *PLoS Pathog.* **2015**, *11*, e1005114. [CrossRef]
62. Weil, M.; Shulman, L.M.; Heiman, S.; Stauber, T.; Alfandari, J.; Weiss, L.; Silberstein, I.; Indenbaum, V.; Mendelson, E.; Sofer, D. Prolonged Excretion of Type-2 Poliovirus from a Primary Immune Deficient Patient during the Transition to a Type-2 Poliovirus-Free World, Israel, 2016. *Eurosurveillance* **2016**, *21*, 30408. [CrossRef]
63. Roulstone, V.; Khan, K.; Pandha, H.S.; Rudman, S.; Coffey, M.; Gill, G.M.; Melcher, A.A.; Vile, R.; Harrington, K.J.; de Bono, J.; et al. Phase I Trial of Cyclophosphamide as an Immune Modulator for Optimizing Oncolytic Reovirus Delivery to Solid Tumors. *Clin. Cancer Res.* **2015**, *21*, 1305–1312. [CrossRef] [PubMed]
64. Harrington, K.J.; Hingorani, M.; Tanay, M.A.; Hickey, J.; Bhide, S.A.; Clarke, P.M.; Renouf, L.C.; Thway, K.; Sibtain, A.; McNeish, I.A.; et al. Phase I/II Study of Oncolytic HSV GM-CSF in Combination with Radiotherapy and Cisplatin in Untreated Stage III/IV Squamous Cell Cancer of the Head and Neck. *Clin. Cancer Res.* **2010**, *16*, 4005–4015. [CrossRef] [PubMed]
65. Hu, J.C.C.; Coffin, R.S.; Davis, C.J.; Graham, N.J.; Groves, N.; Guest, P.J.; Harrington, K.J.; James, N.D.; Love, C.A.; McNeish, I.; et al. A Phase I Study of OncoVEXGM-CSF, a Second-Generation Oncolytic Herpes Simplex Virus Expressing Granulocyte Macrophage Colony-Stimulating Factor. *Clin. Cancer Res.* **2006**, *12*, 6737–6747. [CrossRef] [PubMed]
66. Senzer, N.N.; Kaufman, H.L.; Amatruda, T.; Nemunaitis, M.; Reid, T.; Daniels, G.; Gonzalez, R.; Glaspy, J.; Whitman, E.; Harrington, K.; et al. Phase II Clinical Trial of a Granulocyte-Macrophage Colony-Stimulating Factor-Encoding, Second-Generation Oncolytic Herpesvirus in Patients with Unresectable Metastatic Melanoma. *J. Clin. Oncol.* **2009**, *27*, 5763–5771. [CrossRef] [PubMed]
67. Chiocca, E.A.; Smith, K.M.; McKinney, B.; Palmer, C.A.; Rosenfeld, S.; Lillehei, K.; Hamilton, A.; DeMasters, B.K.; Judy, K.; Kirn, D. A Phase I Trial of Ad.HIFN-Beta Gene Therapy for Glioma. *Mol. Ther.* **2008**, *16*, 618–626. [CrossRef]
68. Nemunaitis, J.; Tong, A.W.; Nemunaitis, M.; Senzer, N.; Phadke, A.P.; Bedell, C.; Adams, N.; Zhang, Y.-A.; Maples, P.B.; Chen, S.; et al. A Phase I Study of Telomerase-Specific Replication Competent Oncolytic Adenovirus (Telomelysin) for Various Solid Tumors. *Mol. Ther.* **2010**, *18*, 429–434. [CrossRef]
69. Imlygic®®Clinical Overview and Handling Guide (USA, 2019). Available online: https://cdn.imlygichcp.com/cdn/917dac5d-ff46-4382-bb1e-8a4041ae951b/en/1/20201222t152404z/imlygic-clinical-overview.pdf (accessed on 11 July 2023).
70. U.S. National Institutes of Health, ClinicalTrials.gov. Postmarketing Prospective Study of Melanoma Patients Treated With IMLYGIC®® to Characterize Risk of Herpetic Infection. Identifier: NCT02910557. Available online: https://www.clinicaltrials.gov/study/NCT02910557 (accessed on 11 July 2023).
71. Laurie, S.A.; Bell, J.C.; Atkins, H.L.; Roach, J.; Bamat, M.K.; O'Neil, J.D.; Roberts, M.S.; Groene, W.S.; Lorence, R.M. A Phase 1 Clinical Study of Intravenous Administration of PV701, an Oncolytic Virus, Using Two-Step Desensitization. *Clin. Cancer Res.* **2006**, *12*, 2555–2562. [CrossRef]
72. Hotte, S.J.; Lorence, R.M.; Hirte, H.W.; Polawski, S.R.; Bamat, M.K.; O'Neil, J.D.; Roberts, M.S.; Groene, W.S.; Major, P.P. An Optimized Clinical Regimen for the Oncolytic Virus PV701. *Clin. Cancer Res.* **2007**, *13*, 977–985. [CrossRef]
73. Pecora, A.L.; Rizvi, N.; Cohen, G.I.; Meropol, N.J.; Sterman, D.; Marshall, J.L.; Goldberg, S.; Gross, P.; O'Neil, J.D.; Groene, W.S.; et al. Phase I Trial of Intravenous Administration of PV701, an Oncolytic Virus, in Patients with Advanced Solid Cancers. *J. Clin. Oncol.* **2002**, *20*, 2251–2266. [CrossRef]
74. Tell, J.G.; Coller, B.-A.G.; Dubey, S.A.; Jenal, U.; Lapps, W.; Wang, L.; Wolf, J. Environmental Risk Assessment for RVSVΔG-ZEBOV-GP, a Genetically Modified Live Vaccine for Ebola Virus Disease. *Vaccines* **2020**, *8*, 779. [CrossRef]
75. European Commission GMO: Deliberate Release into the Environment of Other than Plants GMOs for Any Other Purposes than Placing on the Market (Experimental Releases). List of SNIFs Submitted to the Member State's Competent Authorities under Directive 2001/18/EC (after 17 October 2002). Keyword VSV. Available online: https://webgate.ec.europa.eu/fip/GMO_Registers/GMO_Part_B_Others.php?Keyword=VSV (accessed on 11 July 2023).
76. Pérez-Losada, M.; Arenas, M.; Galán, J.C.; Palero, F.; González-Candelas, F. Recombination in Viruses: Mechanisms, Methods of Study, and Evolutionary Consequences. *Infect. Genet. Evol.* **2015**, *30*, 296–307. [CrossRef] [PubMed]
77. Buijs, P.R.A.; Verhagen, J.H.E.; van Eijck, C.H.J.; van den Hoogen, B.G. Oncolytic Viruses: From Bench to Bedside with a Focus on Safety. *Hum. Vaccin. Immunother.* **2015**, *11*, 1573–1584. [CrossRef] [PubMed]

vaccines

MDPI

Review

Regulatory T Cells (Tregs) and COVID-19: Unveiling the Mechanisms, and Therapeutic Potentialities with a Special Focus on Long COVID

Manish Dhawan [1,2,*], Ali A. Rabaan [3,4,5], Sara Alwarthan [6], Mashael Alhajri [6], Muhammad A. Halwani [7], Amer Alshengeti [8,9], Mustafa A. Najim [10], Ameen S. S. Alwashmi [11], Ahmad A. Alshehri [12], Saleh A. Alshamrani [12], Bashayer M. AlShehail [13], Mohammed Garout [14], Saleh Al-Abdulhadi [15,16], Shamsah H. Al-Ahmed [17], Nanamika Thakur [18] and Geetika Verma [19]

1 Department of Microbiology, Punjab Agricultural University, Ludhiana 141004, India
2 Trafford College, Altrincham, Manchester WA14 5PQ, UK
3 Molecular Diagnostic Laboratory, Johns Hopkins Aramco Healthcare, Dhahran 31311, Saudi Arabia
4 College of Medicine, Alfaisal University, Riyadh 11533, Saudi Arabia
5 Department of Public Health and Nutrition, The University of Haripur, Haripur 22610, Pakistan
6 Department of Internal Medicine, College of Medicine, Imam Abdulrahman Bin Faisal University, Dammam 34212, Saudi Arabia
7 Department of Medical Microbiology, Faculty of Medicine, Al Baha University, Al Baha 4781, Saudi Arabia
8 Department of Pediatrics, College of Medicine, Taibah University, Al-Madinah 41491, Saudi Arabia
9 Department of Infection Prevention and Control, Prince Mohammad Bin Abdulaziz Hospital, National Guard Health Affairs, Al-Madinah 41491, Saudi Arabia
10 Department of Medical Laboratories Technology, College of Applied Medical Sciences, Taibah University, Al-Madinah 41411, Saudi Arabia
11 Department of Medical Laboratories, College of Applied Medical Sciences, Qassim University, Buraydah 51452, Saudi Arabia
12 Department of Clinical Laboratory Sciences, College of Applied Medical Sciences, Najran University, Najran 61441, Saudi Arabia
13 Pharmacy Practice Department, College of Clinical Pharmacy, Imam Abdulrahman Bin Faisal University, Dammam 31441, Saudi Arabia
14 Department of Community Medicine and Health Care for Pilgrims, Faculty of Medicine, Umm Al-Qura University, Makkah 21955, Saudi Arabia
15 Department of Medical Laboratory Sciences, College of Applied Medical Sciences, Prince Sattam Bin Abdulaziz University, Riyadh 11942, Saudi Arabia
16 Dr. Saleh Office for Medical Genetic and Genetic Counseling Services, The House of Expertise, Prince Sattam Bin Abdulaziz University, Dammam 32411, Saudi Arabia
17 Specialty Paediatric Medicine, Qatif Central Hospital, Qatif 32654, Saudi Arabia
18 University Institute of Biotechnology, Department of Biotechnology, Chandigarh University, Mohali 140413, India
19 Department of Experimental Medicine and Biotechnology, Post Graduate Institute of Medical Education and Research (PGIMER), Chandigarh 160012, India
* Correspondence: dhawanmanish501@gmail.com; Tel.: +44-01619287242

Abstract: The COVID-19 pandemic has caused havoc all around the world. The causative agent of COVID-19 is the novel form of the coronavirus (CoV) named SARS-CoV-2, which results in immune system disruption, increased inflammation, and acute respiratory distress syndrome (ARDS). T cells have been important components of the immune system, which decide the fate of the COVID-19 disease. Recent studies have reported an important subset of T cells known as regulatory T cells (Tregs), which possess immunosuppressive and immunoregulatory properties and play a crucial role in the prognosis of COVID-19 disease. Recent studies have shown that COVID-19 patients have considerably fewer Tregs than the general population. Such a decrement may have an impact on COVID-19 patients in a number of ways, including diminishing the effect of inflammatory inhibition, creating an inequality in the Treg/Th17 percentage, and raising the chance of respiratory failure. Having fewer Tregs may enhance the likelihood of long COVID development in addition to contributing to the disease's poor prognosis. Additionally, tissue-resident Tregs provide tissue repair in addition to immunosuppressive and immunoregulatory activities, which may aid in the recovery of COVID-19 patients. The severity of the illness is also linked to abnormalities in the Tregs' phenotype, such as reduced expression of FoxP3 and other immunosuppressive cytokines, including IL-10 and TGF-beta. Hence, in this review, we summarize the immunosuppressive mechanisms and their possible roles in the prognosis of COVID-19 disease. Furthermore, the perturbations in Tregs have been associated with disease severity. The roles of Tregs are also explained in the long COVID. This review also discusses the potential therapeutic roles of Tregs in the management of patients with COVID-19.

Keywords: COVID-19; immune response; SARS-CoV-2; T regulatory cells (Tregs); long COVID; therapeutics

1. Introduction

The so-called COVID-19 pandemic, which has caused severe damage to humankind, was caused by the novel form of the coronavirus named SARS-CoV-2. The SARS-CoV-2 infection has shown variability in the prognosis of the COVID-19 disease, which can cause flu-like symptoms, viral pneumonia, multiple organ damage, or acute respiratory distress syndrome (ARDS) [1–4]. Comparing the SARS-CoV-2 infection to earlier coronavirus infections, one may see unique patterns of cellular and humoral immunological abnormalities [1,4]. In the early and moderate phases, it may cause exhaustion of T cells, dendritic cells (DCs), and natural killer (NK) cells; however, excessive stimulation of such immune cells has been reported in severe instances, leading to a cytokine storm [5]. Cytokine storm has been proposed as the leading cause of death in COVID-19-infected patients [1].

Interestingly, scientists are still unveiling the exact roles of immune cells in deciding the secretion of a balanced number of cytokines and chemokines, which will be essential to elicit the only required immune response despite an exaggerated immune response in the form of uncontrolled release of cytokines and chemokines [4,6]. Numerous researchers hold the view that adaptive immune responses, particularly cell-mediated immune responses, are essential for limiting the SARS-CoV-2 infection by regulating the release of essential cytokines and other anti-inflammatory proteins [6]. Furthermore, the rapid evolution of SARS-CoV-2 into the diverge variants with a plethora of mutations makes scientists think about the cell-mediated immune response seriously [7,8].

Strong T-cell responses have been associated with less severe outcomes in numerous infections. Hyperactivation, however, can potentially have negative effects as the infection spreads [1,9]. Furthermore, in this context, several studies have linked increased levels of effector molecules produced by CD8+ T cells with better clinical outcomes in acute COVID-19 [10,11]. Increased activation of T cells has been linked to a negative outcome of the SARS-CoV-2 infection [12], despite the fact that polyfunctionality peaks in moderate sickness [11]. This suggests that excessive stimulation of immune cells may be deleterious. Virus-specific T-cell responses in asymptomatic infection are characterized by balanced secretion of anti-inflammatory and proinflammatory cytokines such as IL-10 and IL-6 as opposed to symptomatic disease, characterized by more polarized production of inflammatory mediators [13–15]. The scientific community is clearly divided on how many activations of immune cells, such as T cells and NK cells, are required. Such contradictory disputes still exist even after multiple advancements in the field of cellular immunology [14,15].

A fine-tuned immune response is vital in determining the outcome of the SARS-CoV-2 infection, and regulatory T cells (Tregs) have been proven to be crucial in controlling the immune response, according to recent research on immune cells. Along with CD4+ and CD8+ T cells, Tregs play a critical role in immunological tolerance and balance [16,17]. Tregs are significant regulators of the inflammatory response. The role of Tregs specific to SARS-CoV-2 in the progression of the illness is currently unknown [17], but systemic inflammation and intense pneumonitis are the major clinical manifestations of severe COVID-19 disease [17,18]. Additionally, virus-specific T-cell responses, especially those of Tregs, have been shown to have an impact on tissue injury in respiratory diseases [18].

Tregs are indeed key subsets of T cells that suppress the immune system. Recent research has shown that COVID-19 patients have significantly fewer Tregs than the general population. Such a decline may have an impact on COVID-19 patients in a number of ways, including diminishing the consequence of inflammatory inhibition, creating an imbalance in the Treg/Th17 ratio, and raising the risk of respiratory failure [13,19]. Treg-targeted treatment may help COVID-19 patients with their symptoms and slow down the disease development [19]. Importantly, it is still not clear whether the decline in Tregs in COVID-19 patients leads to a poor prognosis or whether the increased number of Tregs has beneficial effects. Many scientists believe that a balanced amount of Tregs number is essential to containing any adverse effects of severe infection of SARS-CoV-2 [19–21]. Additionally, there are many ways that viral proteins can activate and change T cells. For example, a drop in Foxp3 levels can induce the activation of Tregs or the death of Treg cells. The expression of S-protein on the SARS-CoV-2's surface is required for the invasion into the host. Furin, a pro-protein convertase, activates the S-protein, and its T-cell-specific deletion activity impairs FoxP3 and TBX21, which induce Treg development. CD4+ T cells are hyperactivated in severe COVID-19 patients, although Foxp3 expression is suppressed. Before developing into Tregs, a significant fraction of T cells get activated, multiply, and expire quickly [19]. However, how S-protein and other viral proteins can lead to the generation of specific Tregs is still unclear.

It is also worth noting that recent research has proposed that the pathophysiology of COVID-19 may be influenced by changes in Tregs, important regulators of immunological homeostasis, but how much change is required to induce a controlled secretion of cytokines is yet to be uncovered. Severely infected patients with COVID-19 have shown unique Treg phenotype and increased expression of its characteristic transcription factor FoxP3 [20,21]. Such Tregs have shown a distinctive transcriptional profile, with upregulation of a number of suppressive effectors as well as proinflammatory molecules, including IL-32, and remarkable similarities to tumor-infiltrating Tregs that inhibit antitumor responses [20]. These characteristics were most obvious during acute, severe illness, and some of them continued in recovering individuals. IL-6 and IL-18 may each contribute various aspects of these COVID-19-linked perturbations, according to a screen for potential agents [20,21]. These findings imply that Tregs may have negative effects on COVID-19 by directly promoting inflammation and inhibiting antiviral T-cell responses during the disease's acute phase [20–22].

Hence, the immunological cells such as Tregs, which are intended to moderate hyperactivated immune responses, should be carefully considered to develop the therapeutic modalities not only against SARS-CoV-2 but also for the other viral infections [1,3,20]. Therefore, this article focuses on the current knowledge of Tregs' function in the modulation of immune responses to COVID-19. Furthermore, insufficient research has been conducted on regulatory T cells (Tregs) in patients with long COVID and recovering COVID-19 patients [20]. Aspects of Treg function, such as cytokine production or suppressive efficacy in long COVID, have not been investigated in any of the current clinical studies [23]. Due to a dearth of studies addressing Tregs in these aspects, it is hard to draw clear conclusions on the kind of Treg adaptations in long COVID and their potential therapeutic involvement in long COVID management. In this context, we have uncovered recent information on the therapeutic potential of Tregs in the management of COVID-19 and long COVID.

2. Immunoregulatory Functions of Tregs

Tregs are required to ensure immunologic homeostasis and self-tolerance and halt exaggerated immunological responses. All these mechanisms are tightly controlled by the balanced expression of the FoxP3 transcription factor. In human peripheral blood, Tregs make up 10% of CD4+ T cells, and these CD4+ cells express specific markers such as FoxP3, which enable their immunosuppressive activities [24,25]. Through a variety of effector pathways, Tregs control the stimulation of several innate and adaptive immune system pathways [20,21]. Additionally, specific "tissue Treg" populations regulate homeostasis in a number of non-immunological tissues, reducing inflammation and encouraging orderly tissue regeneration [20,26,27]. However, Tregs may also be harmful. This is best shown by the fact that they inhibit powerful cytotoxic responses in tumors, where they take on unique phenotypic characteristics [28]. On antiviral responses, they may potentially have contradictory effects [20,29,30], which can lead to a higher viral load.

Previously, it has been reported that the co-transfer of Tregs cells can prevent autoimmune disease in athymic nude mice [31]. Many studies have shown that FOXP3+ Tregs play an important role in maintaining fetal-maternal tolerance, oral tolerance, transplantation tolerance, and mucosal tissue tolerance via various immune suppressive pathways [30,32–35].

Before understanding the mechanisms by which Tregs imply their suppression, it is essential to note that Tregs can be majorly divided into two categories, including thymic Tregs (tTregs) and peripheral Tregs (pTregs) based on their site of morphogenesis or development. The tTregs develop in the thymus from precursors of CD4+ helper T (Th) cells, whereas peripheral Tregs (pTregs) differentiate from mature CD4+ Th cells in the periphery. Induced Tregs (iTregs) are a third form of Treg that could be developed ex vivo using mature CD4+ Th cells by stimulating the T-cell receptor (TCR) and by administering TGF-beta [36]. It is commonly acknowledged that the characteristic of Treg morphogenesis in humans is the simultaneous expression of Foxp3 and IL-2 receptor alpha-chain (CD25) with a reduced IL-7 receptor (CD127) expression [37] [Figure 1]. Surprisingly, numerous researchers have shown that a low dosage of IL-2 may increase Treg number and function. Some recent studies have revealed that a low dose of IL-2 may grow autologous Treg cells, which can be used to treat a variety of inflammatory disorders [38].

The mechanisms by which Tregs suppress the immune response or regulate the immunological processes can be divided into active and counteractive mechanisms [27]. The active mode involves the production of immune suppressive cytokines by Tregs, including IL-10, TGF-beta, IL-35, and adenosine. At the same time, the counteractive mode entails the removal of components essential for the activation and survival of effector T cells, including peptide-MHC class II, CD80-CD86, and IL-2 [39–41]. Although the exact immunosuppressive mechanisms that operate in vivo are not well understood, it is generally agreed that activation of the Treg TCR occurs before suppressive action [27].

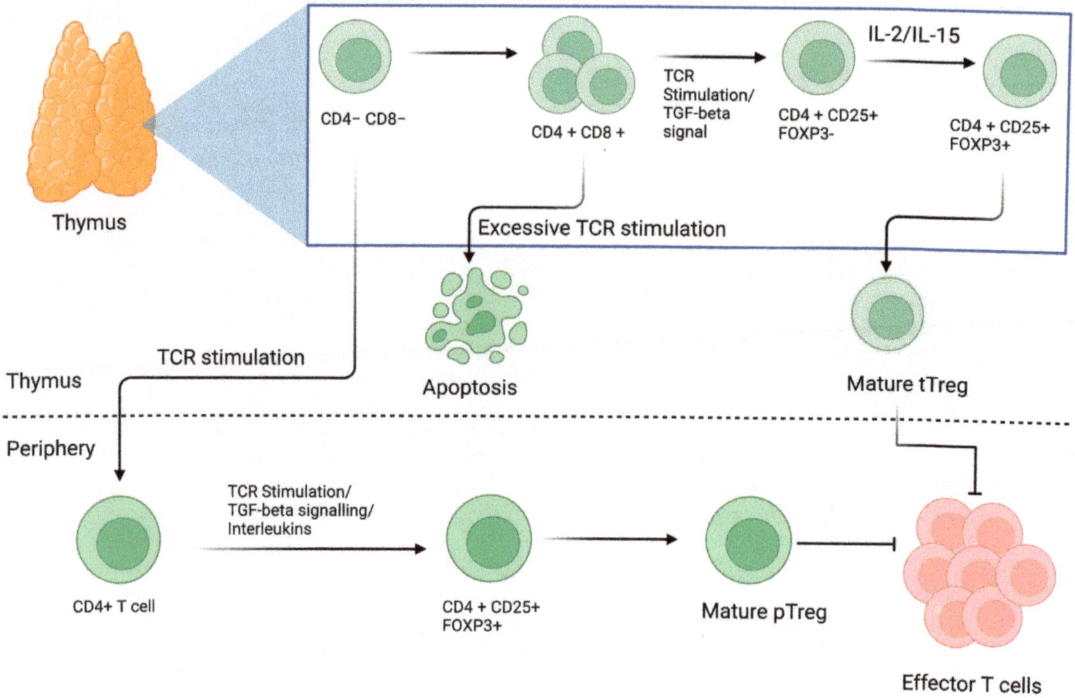

Figure 1. The schematic representation of the morphogenesis and development of Tregs. On the basis of the development and their functional markers, Tregs have been classified into two major categories thymic Tregs (tTregs) and peripheral Tregs (pTregs). Additionally, mature CD4+ Th cells can be induced into Tregs by TCR stimulation.

Additionally, Tregs express CD39, which helps in the metabolism of ATP to AMP, which in turn prevents dendritic cells (DCs) maturation due to the depletion of ATP [42]. Furthermore, co-expressed CD39 and CD73 on Tregs were able to convert ADP into adenosine, which coupled to the effector T cell's adenosine A2A receptor and hindered effector T cells from being activated [43,44]. Consequently, by decreasing the expression of IL-6 and increasing the synthesis of TGF-beta, the stimulation of the adenosine A2A receptor encouraged the development of Tregs [45]. Furthermore, Tregs may suppress the expression of the costimulatory molecules CD80 and CD86 on DCs [20,43]. Antigen-presenting cells (APCs) were unable to get activated as a result of Tregs' production of CTLA-4, which decreased CD86 via transendocytosis [44,46]. Additionally, by increasing the expression of indoleamine 2,3-dioxygenase in DCs through CTLA-4-induced signaling, Tregs might starve effector T cells [47,48], which in turn suppresses the immune response [Figure 2].

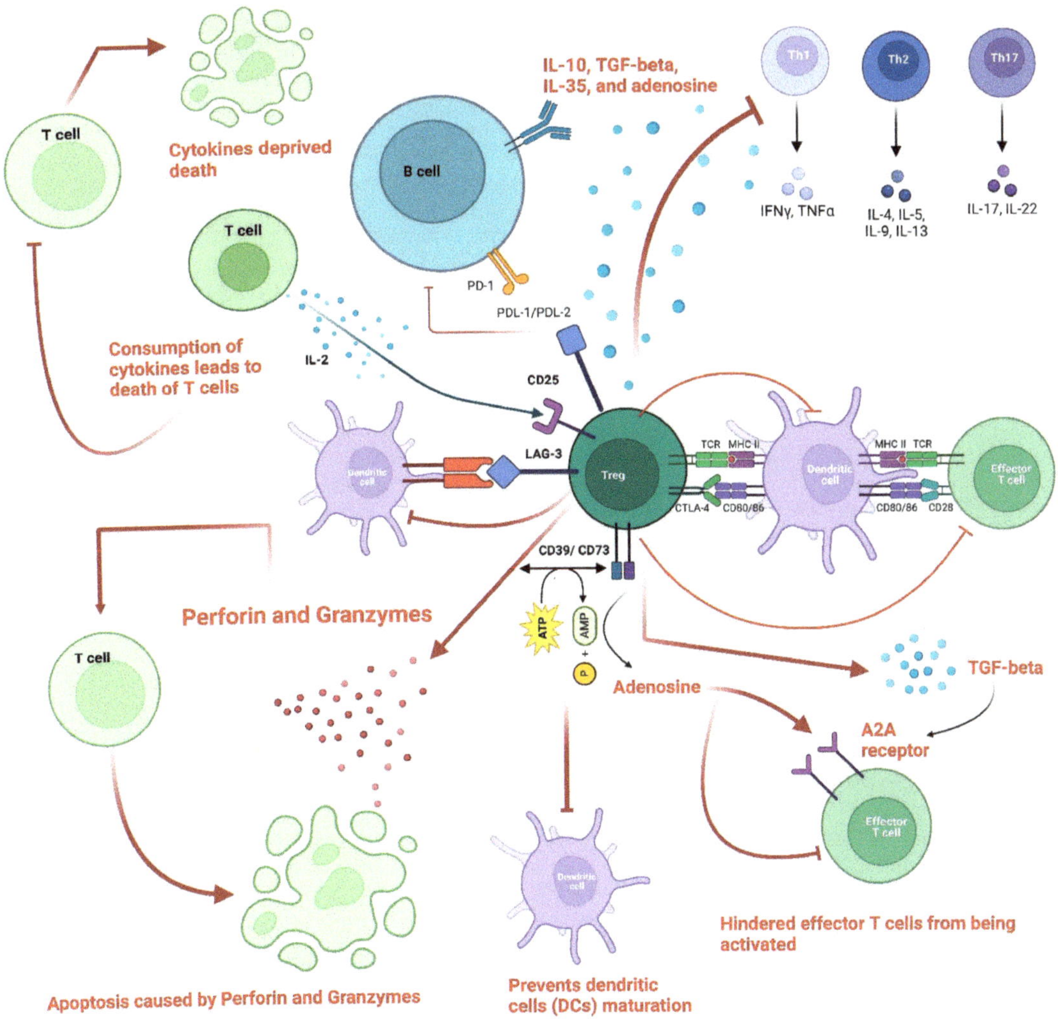

Figure 2. The figure shows various immunosuppressive mechanisms used by Tregs to control the immune system. Cells of both adaptive and innate immune responses are suppressed by Tregs via either direct or indirect mechanisms. Tregs have the ability to generate TGF-beta, IL-10, and IL-35, which have an inhibitory effect on T cells. This can lead to suppressed actions of Th1, Th2, and Th17 type T cells. Due to the strong expression of IL-2 receptors, i.e., CD25, Tregs can cause cytokine-deprived death of effector T cells. Additionally, the lack of IL-2 prevents natural killer cells from multiplying and acting as effector cells. Tregs have been shown to directly affect B cells through the PDL1/PD-1 interaction. Tregs can inhibit the macrophages by increasing CD80/CD86 expression, which gets stimulated through CTLA-4. The proliferation of T effectors is decreased by the expression of CD39 on Tregs, which mediates the conversion of ATP to adenosine and AMP. A2A receptors on T cells get stimulated by AMP and hinder the activation of effector T cells. Additionally, the usage of ATP and its conversion into AMP inhibits the activation of dendritic cells. Moreover, Tregs also produce granzyme and perforin, which damage the T cells' membrane, which in turn leads to cell death or apoptosis.

Aside from that, Tregs produced the lymphocyte activation gene 3 (LAG-3), which competitively bonded to the major histocompatibility complex class II (MHC-II) and prevented dendritic cells (DCs) from maturing [49]. The cytolysis of CD8+ T cells and NK cells by Granzymes- and Perforin-dependent means constituted another significant Treg-mediated suppressive pathway [41]. According to Gotot et al. (2012), in addition to apoptosis caused by Perforin and Granzymes, programmed death-ligand 1(PD-L1) of Tregs and programmed death-1 (PD-1) of autoreactive B lymphocytes interfere with the proliferation and functionality of autoreactive B lymphocytes [50] [Figure 2].

3. Possible Roles of Tregs in COVID-19 Pathogenesis and Disease Severity

While the pandemic was at its peak, numerous studies have discussed the possible connection between Treg and the severity of COVID-19. According to some studies, the percentage of Tregs is rising, or their functional markers are being expressed more strongly in severely infected patients with COVID-19 [51,52]. For instance, one recent research found that severe COVID-19 patients had greater levels of CD25+ FOXP3+ Tregs among CD4+ T cells, increased FOXP3 expression, and elevated production of activated Treg markers including KLRG1 and PD-1, all of which returned to normal levels in the recovering individuals or convalescent patients [51]. Likewise, another recent observation found that the number, multiplication, and expression of certain proteins of CD25+ CD127+ FOXP3+ Tregs increased, along with their growing suppressive activity, in severely infected patients with COVID-19 [52]. Scientists discovered increased Tregs and Th17 cells as well as decreased T-cell numbers in the bronchoalveolar lavage fluid (BALF) of COVID-19 patients with ARDS [53].

In contrast to the healthy donor population and convalescent patients, the percentage of CD25+ CD127− Tregs among all CD4+ T cells was found to increase significantly in patients with persistent SARS-CoV-2 infection. Additionally, the increased expression of CTLA-4 on Tregs was reported in patients with persistent antigen expression [54]. Intriguingly, most of the patients have been reported to have an increased number of naive Tregs (CD45RA+ CCR7+). Additionally, central memory Tregs (CD45RA− CCR7+) with strong expression of PD-1 were reported in the patients with COVID-19 [55]. Additionally, the CD4+ FOXP3+ Tregs of the lung and PBMC showed a rising trend on day five after infection in the nonhuman model of COVID-19 pathogenesis [56]. There has not been much research done on the composition of T-cell subsets in SARS-CoV-2-infected convalescent patients. Based on the number of days following RT-PCR confirmation of SARS-Co-V2 infection, researchers calculated the lymphocyte absolute numbers, the frequency of memory T-cell subsets, and the plasma levels of common gamma-chain in seven groups of COVID-19 patients. The findings demonstrate that CD4+ naive T cells, regulatory T cells, transitional memory, and stem cell memory T-cell frequencies decreased from Days 15–30 to Days 61–90 and then remained steady. Conversely, CD4+ naive, transitional, and stem cell memory T-cell frequencies declined from Days 15–30 to Days 61–90 and then decreased again. Patients with severe COVID-19 had reduced lymphocyte numbers and frequency levels; greater naive cells (Tregs); lower frequencies of central memory, effector memory, and stem cell memory, and higher plasma levels of IL2, IL7, IL15, and IL21. As a result, the research suggests that convalescent COVID-19 people had altered memory T-cell subset frequencies, which will be clarified in the future [57]. Further investigations are needed to confirm this idea, but it is possible that an increase in the cell percentage and the number of functional indicators would result in higher Treg suppression, which can be detrimental to COVID-19 patients [54,56] [Figure 3].

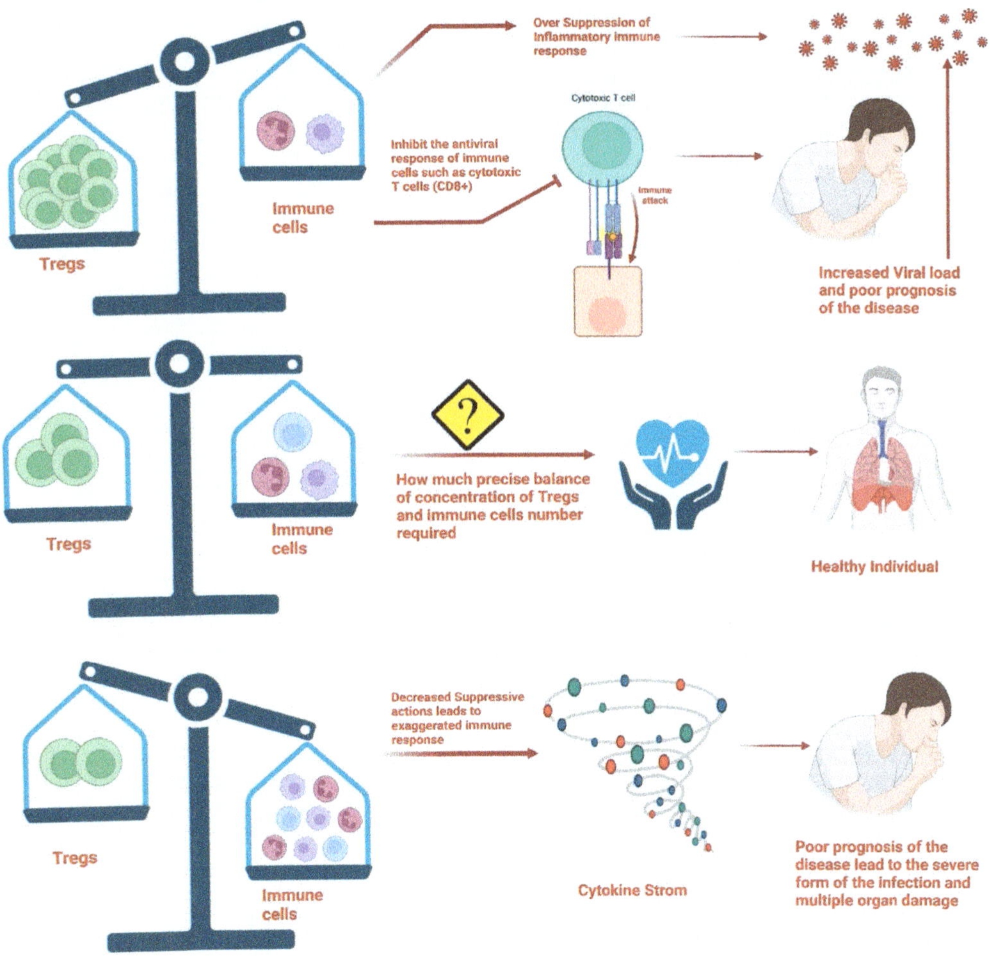

Figure 3. The figure represents the Treg involvement in the pathophysiology of COVID-19. The increased number of Tregs in severely infected patients can play deleterious effects by limiting the antiviral effects of effector T cells. Additionally, the overly expressed FoxP3 in Tregs can lead to excessive immunosuppressive activities, which lead to a poor prognosis of the disease. On the other hand, the substantial decrease in the number of Tregs cannot alleviate the excessively stimulated immune response in severely infected patients. Moreover, a balanced number of Tregs compared to Th1/Th17 T cells and other immune cells can prevent the poor prognosis of the disease.

Considering the biphasic functions of Tregs throughout the SARS-CoV-2 infection, it is still debatable how the fraction of Tregs in COVID-19 changed. The number of Tregs has decreased in COVID-19 patients, according to many researchers. For instance, one study found that the Th17/Treg ratio was substantially enhanced while the number of Tregs in ICU-hospitalized patients was reduced significantly [58]. It is interesting to note that the immunomodulatory and immunosuppressive functions of Tregs isolated from severely infected COVID-19 patients were found to be compromised. Another study found a comparable rise in the Th17/Treg ratio in the PBMC of COVID-19 patients, which was associated with a negative outcome and lower levels of TGF-beta and IL-10, cytokines that are important for Tregs [59]

[Figure 3]. Additionally, a single-cell transcriptomic evaluation of viral antigen-reactive CD4+ T cells of patients with SARS-CoV-2 infection found that the percentages of SARS-CoV-2-reactive Tregs, T follicular helper cells (Tfh), and cytotoxic T helper cells responsive to the viral infection were enhanced in hospitalized COVID-19 patients [60].

Another comparative analysis reported a reduced number of Tregs in severely infected patients with SARS-CoV-2 as compared to the patients with mild symptoms. It has been concluded that the proportion of Tregs was negatively correlated with viral load, indicating that lower Treg levels can be associated with a higher risk of illness, especially in hospitalized patients with COVID-19 [61]. According to another study, individuals with severe COVID-19 had a lower percentage of regulatory T cells (CD3+ CD25+) [62]. Another research that evaluated the PBMCs of COVID-19 patients found that the Tregs ratio increased as the disease progressed from moderate to severe but decreased as it progressed to critical [63]. This suggests that the Tregs underwent a dynamic shift as COVID-19 progressed.

Intriguingly, a study that examined the gene expression patterns of CD4+ T cells of patients with SARS-CoV-2 infection discovered that CD25 was significantly upregulated [63,64]. It is quite interesting to observe that the Tregs of severely infected patients reported having a reduced level of master transcription factor (FOXP3+). The increased level of FURIN appeared to be related to the increased level of CD25, which may facilitate SARS-CoV-2 entry into lung epithelial cells and reduce the immunosuppressive activities of Tregs in patients with poor disease prognoses. Tregs seem to have decreased during the acute phase of the SARS-CoV-2 infection in children and returned to baseline after recovery [64]. Surprisingly, a high-dimensional flow cytometry examination of the airways of severely infected COVID-19 patients revealed decreased Treg frequency as compared to healthy individuals [65]. This finding raises the possibility that the functionality of tissue-resident Tregs, especially residential to lungs, was compromised in severely infected patients with COVID-19. It is well-established that pro-inflammatory cytokines such as IL-6 may cause Tregs to lose their stability in vitro [66]. Therefore, under the inflammatory conditions brought on by COVID-19, high levels of IL-1, IL-6, and IL-23 may promote the downregulation of FOXP3 [67], resulting in decreased functionality of Tregs.

Additionally, it was shown that COVID-19 patients' Treg subset composition varied. For instance, the research found that in adult patients with more severe illnesses, the ratio of CD39+ Tregs in PBMCs increased, but in young patients, the ratio of CD39+ Tregs dropped in an age-dependent way [68]. According to another research, only CCR4Hi Tregs in hospitalized COVID-19 patients elevated, while total Tregs remained unchanged [69]. According to Chen et al. (2020), when compared to moderately infected COVID-19 patients, the severely infected subjects demonstrated a substantially decreased proportion of CD45RA+ memory Tregs and a fractionally greater percentage of CD45RO+ naive Tregs, implying that the proportion of Treg subsets may be able to anticipate the prognosis of the disease cases [70]. Other research found a similar pattern, particularly in severely infected patients with COVID-19, as compared to moderately infected ones [20,21].

According to reports, individuals who had COVID-19 and lymphopenia had a worse prognosis; lower blood lymphocyte percentages suggested this [71]. Multiple possible processes might be at work in lymphopenia. Additionally, via single-cell RNA-sequencing, the SARS-CoV-2 RNA was also found in immune cells [72], and it has been postulated that SARS-CoV-2 may have the capability of infecting Treg through ACE2-independent receptors [30,73]. This can substantially affect the functionality of Tregs, which needs to uncover in future studies.

Numerous studies have shown an increase in the percentage or quantity of Tregs in COVID-19 patients (particularly those with the milder condition), but they have also found a decrease in the amount of Tregs in the individuals. For instance, it has been shown that severe COVID-19 patients had significantly fewer Tregs (CD3+ CD4+ CD25hi CD127lo FoxP3+) in their PBMCs [60,74,75]. Single-cell research revealed that FoxP3 expression was noticeably lower in severe COVID-19 patients, despite greater expression of CD25 [76]. In PBMC generated from COVID-19 patients receiving ICU care, recent research looked at

Tregs and discovered a sharp fall in the proportion of Tregs along with lower production of FoxP3 and inhibitory cytokines such as IL-10 and TGF-beta [59] [Figure 3].

Furthermore, Mohebbi et al. (2020) also reported the reduced expression of important markers such as CD25 and FOXP 3 in Tregs of severely infected patients with COVID-19 as compared to healthy donors [75]. It is important to consider that following SARS-CoV-2 infection, the number of Tregs (CD3+ CD4+ CD25+) considerably decreased throughout the development of infection and symptoms [21]. Scientists are still figuring out the reasons behind the increase in the number of Tregs in moderate conditions of infection and then rapidly decreased as the infection progressed. In adults and children with severe COVID-19, the fraction of Tregs was observed to be lower in other studies as well [60,64]. Such data suggest that the excessive inflammation and pathophysiology of COVID-19 may be responsible for a decreased number of Tregs as well as enhanced Th17 responses. Additionally, recent research found that patients with COVID-19 had higher proportions of Tregs (characterized by the presence of CD3+ CD4+ CD25+ markers) and higher levels of FoxP3 expression by Tregs, which were associated with a poor prognosis of the disease [20]. Such Tregs are reported to secrete a range of immunosuppressive molecules along with inflammatory cytokines such as IL-32, which in turn can limit anti-viral T-cell responses, simultaneously increasing inflammatory responses in severely infected patients with COVID-19 [20,21].

It is important to note that certain investigations, such as those in cancer patients infected with SARS-CoV-2 [77], did not notice any variation in the number of Tregs in the peripheral blood of COVID-19 patients [78]. Additionally, many other studies could not conclude the exact change in the number of Tregs in severely and moderately infected patients with SARS-CoV-2 [20,21]. As a result, there is still debate around recent data on the absolute and relative numbers of Treg cells in COVID-19 patients [21]. This is likely due to the various parameters employed to identify Tregs and the fact that the observation was taken at various phases of the illness [21,22].

Moreover, the patients with reduced or less amount of Tregs along with the low concentration of master regulator FoxP3 were reported to have less severe outcomes of the SARS-CoV-2 infection. Importantly, there are possibilities that these Tregs are advantageous, especially in regulating the cytokine storm that can be severe without the immunosuppressive activities of such Tregs [21]. Nevertheless, insufficient cell numbers made it impossible to directly evaluate their immunosuppression capabilities [79]. Contradictorily, the increased number of Tregs and increased expression of FoxP3 and other effector molecules can interfere with the antiviral response of immune cells such as cytotoxic T cells (CD8+) in the severe phase of the infection [80] [Figure 3] as compared to the initial phase of the infection which in turn can lead to the secondary re-expansion of disease [20,79,81]. However, the exact reasons behind such a shift are yet to be resolved clearly. However, this can be associated with enhanced levels of FoxP3 and other Treg effector molecules along with phenotypic similarities with the immunosuppressive tumor Tregs [20,21].

It is also quite fascinating since the wide community of scientists suggests that Tregs during the SARS-CoV-2 infection get activated, suggesting their immunoregulatory or immunosuppressive activities to prevent immune cells of both innate and adaptive immune response from damaging self-tissues mainly by limiting the excessive release of pro-inflammatory cytokines and chemokines [20,82]. However, it is also possible that in the early stages of infection, a greater proportion of activated Tregs might weaken the immune system's ability to fight off viruses such as SARS-CoV-2 [9,20]. The excessive production of pro-inflammatory cytokines that causes ARDS, however, may be caused by a decrease in the number of Tregs with compromised functions in severe instances or later stages of the illness [21]. However, a significant amount of research has been done in this field; these ambiguities are yet to be resolved with non-human or human models to understand the immunological response to SARS-CoV-2.

4. Perturbations in Tregs and Disease Severity

A significant number of variations in the phenotypic characteristics of Tregs have been reported in severely infected patients with COVID-19, along with increased FoxP3 expression with a unique transcriptional pattern that is very similar to tumor Tregs [83,84]. A broad range of transcriptional patterns have been observed in Tregs, which includes an elevation of interferon-stimulated genes, and these changes have been reported in various other viral infections. However, unusual cell proliferation and heightened effector functions, including ENTPD1, LAG3, and LRRC32, have been observed in Tregs of severely infected patients with COVID-19. Among many of the increased "Severe COVID-19 Treg Signature" (SCTS) transcripts are several members of the tumor necrosis factor (TNF) receptor family, which play crucial roles in Treg function and homeostasis [84,85]. Additionally, increased expression of CXCR3 has been observed in the Tregs of severely infected patients with COVID-19 [85]. CXCR3 receptor for binds to CXCL10 chemokine (member of the CXC chemokine family) to exert its biological effects. CXCL10 has been shown to be a key biological marker modulating illness severity and may be used as a prognostic marker for a number of disorders [86].

Recent findings raise two very important questions. First, where do such perturbations/variations come from? They are not brought on by infecting Tregs with viral particles. Since none of the treatments given to these individuals are correlated with the Treg features, they seem to be unrelated to therapeutic interventions [20,87]. The immunologic environment in such individuals is more likely to be the cause of the phenotypic changes, which is unique to Tregs since Tconvs are much less labeled [87,88]. Additionally, TCR-mediated stimulation is unlike to stimulate the phenotypic changes, given the extensive impact on Tregs in the single-cell data [88], which presumably transcends clonotypic specificity, and the significant loss of Nur77 (NR4A1) [20].

Previous findings indicate that a number of variables are involved, namely IL-6 and IL-18 (although other variables may also be involved), each of which contributes to a different feature of the disturbed Treg phenotype. Since IL-6 is often considered a Treg antagonist and prevents FoxP3 expression by TGF-beta/IL-2 in culture, its effect in this situation first seems counterintuitive [89]. Recent research has provided a more nuanced picture of the role of IL-6 in Treg cells, showing that it is necessary for the development of the RORγ+ Treg subsets and may enhance their suppressive properties [90–92]. Tregs with effective inhibitory functionality is considerably more prevalent in transgenic mice with persistently higher serum IL-6 concentrations [93], as the recent findings found perturbations in Tregs of rheumatoid arthritis patients, which might play an important role in the clinical manifestation of the disease [94]. Hence, direct evaluation of Tregs from the lungs of COVID-19 patients would have been beneficial.

Additionally, there are other cytokines, such as IL-18, which determine the phenotypic and functional characteristics of Tregs. IL-18 signaling from epithelial cells to Tregs is necessary for defense against colitis in the RAG transfer paradigm, and it has been shown that IL-18 promotes Treg reparative activity through amphiregulin [95,96]. Recent research suggests that Notch4 and IL-18 signaling work together to regulate pro-reparative effects in Tregs [97]. A subfraction of Tregs with a preference for thymus-homing exhibits the IL-18 receptor predominantly [98]. Recent research suggests that IL-18 has a larger influence on Treg cells than only pro-reparative pathways, including a greater range of Treg effector activities that are represented in module M5 (typical Treg transcripts, such as TNFRSF18 or LRRC32) [20]. Additionally, circulating Tregs from patients with severe COVID-19 exhibit decreased amphiregulin expression, suggesting that some of IL-18's effects may be mitigated by other COVID-19 cytokine storm components [20,21].

Second, it is important to note that, these abnormal Tregs contribute to the physiopathology of COVID-19. Patients who had lower levels of FoxP3, fewer Tregs, and less severe SCTS did better, which brings up the traditional problem of inferring causality from the association. However, it might be possible that these Tregs are advantageous, regulating a cytokine storm that would not have been as bad without their extraordinary contribution. In context to this, a recent investigation on CD8+ T cells from the same patients revealed a lack of SARS-CoV2-reactive cells in the blood throughout the acute stage, which supports this theory [51,99]. However, in the absence of FoxP3 expression, Tregs have been shown to have pro-inflammatory properties [100], which can be detrimental. Hence, it is difficult to conclude the exact roles of Tregs' perturbations during the SARS-CoV-2 infection.

Asymptomatic COVID-19 patients, along with controls, were examined in a recent study for the expression levels of CTLA4 on the Tregs. CTLA4 is an important immunosuppressive activity marker. The research found that CD45RA+FoxP3+ resting Tregs, activated Tregs, and total Tregs dynamics all were identical [101]. A further investigation examined the surface expression of the Treg inhibitory marker CD127. When compared to healthy donors, they discovered that the expression of CD127 was considerably downregulated in both moderately and severely infected patients with COVID-19. Severely infected patients who recovered afterward were reported to have decreased levels of CD127 on Tregs [70].

Recently, Benamar et al. (2023) have brought attention to the fact that Multisystem Inflammatory Syndrome in Children (MIS-C) develops in certain pediatric patients after acute infection with SARS-CoV-2 via unidentified pathways. They have demonstrated that Tregs in MIS-C were destabilized through a Notch1-dependent pathway, while acute COVID-19 severity and outcomes were previously associated with Notch4 expression on Tregs. Due to dominant-negative mutations in the Notch1 regulators NUMB and NUMBL, which result in Notch1 overexpression, patients with MIS-C displayed enrichment of uncommon detrimental variations impacting the inflammatory and autoimmune pathways, according to genetic analyses [102]. Tregs that had been stimulated by Notch1 signaling produced CD22, which was then destabilized by mTORC1 and promoted systemic inflammation. These findings suggest unique immunological checkpoints regulated by individual Treg Notch receptors that influence the inflammatory outcome in SARS-CoV-2 infection and reveal a Notch1/CD22 signaling pathway that affects Treg function in MIS-C [102]. These studies suggest that additional studies are required to uncover the vast number of variations/perturbations in the Tregs of severely infected patients with COVID-19.

5. Tregs Association with Long COVID

According to Guan et al. (2020), the clinical manifestations of SARS-CoV-2 infection vary from asymptomatic/mild illness to severe pneumonia and respiratory distress syndrome, which may eventually result in death [103]. It has been noted that COVID-19 could encompass multi-system comorbidities, such as thrombotic events, vasculitis, and myocarditis, despite the fact that most patients only perceive mild symptoms such as fever, sore throat, breathing difficulties, loss of smell and taste, or cough [104,105].

Apart from the above-mentioned manifestations of the COVID-19 disease, severe immunopathology has been considered an important characteristic in various cases. The poor prognosis of the SARS-CoV-2 infection or the multiple organ damage is specifically associated with defective T-cell-mediated immune response, which is characterized by excessive proinflammatory cytokines, reduced number of lymphocytes, and newly developed or worsened autoimmune response [23,106]. According to a recent observational cohort research, one in eight individuals who caught COVID-19 is thought to have symptoms that last longer than the acute symptomatic period [107]. The World Health Organization (WHO) describes these sequelae, also known as "long COVID" in common usage today, as a post-COVID-19 condition that typically manifests three months following a confirmed or suspected SARS-CoV-2 infection and includes a group of new-onset, prolonged, or varying ailments that persists for at least two months [108]. According to several studies, the most prevalent symptoms in this situation include exhaustion, breathlessness, post-exertional malaise, chronic cough, headache, muscle aches, tachycardia, concentration deficits, and a decreased quality of life [23,109–111].

Numerous possibilities are now being discussed; however, it is still unclear what pathophysiological pathways contribute to the emergence and progression of long COVID. Moreover, Merad et al. (2022) proposed that immunopathological mechanisms, including systemic inflammation with viral persistence, post-viral autoimmune response, microbiome dysbiosis, and unrepaired tissue damage, may be involved in the pathogenesis of long COVID [112]. Accordingly, it has been shown that impacted individuals show a considerable increase in the number of inflammatory markers when compared to those who have recovered, suggesting a hyperactive and disrupted immune response, especially consisting of T cells [113,114]. But the interesting fact is that only a few studies have been done on the involvement of Tregs in patients suffering from long COVID or recovering patients from long COVID. Tregs can be important components of the immune system that may control and fine-tune autoimmune responses, promoting immunological homeostasis in the long COVID [23].

Recent investigations examined the percentage of Tregs among CD4+ cells in patients who still have COVID-19 symptoms and contrasted these to seronegative controls and COVID-19 survivors [115–117]. The patients who were part of the long COVID group reported a wide range of symptoms, including headaches, palpitations, insomnia, myalgia, fatigue, and shortness of breath. It has been postulated that Tregs can play important roles in the progression of long COVID. Contradictory findings were seen in the two trials that examined individuals who had persistent symptoms almost a year after the illness. A recent study found that patients with long COVID have more than two times the number of Tregs as compared to the fully recovered subjects from COVID-19 [115]. At the same time, a contradictory observation has recorded a considerable decrease in Tregs concentration in patients with long COVID [117]. The proportions of Tregs expressing FoxP3 were recorded in more than 100 patients with long COVID and found to have a reduced number of Tregs compared to the seronegative controls [116]. However, apart from the change in number, none of these studies investigated the immunosuppressive activities of Treg cells.

The above studies that collected various samples of blood while recovering from COVID-19 provide additional evidence for the aforementioned; they found that the intensity of Tregs displayed by subjects at the second and third follow-ups seemed to be comparable to the frequency of seronegative subjects than it was during the first analysis [118–120]. In addition, FoxP3 expression was upregulated in the Tregs obtained from the recovering patients [58]. Although the recruited participants recovered from asymptomatic infections, which may have initially caused less severe Treg alterations, as suggested by other studies [19,23], the relevance of this discovery is still unclear. Accordingly, convalescent patients did not exhibit considerably different Treg levels from acute non-hospitalized subjects [20,121].

The lack of research examining Tregs in a particular cohort makes it impossible to draw any definitive inferences on the kind of Treg adaptations in long COVID [23]. Nevertheless, these investigated analyses revealed that Treg dysregulations/perturbations persist in long COVID patients even years after their original SARS-CoV-2 infection [115]. Furthermore, other comparative studies found a higher and lower proportion of Tregs among CD4+ cells in patients with residual symptoms compared to recovered subjects [23]. The number of cells was found to be comparable in terms of the time elapsed from disease onset to follow-up sampling [23,115].

It is important to keep this in mind while understanding such findings because long COVID is a heterogeneous and multidimensional condition with a variety of clinical signs [122]. Previous studies have hypothesized that long COVID may include a number of symptoms and various sub-diagnoses, many of which have no immunological basis [123–125]. It is plausible that Treg dysregulation leads to a long COVID-associated immunopathology in numerous ways, as a particular pathophysiological mechanism cannot explain the post-acute consequences of COVID-19 [23,125]. Further, it becomes increasingly clear that long COVID is not a single diagnosis but rather a group of illnesses with various pathophysiology components. Therefore, it may be considered that the abovementioned studies looking at long COVID depicted a mix of distinct illnesses considering the variety of symptoms shown by the recruited individuals [20,23]. Additional research should explore whether Treg frequencies and the Th17/Treg ratio are correlated with certain symptom combinations, as previously suggested, or with laboratory variables like immunological status, cytokine levels, or autoantibody titers [23].

6. Tregs-Based Therapies and Their Therapeutic Potentials

Many studies have implied that Tregs play a protective role by regulating the exaggerated immune response reported in severely infected patients with COVID-19. The deleterious consequences associated with the uncontrolled release of cytokines in severely infected patients with COVID-19 may be managed by using Tregs' immunosuppressive capabilities [21] [Figure 4].

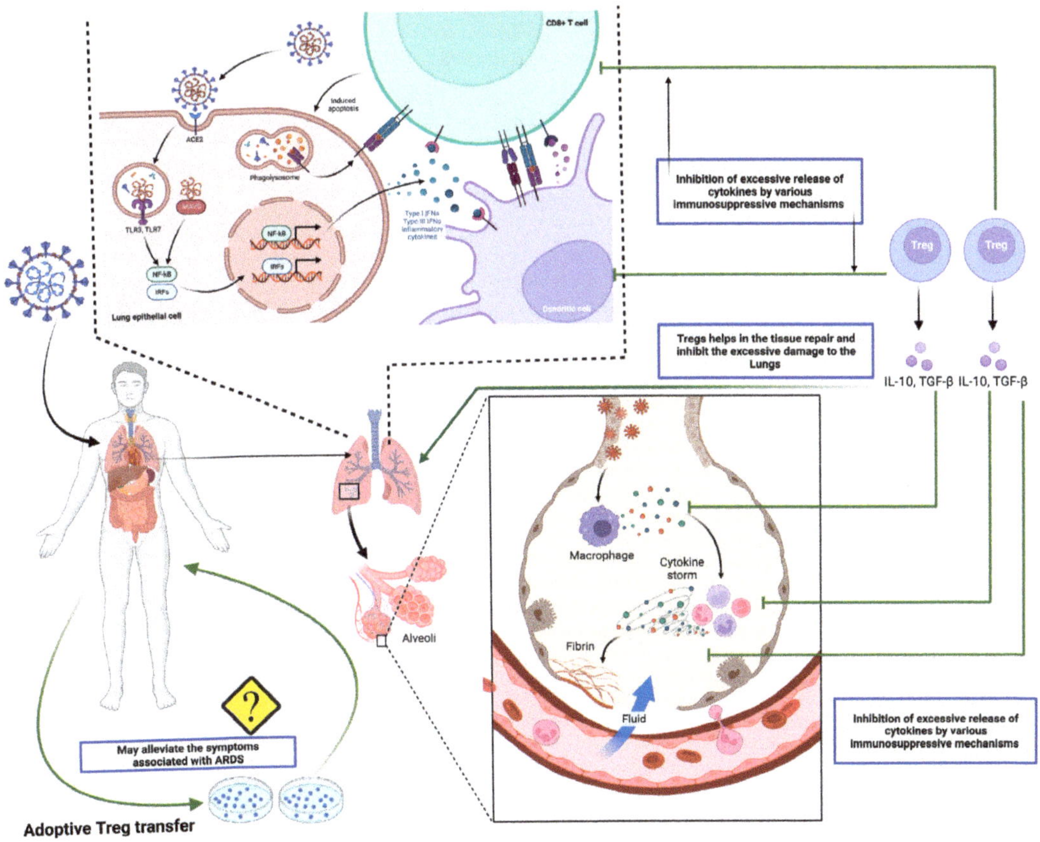

Figure 4. The figure shows the therapeutic potential of Tregs by suppressing the exaggerated immune response. SARS-CoV-2 infects the lung epithelial cells by entering through ACE2 receptors. SARS-CoV-2 infects lung epithelial cells by using ACE2 receptors. As viral RNA enters the cell, it activates endosomal and cytoplasmic sensors, including TLR3/7 and MAVS. Further, these endosomal and cytoplasmic receptors activate IRFs and NFkB, resulting in the production of inflammatory cytokines such as interferons (IFN). Dendritic cells acquire antigen before migrating to lymphoid organs to activate adaptive immunity. Following the recognition of antigens on antigen-presenting cells (APCs) or infected cells, CD8 T lymphocytes trigger apoptosis. Additionally, the viral antigens present to the T cells through antigen processing. Antigen processing is the process through which APCs, such as dendritic cells and alveolar macrophages, endocytose and kill the SARS-CoV-2 virus. MHC proteins then express antigen fragments on the cell membrane, enabling T lymphocytes to identify them. The overstimulated T cells and APCs in severely infected patients lead to excessive secretion of cytokines/chemokines, which leads to lung damage and ARDS. The balanced concentration of Tregs can suppress the exaggerated immune response through its immunoregulatory and immunosuppressive activities. In this context, recent studies suggested the beneficial effects of the adoptive transfer of Tregs in severely infected patients, which is yet to be approved for its clinical safety.

A potential cellular therapeutic approach for the management of autoimmune disorders and graft-versus-host disease is adoptive Treg transfer [126]. It is crucial to note that earlier research has shown the efficacy of such an intervention in several preclinical ARDS models [127]. Additionally, according to mouse models, the transfer of Tregs may increase the chance that a mouse infected with coronavirus-induced encephalitis would survive and decrease the amount of cardiac fibrosis that the virus causes [128]. Ex vivo expanded Treg cells may therefore be able to restore Treg balance in patients with decreased Treg activity brought along by SARS-CoV-2 infection and subsequently lessen the severity of life-threatening symptoms by reducing excessive inflammation and suppressing the uncontrolled release of cytokines/chemokines [21] [Figure 4].

The effectiveness of the adoptive transfer of Tregs derived from allogeneic HLA-matched umbilical cord was reported, which provided directions for the implementation of the adoptive transfer of Tregs to manage COVID-19 [129]. In this research, intravenous allogeneic cord blood-derived Tregs were given to two severely infected patients having ARDS. The patients were given tocilizumab and vasopressors, while only the first patient received hydroxychloroquine and broad-spectrum antibiotics before receiving therapy with Tregs [21,128,129]. The circumstances of both patients significantly improved after two rounds of cell infusion, which was associated with lower levels of proinflammatory cytokines such as IL-6, TNF-alpha, IFN-gamma, IL-8, IL-12, and MCP-4 in the blood. Interestingly, there were no symptoms of an infusion reaction, a resurgence of inflammatory response, or any additional negative repercussions [129].

Hence, the infusion of Tregs derived from cord blood can be an effective therapeutic intervention to manage severely infected patients with COVID-19. Another current clinical study (NCT04468971) is evaluating the effectiveness and safety of Tregs usage in the management of COVID-19 patients [130]. Additionally, hybrid Tregs having characteristics of TREG/Th2 cells are being investigated in another clinical investigation to alleviate the inflammatory response in severely infected patients showing the symptoms of multiple organ damage [130]. These hybrid cells have shown the capability to reduce the inflammatory response and mediate a beneficial impact on respiratory tissues [130,131].

Circulating soluble IL-2 receptor concentrations have been shown to be higher in severely infected patients with COVID-19 [131,132]. By lowering the bioavailability of IL-2 to Treg cells, soluble IL-2 receptors may limit the development of Treg cells in COVID-19 patients [131]. Previous research has shown that in vivo administration of low-dose IL-2 was able to precisely stimulate Treg expansions in patients with type 1 diabetes and graft-versus-host disease [133,134]. Such investigations led to the registration of a clinical trial to examine the effectiveness of low-dose IL-2 in the management of COVID-19 patients with ARDS [124]. Additionally, a recent study reported that the administration of recombinant IL-2 (rIL-2) might significantly enhance the frequency of lymphocytes, including Tregs, in the peripheral blood [135]. Additionally, after receiving rIL-2 therapy, the concentration of CRP dropped [135], which may contain the deleterious consequences of severe viral infection.

Additionally, a phase 3 clinical research (NCT04724629) investigating the effectiveness and durability of treatment using IL-2 or an inhibitor of IL-17 has just been filed for patients with COVID-19. Nevertheless, clinical observation revealed that patients with severe and critical conditions had higher levels of soluble IL-2R. This led to the development of soluble IL-2R as a biomarker for early detection of severe COVID-19 and for estimating clinical progression [30,136,137]. An elevated concentration of soluble IL-2R may be able to scavenge IL-2, indicating that low-dose IL-2 therapy was not the best course of action for treating COVID-19 [138]. According to reports, an anti-human IL-2 (hIL-2) antibody may change the ratio of effector T cells (Teff) to regulatory T cells (Treg) when it is attached to hIL-2 [139].

In a mouse model of experimental autoimmune encephalomyelitis (EAE), the IL-2 monoclonal antibody JES6-1 selectively expanded Tregs and reduced inflammation [140]. Autoimmune disorders and inflammatory conditions are caused by an imbalance of Tregs vs. other immune cells in living organisms. A JAK 1/2 inhibitor called ruxolitinib has been shown to boost FOXP3 abundance and Treg frequency while decreasing Th17 frequency [141]. Ruxolitinib therapy in the Phase I/II study for COVID-19 was finished in 2021. According to recent research, the transitory breakdown of Treg tolerance may stimulate DCs and cause them to produce an effective adaptive immune response against SARS-CoV-2 [142]. Therefore, balancing Tregs and DCs may be a potential approach for treating COVID-19 [30].

Additionally, several small-molecule-based medications that potentially enhance Tregs activity may be employed to stave off the cytokine storm brought on by severe viral infection. Recently, it has been discovered that the GSK3 inhibitor SB216763 might improve the suppressive effect of hiTregs by increasing the release of IL-10 and reducing proinflammatory iTregs [143]. Another research proposed GSK3 inhibition as a viable treatment strategy against SARS-CoV-2 [144]. Tregs formation required the PI3K-Akt-mTOR signaling pathway [145]. In the treatment of Type 1 diabetic patients, rapamycin, an inhibitor of mTOR, promotes the development of Tregs, simultaneously inhibiting the growth of effector T cells [146,147]. In this context, rapamycin therapy has the ability to stop the excessive release of cytokines/chemokines in severely infected patients with COVID-19 [148].

Furthermore, a metabolite of vitamin A called all-trans retinoic acid (atRA) has been shown to decrease the de novo production of Th17 from naive CD4+ T cells and to promote the development of Tregs from naive CD4+ T cells [149,150]. AtRA might preserve the stability and functionality of nTregs in an inflammatory environment in addition to controlling the balance of Tregs/Th17 [151]. By suppressing 3CLpro activity, AtRA was also found to have antiviral effects against SARS-CoV-2 [152].

Treg-based treatment has the possibility of using antigen-specific TCR, which might be guided in the direction of a desired antigen [153]. In animal models of Type 1 diabetes, arthritis, and transplantation, TCR-Tregs could be grown ex vivo and performed better than polyclonal Tregs [154–156]. TCR-Treg treatment may offer benefits of a lower dose but greater effectiveness and has therapeutic benefits in COVID-19 patients by attacking a distinct antigen of SARS-CoV-2 [30]. Another tactic is the use of CAR-Tregs, which may attach to tissue-specific self-antigens and focus on suppressive activities on the location of the illness [157]. In several preclinical models, such as experimental autoimmune encephalomyelitis and experimental allergic asthma, CAR-Treg treatment has been shown to be effective [158–160]. CAR-Treg treatment for renal transplantation is currently the subject of Phase I/II investigation. Despite receiving a lot of interest in treating tumors and a number of autoimmune illnesses, COVID-19 has not yet been treated with CAR-Treg therapy. Potential uses for CAR-Treg in the treatment of SARS-CoV-2 are made possible by its capacity to generate immunological tolerance [30].

Furthermore, CTLA-4, which is an important functional marker of Tregs, has been studied to manage COVID-19. The stimulatory receptor CD28's ligands CD80 and CD86 interact with CTLA-4 and lessen co-stimulatory signals for T-cells via boosting trans-endocytosis and the degradation of two ligands [46]. Abatacept, a recombinant Fc-fused form of CTLA-4 protein, has been used for many years as an immunotherapy for a variety of autoimmune illnesses since it has been shown to interfere with T-cell signaling and stimulation [138]. A clinical study using Abatacept for the treatment of COVID-19 patients was just finished and reported beneficial effects in reducing the inflammatory response.

Recently a clinical study employing the combination of Abatacept and the COVID-19 vaccine was conducted by the University of Alabama. Abatacept may reduce the persistence of viral infection and result in milder symptoms, according to an epidemiological study [161]. This implies that the use of CTLA-4-based therapy can be an effective approach to managing patients with COVID-19. TGF-beta, an immunoregulatory molecule generated from Tregs, is also thought to be a target for SARS-CoV-2 therapy in addition to CTLA-4. According to Vaz de Paula et al. (2021), TGF-beta may have a role in both the fluid balance of the lung and the development of lung fibrosis [162]. In order to prevent the establishment of inflammation in the lungs, inhibiting TGF-beta by neutralizing and eliminating TGF-beta using antibodies and/or TGF-beta inhibitors becomes a potential strategy [163], and this can be employed in the management of COVID-19 patients with severe lung damage [164].

A range of studies consisting of COVID-19 patients showed that Notch4 expression was elevated on Tregs and correlated with illness severity, death, and healing. In viral respiratory illnesses, such as SARS-CoV-2 and influenza, the Notch4-amphiregulin nexus has been discovered as a presumed target of treatment [165,166]. In order to stabilize FOXP3 expression and further control the development and function of Tregs, the pathway of Notch4 and Notch ligand delta-like ligand 4 (DLL4) is discovered to elevate H3K4me3 around the *foxp3* locus [167]. The above information shows that disturbing or interfering along the Notch4-DLL4 axis can be a potential therapeutic approach to treat COVID-19. It is also important to remember the multiple functions of FOXP3+ Tregs during viral infection [168,169]. Prior to Treg-based treatment, it is important to thoroughly understand the continuous fluctuations of Tregs, especially their percentage, suppressive function, and FOXP3 stability during various phases of COVID-19 [30,170].

7. Conclusions and Future Perspectives

It has been shown that virus-specific T-cell responses, particularly those of regulatory T cells (Tregs), affect tissue damage in respiratory illnesses. Tregs have been shown to play an important role in the pathogenesis of COVID-19 because of their wide range of immunosuppressive activities. Tregs inhibit not only the cells of the innate immune response, such as dendritic cells, natural killer cells, and macrophages, but also the cells of the adaptive immune response, including B and T cells. One of the most important aspects of Tregs in COVID-19 is their capability to limit the excessive release of cytokines which is the major reason for mortality and morbidity in COVID-19 patients. Increases in Tregs have been discovered to be a critical feature during the early stages of SARS-CoV-2 infection because they may reduce CD8+ T cells' ability to mount an effective antiviral immune response, which can have a negative impact on COVID-19 disease prognosis. Nevertheless, Tregs have been found to be decreased or non-functional in severely infected patients with COVID-19. According to many studies, Tregs were elevated in COVID-19 patients and were detrimental to the disease's development. Contradictorily, cytokine storm or exaggerated immune response has been linked to lower Treg levels, which leads to a poor prognosis of the disease. It is currently unclear how the proportion of regulatory T cells in COVID-19 changed, particularly when taking into account the biphasic roles of Tregs during the course of the SARS-CoV-2 infection. Tregs are helpful in suppressing inflammation as the illness advances. Hence, to re-establish antiviral immune responses, strategies that target Tregs and lessen their suppressive activity may be helpful, particularly in elderly individuals with immuno-compromised immunity. It is essential to make use of methods that either induce or enlarge Tregs in these individuals in order to bring down the level of hyperinflammation and tissue damage.

Severely infected individuals with COVID-19 have also been shown to have alterations in the phenotypic traits of their Tregs, as well as elevated FoxP3 expression and a distinct transcriptional pattern that is strikingly similar to that of tumor Tregs. In severely infected patients with COVID-19, typical cell growth and enhanced effector functions, particularly ENTPD1, LAG3, and LRRC32, have been noted. Scientists are still figuring out the precise relevance of such perturbations in the Tregs of severely infected patients. Additionally, why such perturbations arise is yet to be resolved. Interestingly, the roles of Tregs have been studied in patients with long COVID. Recent analysis has revealed that Treg dysregulations/perturbations persist in long COVID patients even years after their original SARS-CoV-2 infection. However, the exact roles are still not clear. However, there is no doubt that several studies reported the positive results of several Tregs-based therapeutic interventions. The effectiveness of the adoptive transfer of Tregs has been reported to alleviate the disease severity. Additionally, a low dose of IL-2 has been found to be effective in the generation and stimulation of Tregs in severely infected COVID-19 patients. Many studies have reported the potential uses of CAR-Treg in the treatment of SARS-CoV-2. Furthermore, many small molecules have been found to induce Tregs, which can alleviate the cytokine storm. While many studies have shown the therapeutic potentialities of Tregs-mediated therapies, it is essential to study the effectiveness of Tregs in detail. Tregs should be investigated further as possible treatment targets and prognostic indicators in COVID-19. To draw firmer findings, more research is necessary. This research should include more patients with moderate and severe disorders as well as proven techniques for Treg characterization and Tregs' concentration measurement. Likewise, studies on individuals who received various COVID-19 immunizations are desperately required to ascertain if Tregs in blood fluctuate after vaccinations and whether these alterations may link to the beneficial effects of immunizations.

Author Contributions: Conceptualization, M.D.; investigation and resources, M.D., A.A.R., S.A., M.A., M.A.H., A.A., M.A.N., A.S.S.A., A.A.A., S.A.A., N.T. and G.V.; writing—original draft preparation, M.D.; writing—review and editing, M.D., A.A.R., A.A., M.A.N., A.S.S.A., A.A.A., B.M.A., M.G., S.A.-A., S.H.A.-A., N.T. and G.V. visualization and supervision, M.D. and A.A.R.; project administration, M.D. and A.A.R. All authors have read and agreed to the published version of the manuscript.

Funding: This research received no external funding.

Institutional Review Board Statement: Not applicable.

Informed Consent Statement: Not applicable.

Data Availability Statement: All data are available in this manuscript.

Acknowledgments: All authors acknowledge their respective institutions and universities.

Conflicts of Interest: The authors declare no conflict of interest.

Abbreviations

ACE2	angiotensin converting enzyme 2
APCs	antigen-presenting cells
BCR	B cell receptor
BALF	bronchoalveolar lavage fluid
COVID-19	coronavirus disease 19
CTLA-4	cytotoxic T lymphocyte associated antigen-4
FoxP3	Forkhead box P3
LAG-3	lymphocyte activation gene 3
MHC	major histocompatibility complex
MHC II	major histocompatibility complex class II
mAbs	monoclonal antibodies
nAbs	neutralizing antibodies
pTregs	peripheral Tregs
PD-L1	programmed death -ligand 1
SARS-CoV-2	severe acute respiratory syndrome coronavirus 2
Tregs	T regulatory cells
tTregs	thymic Tregs
TGF-beta	transforming growth factor-beta 1
TLRs	Toll like receptors
Th1	T helper 1
Th2	T helper 2
Th17	T helper 17
TCR	T cell receptor

References

1. Alahdal, M.; Elkord, E. Exhaustion and Over-Activation of Immune Cells in COVID-19: Challenges and Therapeutic Opportunities. *Clin. Immunol.* **2022**, *245*, 109177. [CrossRef] [PubMed]
2. Dhawan, M.; Saied, A.A.; Mitra, S.; Alhumaydhi, F.A.; Emran, T.B.; Wilairatana, P. Omicron Variant (B.1.1.529) and Its Sublineages: What Do We Know so Far amid the Emergence of Recombinant Variants of SARS-CoV-2? *Biomed. Pharmacother.* **2022**, *154*, 113522. [CrossRef]
3. Ahmad, S.; Hatmal, M.M.; Lambuk, L.; Al-Hatamleh, M.A.I.; Alshaer, W.; Mohamud, R. The Role of TNFR2$^+$ Tregs in COVID-19: An Overview and a Potential Therapeutic Strategy. *Life Sci.* **2021**, *286*, 120063. [CrossRef] [PubMed]
4. Ahmed, J.Q.; Maulud, S.Q.; Dhawan, M.; Priyanka; Choudhary, O.P.; Jalal, P.J.; Ali, R.K.; Tayib, G.A.; Hasan, D.A. MicroRNAs in the Development of Potential Therapeutic Targets against COVID-19: A Narrative Review. *J. Infect. Public Health* **2022**, *15*, 788–799. [CrossRef] [PubMed]
5. Tandel, N.; Negi, S.; Dalai, S.K.; Tyagi, R.K. Role of natural killer and B cell interaction in inducing pathogen specific immune responses. *Int. Rev. Immunol.* **2023**. *advance online publication*. [CrossRef]
6. Kudlay, D.; Kofiadi, I.; Khaitov, M. Peculiarities of the T Cell Immune Response in COVID-19. *Vaccines* **2022**, *10*, 242. [CrossRef]
7. Moss, P. The T Cell Immune Response against SARS-CoV-2. *Nat. Immunol.* **2022**, *23*, 186–193. [CrossRef] [PubMed]
8. Chavda, V.P.; Mishra, T.; Vuppu, S. Immunological Studies to Understand Hybrid/Recombinant Variants of SARS-CoV-2. *Vaccines* **2022**, *11*, 45. [CrossRef] [PubMed]
9. Arish, M.; Qian, W.; Narasimhan, H.; Sun, J. COVID-19 Immunopathology: From Acute Diseases to Chronic Sequelae. *J. Med. Virol.* **2022**, *95*, e28122. [CrossRef]
10. Liu, J.; Chandrashekar, A.; Sellers, D.; Barrett, J.; Jacob-Dolan, C.; Lifton, M.; McMahan, K.; Sciacca, M.; VanWyk, H.; Wu, C.; et al. Vaccines Elicit Highly Conserved Cellular Immunity to SARS-CoV-2 Omicron. *Nature* **2022**, *603*, 493–496. [CrossRef]
11. Su, Y.; Chen, D.; Yuan, D.; Lausted, C.; Choi, J.; Dai, C.L.; Voillet, V.; Duvvuri, V.R.; Scherler, K.; Troisch, P.; et al. Multi-Omics Resolves a Sharp Disease-State Shift between Mild and Moderate COVID-19. *Cell* **2020**, *183*, 1479–1495.e20. [CrossRef]
12. Mathew, D.; Giles, J.R.; Baxter, A.E.; Oldridge, D.A.; Greenplate, A.R.; Wu, J.E.; Alanio, C.; Kuri-Cervantes, L.; Pampena, M.B.; D'Andrea, K.; et al. Deep Immune Profiling of COVID-19 Patients Reveals Distinct Immunotypes with Therapeutic Implications. *Science* **2020**, *369*, eabc8511. [CrossRef]
13. Dhawan, M.; Rabaan, A.A.; Fawarah, M.M.A.; Almuthree, S.A.; Alsubki, R.A.; Alfaraj, A.H.; Mashraqi, M.M.; Alshamrani, S.A.; Abduljabbar, W.A.; Alwashmi, A.S.S.; et al. Updated Insights into the T Cell-Mediated Immune Response against SARS-CoV-2: A Step towards Efficient and Reliable Vaccines. *Vaccines* **2023**, *11*, 101. [CrossRef]
14. Le Bert, N.; Clapham, H.E.; Tan, A.T.; Chia, W.N.; Tham, C.Y.L.; Lim, J.M.; Kunasegaran, K.; Tan, L.W.L.; Dutertre, C.-A.; Shankar, N.; et al. Highly Functional Virus-Specific Cellular Immune Response in Asymptomatic SARS-CoV-2 Infection. *J. Exp. Med.* **2021**, *218*, e20202617. [CrossRef]
15. Grau-Expósito, J.; Sánchez-Gaona, N.; Massana, N.; Suppi, M.; Astorga-Gamaza, A.; Perea, D.; Rosado, J.; Falcó, A.; Kirkegaard, C.; Torrella, A.; et al. Peripheral and Lung Resident Memory T Cell Responses against SARS-CoV-2. *Nat. Commun.* **2021**, *12*, 3010. [CrossRef] [PubMed]
16. Goswami, T.K.; Singh, M.; Dhawan, M.; Mitra, S.; Emran, T.B.; Rabaan, A.A.; Mutair, A.A.; Alawi, Z.A.; Alhumaid, S.; Dhama, K. Regulatory T Cells (Tregs) and Their Therapeutic Potential against Autoimmune Disorders—Advances and Challenges. *Hum. Vaccines Immunother.* **2022**, *18*, 2035117. [CrossRef]
17. Gao, M.; Liu, Y.; Guo, M.; Wang, Q.; Wang, Y.; Fan, J.; Shen, Y.; Hou, J.; Wan, Y.; Zhu, Z. Regulatory CD4$^+$ and CD8$^+$ T Cells Are Negatively Correlated with CD4$^+$/CD8$^+$ T Cell Ratios in Patients Acutely Infected with SARS-CoV-2. *J. Leukoc. Biol.* **2020**, *109*, 91–97. [CrossRef] [PubMed]
18. Hillaire, M.; Rimmelzwaan, G.; Kreijtz, J. Clearance of Influenza Virus Infections by T Cells: Risk of Collateral Damage? *Curr. Opin. Virol.* **2013**, *3*, 430–437. [CrossRef]
19. Wang, H.; Wang, Z.; Cao, W.; Wu, Q.; Yuan, Y.; Zhang, X. Regulatory T Cells in COVID-19. *Aging Dis.* **2021**, *12*, 1545. [CrossRef]
20. Galván-Peña, S.; Leon, J.; Chowdhary, K.; Michelson, D.A.; Vijaykumar, B.; Yang, L.; Magnuson, A.M.; Chen, F.; Manickas-Hill, Z.; Piechocka-Trocha, A.; et al. Profound Treg Perturbations Correlate with COVID-19 Severity. *Proc. Natl. Acad. Sci. USA* **2021**, *118*, e2111315118. [CrossRef] [PubMed]
21. Wang, Y.; Zheng, J.; Islam, M.S.; Yang, Y.; Hu, Y.; Chen, X. The Role of CD4$^+$FoxP3$^+$ Regulatory T Cells in the Immunopathogenesis of COVID-19: Implications for Treatment. *Int. J. Biol. Sci.* **2021**, *17*, 1507–1520. [CrossRef] [PubMed]
22. Seepathomnarong, P.; Ongarj, J.; Sophonmanee, R.; Seeyankem, B.; Chusri, S.; Surasombatpattana, S.; Pinpathomrat, N. Regulatory T Cells Decreased during Recovery from Mild COVID-19. *Viruses* **2022**, *14*, 1688. [CrossRef]
23. Haunhorst, S.; Bloch, W.; Javelle, F.; Krüger, K.; Baumgart, S.; Drube, S.; Lemhöfer, C.; Reuken, P.; Stallmach, A.; Müller, M.; et al. A Scoping Review of Regulatory T Cell Dynamics in Convalescent COVID-19 Patients—Indications for Their Potential Involvement in the Development of Long COVID? *Front. Immunol.* **2022**, *13*, 107099. [CrossRef]
24. Baecher-Allan, C.; Brown, J.A.; Freeman, G.J.; Hafler, D.A. CD4$^+$CD25high Regulatory Cells in Human Peripheral Blood. *J. Immunol.* **2001**, *167*, 1245–1253. [CrossRef]
25. Maekawa, D.; Riblet, S.M.; Whang, P.; Hurley, D.J.; Garcia, M. Activation of Cytotoxic Lymphocytes and Presence of Regulatory T Cells in the Trachea of Non-Vaccinated and Vaccinated Chickens as a Recall to an Infectious Laryngotracheitis Virus (ILTV) Challenge. *Vaccines* **2021**, *9*, 865. [CrossRef]

26. Panduro, M.; Benoist, C.; Mathis, D. Tissue Tregs. *Annu. Rev. Immunol.* **2016**, *34*, 609–633. [CrossRef]
27. McRitchie, B.R.; Akkaya, B. Exhaust the Exhausters: Targeting Regulatory T Cells in the Tumor Microenvironment. *Front. Immunol.* **2022**, *13*, 5820. [CrossRef]
28. Magnuson, A.M.; Kiner, E.; Ergun, A.; Park, J.S.; Asinovski, N.; Ortiz-Lopez, A.; Kilcoyne, A.; Paoluzzi-Tomada, E.; Weissleder, R.; Mathis, D.; et al. Identification and Validation of a Tumor-Infiltrating Treg Transcriptional Signature Conserved across Species and Tumor Types. *Proc. Natl. Acad. Sci. USA* **2018**, *115*, E10672–E10681. [CrossRef]
29. Lund, J.M.; Hsing, L.; Pham, T.T.; Rudensky, A.Y. Coordination of Early Protective Immunity to Viral Infection by Regulatory T Cells. *Science* **2008**, *320*, 1220–1224. [CrossRef]
30. Xu, Z.; Jiang, X.; Dai, X.; Li, B. The Dynamic Role of FOXP3$^+$ Tregs and Their Potential Therapeutic Applications During SARS-CoV-2 Infection. *Front. Immunol.* **2022**, *13*, 916411. [CrossRef]
31. Sakaguchi, S.; Sakaguchi, N.; Asano, M.; Itoh, M.; Toda, M. Immunologic Self-Tolerance Maintained by Activated T Cells Expressing IL-2 Receptor Alpha-Chains (CD25). Breakdown of a Single Mechanism of Self-Tolerance Causes Various Autoimmune Diseases. *J. Immunol.* **1995**, *155*, 1151–1164. [CrossRef]
32. Zenclussen, A.C.; Gerlof, K.; Zenclussen, M.L.; Ritschel, S.; Zambon Bertoja, A.; Fest, S.; Hontsu, S.; Ueha, S.; Matsushima, K.; Leber, J.; et al. Regulatory T Cells Induce a Privileged Tolerant Microenvironment at the Fetal-Maternal Interface. *Eur. J. Immunol.* **2006**, *36*, 82–94. [CrossRef] [PubMed]
33. Palomares, O.; Rückert, B.; Jartti, T.; Kücüksezer, U.C.; Puhakka, T.; Gomez, E.; Fahrner, H.B.; Speiser, A.; Jung, A.; Kwok, W.W.; et al. Induction and Maintenance of Allergen-Specific FOXP3$^+$ Treg Cells in Human Tonsils as Potential First-Line Organs of Oral Tolerance. *J. Allergy Clin. Immunol.* **2012**, *129*, 510–520.e9. [CrossRef]
34. Di Ianni, M.; Falzetti, F.; Carotti, A.; Terenzi, A.; Castellino, F.; Bonifacio, E.; Del Papa, B.; Zei, T.; Ostini, R.I.; Cecchini, D.; et al. Tregs Prevent GVHD and Promote Immune Reconstitution in HLA-Haploidentical Transplantation. *Blood* **2011**, *117*, 3921–3928. [CrossRef] [PubMed]
35. Traxinger, B.R.; Richert-Spuhler, L.E.; Lund, J.M. Mucosal Tissue Regulatory T Cells Are Integral in Balancing Immunity and Tolerance at Portals of Antigen Entry. *Mucosal Immunol.* **2022**, *15*, 398–407. [CrossRef]
36. Shevach, E.M.; Thornton, A.M. tTregs, pTregs, and iTregs: Similarities and Differences. *Immunol. Rev.* **2014**, *259*, 88–102. [CrossRef] [PubMed]
37. Liu, W.; Putnam, A.L.; Xu-yu, Z.; Szot, G.L.; Lee, M.R.; Zhu, S.; Gottlieb, P.A.; Kapranov, P.; Gingeras, T.R.; de St. Groth, B.F.; et al. CD127 Expression Inversely Correlates with FoxP3 and Suppressive Function of Human CD4$^+$ T Reg Cells. *J. Exp. Med.* **2006**, *203*, 1701–1711. [CrossRef]
38. Tyagi, R.K.; Jacobse, J.; Li, J.; Allaman, M.M.; Otipoby, K.L.; Sampson, E.R.; Wilson, K.T.; Goettel, J.A. HLA-Restriction of Human Treg Cells Is Not Required for Therapeutic Efficacy of Low-Dose IL-2 in Humanized Mice. *Front. Immunol.* **2021**, *12*, 630204. [CrossRef] [PubMed]
39. Akkaya, B.; Shevach, E.M. Regulatory T Cells: Master Thieves of the Immune System. *Cell. Immunol.* **2020**, *355*, 104160. [CrossRef] [PubMed]
40. Shevach, E.M. Mechanisms of Foxp3$^+$ T Regulatory Cell-Mediated Suppression. *Immunity* **2009**, *30*, 636–645. [CrossRef] [PubMed]
41. Cao, X.; Cai, S.F.; Fehniger, T.A.; Song, J.; Collins, L.I.; Piwnica-Worms, D.R.; Ley, T.J. Granzyme B and Perforin Are Important for Regulatory T Cell-Mediated Suppression of Tumor Clearance. *Immunity* **2007**, *27*, 635–646. [CrossRef]
42. Borsellino, G.; Kleinewietfeld, M.; Di Mitri, D.; Sternjak, A.; Diamantini, A.; Giometto, R.; Höpner, S.; Centonze, D.; Bernardi, G.; Dell'Acqua, M.L.; et al. Expression of Ectonucleotidase CD39 by Foxp3$^+$ Treg Cells: Hydrolysis of Extracellular ATP and Immune Suppression. *Blood* **2007**, *110*, 1225–1232. [CrossRef] [PubMed]
43. Deaglio, S.; Dwyer, K.M.; Gao, W.; Friedman, D.; Usheva, A.; Erat, A.; Chen, J.-F.; Enjyoji, K.; Linden, J.; Oukka, M.; et al. Adenosine Generation Catalyzed by CD39 and CD73 Expressed on Regulatory T Cells Mediates Immune Suppression. *J. Exp. Med.* **2007**, *204*, 1257–1265. [CrossRef] [PubMed]
44. Tyagi, R.K.; Miles, B.; Parmar, R.; Garg, N.K.; Dalai, S.K.; Baban, B.; Cutler, C.W. Human IDO-competent, long-lived immunoregulatory dendritic cells induced by intracellular pathogen, and their fate in humanized mice. *Sci. Rep.* **2017**, *7*, 41083. [CrossRef]
45. Zarek, P.E.; Huang, C.-T.; Lutz, E.R.; Kowalski, J.; Horton, M.R.; Linden, J.; Drake, C.G.; Powell, J.D. A2A Receptor Signaling Promotes Peripheral Tolerance by Inducing T-Cell Anergy and the Generation of Adaptive Regulatory T Cells. *Blood* **2008**, *111*, 251–259. [CrossRef]
46. Qureshi, O.S.; Zheng, Y.; Nakamura, K.; Attridge, K.; Manzotti, C.; Schmidt, E.M.; Baker, J.; Jeffery, L.E.; Kaur, S.; Briggs, Z.; et al. Trans-Endocytosis of CD80 and CD86: A Molecular Basis for the Cell-Extrinsic Function of CTLA-4. *Science* **2011**, *332*, 600–603. [CrossRef]
47. Fallarino, F.; Grohmann, U.; Hwang, K.W.; Orabona, C.; Vacca, C.; Bianchi, R.; Belladonna, M.L.; Fioretti, M.C.; Alegre, M.-L.; Puccetti, P. Modulation of Tryptophan Catabolism by Regulatory T Cells. *Nat. Immunol.* **2003**, *4*, 1206–1212. [CrossRef]
48. Yan, Z.; Garg, S.K.; Banerjee, R. Regulatory T Cells Interfere with Glutathione Metabolism in Dendritic Cells and T Cells. *J. Biol. Chem.* **2010**, *285*, 41525–41532. [CrossRef]
49. Liang, B.; Workman, C.; Lee, J.; Chew, C.; Dale, B.M.; Colonna, L.; Flores, M.; Li, N.; Schweighoffer, E.; Greenberg, S.; et al. Regulatory T Cells Inhibit Dendritic Cells by Lymphocyte Activation Gene-3 Engagement of MHC Class II. *J. Immunol.* **2008**, *180*, 5916–5926. [CrossRef] [PubMed]

50. Gotot, J.; Gottschalk, C.; Leopold, S.; Knolle, P.A.; Yagita, H.; Kurts, C.; Ludwig-Portugall, I. Regulatory T Cells Use Programmed Death 1 Ligands to Directly Suppress Autoreactive B Cells in Vivo. *Proc. Natl. Acad. Sci. USA* **2012**, *109*, 10468–10473. [CrossRef]
51. Samaan, E.; Elmaria, M.O.; Khedr, D.; Gaber, T.; Elsayed, A.G.; Shenouda, R.N.; Gamal, H.; Shahin, D.; Abousamra, N.K.; Shemies, R. Characterization of Regulatory T Cells in SARS-CoV-2 Infected Hemodialysis Patients: Relation to Clinical and Radiological Severity. *BMC Nephrol.* **2022**, *23*, 391. [CrossRef] [PubMed]
52. Vick, S.C.; Frutoso, M.; Mair, F.; Konecny, A.J.; Greene, E.; Wolf, C.R.; Logue, J.K.; Franko, N.M.; Boonyaratanakornkit, J.; Gottardo, R.; et al. A Regulatory T Cell Signature Distinguishes the Immune Landscape of COVID-19 Patients from Those with Other Respiratory Infections. *Sci. Adv.* **2021**, *7*, eabj0274. [CrossRef] [PubMed]
53. Ronit, A.; Berg, R.M.G.; Bay, J.T.; Haugaard, A.K.; Ahlström, M.G.; Burgdorf, K.S.; Ullum, H.; Rørvig, S.B.; Tjelle, K.; Foss, N.B.; et al. Compartmental Immunophenotyping in COVID-19 ARDS: A Case Series. *J. Allergy Clin. Immunol.* **2021**, *147*, 81–91. [CrossRef] [PubMed]
54. Yang, J.; Zhong, M.; Hong, K.; Yang, Q.; Zhang, E.; Zhou, D.; Xia, J.; Chen, Y.; Sun, M.; Zhao, B.; et al. Characteristics of T-cell Responses in COVID-19 Patients with Prolonged SARS-CoV-2 Positivity—A Cohort Study. *Clin. Transl. Immunol.* **2021**, *10*, e1259. [CrossRef]
55. De Biasi, S.; Meschiari, M.; Gibellini, L.; Bellinazzi, C.; Borella, R.; Fidanza, L.; Gozzi, L.; Iannone, A.; Lo Tartaro, D.; Mattioli, M.; et al. Marked T Cell Activation, Senescence, Exhaustion and Skewing towards TH17 in Patients with COVID-19 Pneumonia. *Nat. Commun.* **2020**, *11*, 3434. [CrossRef]
56. Zheng, H.; Li, H.; Guo, L.; Liang, Y.; Li, J.; Wang, X.; Hu, Y.; Wang, L.; Liao, Y.; Yang, F.; et al. Virulence and Pathogenesis of SARS-CoV-2 Infection in Rhesus Macaques: A Nonhuman Primate Model of COVID-19 Progression. *PLOS Pathog.* **2020**, *16*, e1008949. [CrossRef] [PubMed]
57. Rajamanickam, A.; Pavan Kumar, N.; Pandiaraj, A.N.; Selvaraj, N.; Munisankar, S.; Renji, R.M.; Venkataramani, V.; Murhekar, M.; Thangaraj, J.W.V.; Muthusamy, S.K.; et al. Characterization of memory T cell subsets and common γ-chain cytokines in convalescent COVID-19 individuals. *J. Leukoc. Biol.* **2022**, *112*, 201–212. [CrossRef]
58. Mahmoud Salehi Khesht, A.; Karpisheh, V.; Qubais Saeed, B.; Olegovna Zekiy, A.; Yapanto, L.M.; Nabi Afjadi, M.; Aksoun, M.; Nasr Esfahani, M.; Aghakhani, F.; Movahed, M.; et al. Different T Cell Related Immunological Profiles in COVID-19 Patients Compared to Healthy Controls. *Int. Immunopharmacol.* **2021**, *97*, 107828. [CrossRef]
59. Sadeghi, A.; Tahmasebi, S.; Mahmood, A.; Kuznetsova, M.; Valizadeh, H.; Taghizadieh, A.; Nazemiyeh, M.; Aghebati-Maleki, L.; Jadidi-Niaragh, F.; Abbaspour-Aghdam, S.; et al. Th17 and Treg Cells Function in SARS-CoV2 Patients Compared with Healthy Controls. *J. Cell. Physiol.* **2020**, *236*, 2829–2839. [CrossRef]
60. Meckiff, B.J.; Ramírez-Suástegui, C.; Fajardo, V.; Chee, S.J.; Kusnadi, A.; Simon, H.; Eschweiler, S.; Grifoni, A.; Pelosi, E.; Weiskopf, D.; et al. Imbalance of Regulatory and Cytotoxic SARS-CoV-2-Reactive $CD4^+$ T Cells in COVID-19. *Cell* **2020**, *183*, 1340–1353.e16. [CrossRef]
61. Caldrer, S.; Mazzi, C.; Bernardi, M.; Prato, M.; Ronzoni, N.; Rodari, P.; Angheben, A.; Piubelli, C.; Tiberti, N. Regulatory T Cells as Predictors of Clinical Course in Hospitalised COVID-19 Patients. *Front. Immunol.* **2021**, *12*, 5143. [CrossRef]
62. Qin, C.; Zhou, L.; Hu, Z.; Zhang, S.; Yang, S.; Tao, Y.; Xie, C.; Ma, K.; Shang, K.; Wang, W.; et al. Dysregulation of Immune Response in Patients With Coronavirus 2019 (COVID-19) in Wuhan, China. *Clin. Infect. Dis.* **2020**, *71*, 762–768. [CrossRef]
63. Wang, W.; Su, B.; Pang, L.; Qiao, L.; Feng, Y.; Ouyang, Y.; Guo, X.; Shi, H.; Wei, F.; Su, X.; et al. High-Dimensional Immune Profiling by Mass Cytometry Revealed Immunosuppression and Dysfunction of Immunity in COVID-19 Patients. *Cell. Mol. Immunol.* **2020**, *17*, 650–652. [CrossRef]
64. Jia, R.; Wang, X.; Liu, P.; Liang, X.; Ge, Y.; Tian, H.; Chang, H.; Zhou, H.; Zeng, M.; Xu, J. Mild Cytokine Elevation, Moderate $CD4^+$ T Cell Response and Abundant Antibody Production in Children with COVID-19. *Virol. Sin.* **2020**, *35*, 734–743. [CrossRef]
65. Szabo, P.A.; Dogra, P.; Gray, J.I.; Wells, S.B.; Connors, T.J.; Weisberg, S.P.; Krupska, I.; Matsumoto, R.; Poon, M.M.L.; Idzikowski, E.; et al. Longitudinal Profiling of Respiratory and Systemic Immune Responses Reveals Myeloid Cell-Driven Lung Inflammation in Severe COVID-19. *Immunity* **2021**, *54*, 797–814.e6. [CrossRef]
66. Feng, Y.; Arvey, A.; Chinen, T.; van der Veeken, J.; Gasteiger, G.; Rudensky, A.Y. Control of the Inheritance of Regulatory T Cell Identity by a Cis Element in the Foxp3 Locus. *Cell* **2014**, *158*, 749–763. [CrossRef]
67. Yang, X.O.; Nurieva, R.; Martinez, G.J.; Kang, H.S.; Chung, Y.; Pappu, B.P.; Shah, B.; Chang, S.H.; Schluns, K.S.; Watowich, S.S.; et al. Molecular Antagonism and Plasticity of Regulatory and Inflammatory T Cell Programs. *Immunity* **2008**, *29*, 44–56. [CrossRef] [PubMed]
68. Simsek, A.; Kizmaz, M.A.; Cagan, E.; Dombaz, F.; Tezcan, G.; Asan, A.; Demir, H.I.; Bal, S.H.; Ermis, D.Y.; Dilektaslı, A.G.; et al. Assessment of CD39 Expression in Regulatory T-cell Subsets by Disease Severity in Adult and Juvenile COVID-19 Cases. *J. Med. Virol.* **2022**, *94*, 2089–2101. [CrossRef]
69. Ahern, D.J.; Ai, Z.; Ainsworth, M.; Allan, C.; Allcock, A.; Angus, B.; Ansari, M.A.; Arancibia-Cárcamo, C.V.; Aschenbrenner, D.; Attar, M.; et al. A Blood Atlas of COVID-19 Defines Hallmarks of Disease Severity and Specificity. *Cell* **2022**, *185*, 916–938.e58. [CrossRef] [PubMed]
70. Chen, G.; Wu, D.; Guo, W.; Cao, Y.; Huang, D.; Wang, H.; Wang, T.; Zhang, X.; Chen, H.; Yu, H.; et al. Clinical and Immunological Features of Severe and Moderate Coronavirus Disease 2019. *J. Clin. Investig.* **2020**, *130*, 2620–2629. [CrossRef] [PubMed]
71. Tan, L.; Wang, Q.; Zhang, D.; Ding, J.; Huang, Q.; Tang, Y.-Q.; Wang, Q.; Miao, H. Lymphopenia Predicts Disease Severity of COVID-19: A Descriptive and Predictive Study. *Signal Transduct. Target. Ther.* **2020**, *5*, 33. [CrossRef]

72. Ren, X.; Wen, W.; Fan, X.; Hou, W.; Su, B.; Cai, P.; Li, J.; Liu, Y.; Tang, F.; Zhang, F.; et al. COVID-19 Immune Features Revealed by a Large-Scale Single-Cell Transcriptome Atlas. *Cell* **2021**, *184*, 5838. [CrossRef] [PubMed]
73. Shen, X.-R.; Geng, R.; Li, Q.; Chen, Y.; Li, S.-F.; Wang, Q.; Min, J.; Yang, Y.; Li, B.; Jiang, R.-D.; et al. ACE2-Independent Infection of T Lymphocytes by SARS-CoV-2. *Signal Transduct. Target. Ther.* **2022**, *7*, 83. [CrossRef] [PubMed]
74. Kratzer, B.; Trapin, D.; Ettel, P.; Körmöczi, U.; Rottal, A.; Tuppy, F.; Feichter, M.; Gattinger, P.; Borochova, K.; Dorofeeva, Y.; et al. Immunological Imprint of COVID-19 on Human Peripheral Blood Leukocyte Populations. *Allergy* **2020**, *76*, 751–765. [CrossRef]
75. Mohebbi, S.R.; Baghaei, K.; Rostami-Nejad, M.; Mojarad, E.N.; Mirjalali, H.; Yadegar, A.; Asri, N.; Abdoulahi, S.; Assadzadeh Aghdaei, H. Significant Changes of CD4, FOXP3, CD25, and IL6 Expression Level in Iranian COVID-19 Patients. *Gastroenterol. Hepatol. Bed Bench* **2020**, *13*, 388–392.
76. Kalfaoglu, B.; Almeida-Santos, J.; Tye, C.A.; Satou, Y.; Ono, M. T-Cell Hyperactivation and Paralysis in Severe COVID-19 Infection Revealed by Single-Cell Analysis. *Front. Immunol.* **2020**, *11*, 589380. [CrossRef] [PubMed]
77. Thibaudin, M.; Fumet, J.-D.; Bon, M.; Hampe, L.; Limagne, E.; Ghiringhelli, F. Immunological Features of Coronavirus Disease 2019 in Patients with Cancer. *Eur. J. Cancer* **2020**, *139*, 70–80. [CrossRef]
78. Gupta, S.; Su, H.; Narsai, T.; Agrawal, S. SARS-CoV-2-Associated T-Cell Responses in the Presence of Humoral Immunodeficiency. *Int. Arch. Allergy Immunol.* **2021**, *182*, 195–209. [CrossRef] [PubMed]
79. Corthay, A. How Do Regulatory T Cells Work? *Scand. J. Immunol.* **2009**, *70*, 326–336. [CrossRef]
80. Dejaco, C.; Duftner, C.; Grubeck-Loebenstein, B.; Schirmer, M. Imbalance of Regulatory T Cells in Human Autoimmune Diseases. *Immunology* **2006**, *117*, 289–300. [CrossRef]
81. Komatsu, N.; Okamoto, K.; Sawa, S.; Nakashima, T.; Oh-hora, M.; Kodama, T.; Tanaka, S.; Bluestone, J.A.; Takayanagi, H. Pathogenic Conversion of Foxp3$^+$ T Cells into TH17 Cells in Autoimmune Arthritis. *Nat. Med.* **2013**, *20*, 62–68. [CrossRef]
82. Jasim, S.A.; Mahdi, R.S.; Bokov, D.O.; Najm, M.A.A.; Sobirova, G.N.; Bafoyeva, Z.O.; Taifi, A.; Alkadir, O.K.A.; Mustafa, Y.F.; Mirzaei, R.; et al. The Deciphering of the Immune Cells and Marker Signature in COVID-19 Pathogenesis: An Update. *J. Med. Virol.* **2022**, *94*, 5128–5148. [CrossRef]
83. Brown, B.; Ojha, V.; Fricke, I.; Al-Sheboul, S.A.; Imarogbe, C.; Gravier, T.; Green, M.; Peterson, L.; Koutsaroff, I.P.; Demir, A.; et al. Innate and Adaptive Immunity during SARS-CoV-2 Infection: Biomolecular Cellular Markers and Mechanisms. *Vaccines* **2023**, *11*, 408. [CrossRef] [PubMed]
84. Neumann, J.; Prezzemolo, T.; Vanderbeke, L.; Roca, C.P.; Gerbaux, M.; Janssens, S.; Willemsen, M.; Burton, O.; Van Mol, P.; Van Herck, Y.; et al. Increased IL-10-producing Regulatory T Cells Are Characteristic of Severe Cases of COVID-19. *Clin. Transl. Immunol.* **2020**, *9*, e1204. [CrossRef] [PubMed]
85. Filbin, M.R.; Mehta, A.; Schneider, A.M.; Kays, K.R.; Guess, J.R.; Gentili, M.; Fenyves, B.G.; Charland, N.C.; Gonye, A.L.K.; Gushterova, I.; et al. Longitudinal Proteomic Analysis of Severe COVID-19 Reveals Survival-Associated Signatures, Tissue-Specific Cell Death, and Cell-Cell Interactions. *Cell Rep. Med.* **2021**, *2*, 100287. [CrossRef] [PubMed]
86. LIU, M.; GUO, S.; STILES, J.K. The Emerging Role of CXCL10 in Cancer (Review). *Oncol. Lett.* **2011**, *2*, 583–589. [CrossRef]
87. Veiga-Parga, T.; Sehrawat, S.; Rouse, B.T. Role of Regulatory T Cells during Virus Infection. *Immunol. Rev.* **2013**, *255*, 182–196. [CrossRef] [PubMed]
88. Sehrawat, S.; Rouse, B.T. Tregs and Infections: On the Potential Value of Modifying Their Function. *J. Leukoc. Biol.* **2011**, *90*, 1079–1087. [CrossRef]
89. Bettelli, E.; Carrier, Y.; Gao, W.; Korn, T.; Strom, T.B.; Oukka, M.; Weiner, H.L.; Kuchroo, V.K. Reciprocal Developmental Pathways for the Generation of Pathogenic Effector TH17 and Regulatory T Cells. *Nature* **2006**, *441*, 235–238. [CrossRef]
90. Sefik, E.; Geva-Zatorsky, N.; Oh, S.; Konnikova, L.; Zemmour, D.; McGuire, A.M.; Burzyn, D.; Ortiz-Lopez, A.; Lobera, M.; Yang, J.; et al. Individual Intestinal Symbionts Induce a Distinct Population of RORγ^+ Regulatory T Cells. *Science* **2015**, *349*, 993–997. [CrossRef]
91. Ohnmacht, C.; Park, J.-H.; Cording, S.; Wing, J.B.; Atarashi, K.; Obata, Y.; Gaboriau-Routhiau, V.; Marques, R.; Dulauroy, S.; Fedoseeva, M.; et al. The Microbiota Regulates Type 2 Immunity through RORγt$^+$ T Cells. *Science* **2015**, *349*, 989–993. [CrossRef] [PubMed]
92. Hagenstein, J.; Melderis, S.; Nosko, A.; Warkotsch, M.T.; Richter, J.V.; Ramcke, T.; Herrnstadt, G.R.; Scheller, J.; Yan, I.; Mittrücker, H.-W.; et al. A Novel Role for IL-6 Receptor Classic Signaling: Induction of RORγt$^+$Foxp3$^+$ Tregs with Enhanced Suppressive Capacity. *J. Am. Soc. Nephrol.* **2019**, *30*, 1439–1453. [CrossRef] [PubMed]
93. Fujimoto, M.; Nakano, M.; Terabe, F.; Kawahata, H.; Ohkawara, T.; Han, Y.; Ripley, B.; Serada, S.; Nishikawa, T.; Kimura, A.; et al. The Influence of Excessive IL-6 Production In Vivo on the Development and Function of Foxp3$^+$ Regulatory T Cells. *J. Immunol.* **2011**, *186*, 32–40. [CrossRef] [PubMed]
94. Mijnheer, G.; Lutter, L.; Mokry, M.; van der Wal, M.; Scholman, R.; Fleskens, V.; Pandit, A.; Tao, W.; Wekking, M.; Vervoort, S.; et al. Conserved Human Effector Treg Cell Transcriptomic and Epigenetic Signature in Arthritic Joint Inflammation. *Nat. Commun.* **2021**, *12*, 2710. [CrossRef]
95. Arpaia, N.; Green, J.A.; Moltedo, B.; Arvey, A.; Hemmers, S.; Yuan, S.; Treuting, P.M.; Rudensky, A.Y. A Distinct Function of Regulatory T Cells in Tissue Protection. *Cell* **2015**, *162*, 1078–1089. [CrossRef]
96. Harrison, O.J.; Srinivasan, N.; Pott, J.; Schiering, C.; Krausgruber, T.; Ilott, N.E.; Maloy, K.J. Epithelial-Derived IL-18 Regulates Th17 Cell Differentiation and Foxp3$^+$ Treg Cell Function in the Intestine. *Mucosal Immunol.* **2015**, *8*, 1226–1236. [CrossRef] [PubMed]

97. Harb, H.; Benamar, M.; Lai, P.S.; Contini, P.; Griffith, J.W.; Crestani, E.; Schmitz-Abe, K.; Chen, Q.; Fong, J.; Marri, L.; et al. Notch4 Signaling Limits Regulatory T-Cell-Mediated Tissue Repair and Promotes Severe Lung Inflammation in Viral Infections. *Immunity* **2021**, *54*, 1186–1199.e7. [CrossRef] [PubMed]
98. Peligero-Cruz, C.; Givony, T.; Sebé-Pedrós, A.; Dobeš, J.; Kadouri, N.; Nevo, S.; Roncato, F.; Alon, R.; Goldfarb, Y.; Abramson, J. IL18 Signaling Promotes Homing of Mature Tregs into the Thymus. *ELife* **2020**, *9*, e58213. [CrossRef]
99. Buckley, P.R.; Lee, C.H.; Pereira Pinho, M.; Ottakandathil Babu, R.; Woo, J.; Antanaviciute, A.; Simmons, A.; Ogg, G.; Koohy, H. HLA-dependent Variation in SARS-CoV-2 $CD8^+$ T Cell Cross-reactivity with Human Coronaviruses. *Immunology* **2022**, *166*, 78–103. [CrossRef]
100. Overacre-Delgoffe, A.E.; Chikina, M.; Dadey, R.E.; Yano, H.; Brunazzi, E.A.; Shayan, G.; Horne, W.; Moskovitz, J.M.; Kolls, J.K.; Sander, C.; et al. Interferon-γ Drives Treg Fragility to Promote Anti-Tumor Immunity. *Cell* **2017**, *169*, 1130–1141.e11. [CrossRef]
101. Yang, J.; Zhang, E.; Zhong, M.; Yang, Q.; Hong, K.; Shu, T.; Zhou, D.; Xiang, J.; Xia, J.; Zhou, X.; et al. Longitudinal Characteristics of T Cell Responses in Asymptomatic SARS-CoV-2 Infection. *Virol. Sin.* **2020**, *35*, 838–841. [CrossRef] [PubMed]
102. Benamar, M.; Chen, Q.; Chou, J.; Julé, A.M.; Boudra, R.; Contini, P.; Crestani, E.; Lai, P.S.; Wang, M.; Fong, J.; et al. The Notch1/CD22 Signaling Axis Disrupts Treg Function in SARS-CoV-2–Associated Multisystem Inflammatory Syndrome in Children. *J. Clin. Investig.* **2023**, *133*, e163235. [CrossRef] [PubMed]
103. Guan, W.; Ni, Z.; Hu, Y.; Liang, W.; Ou, C.; He, J.; Liu, L.; Shan, H.; Lei, C.; Hui, D.S.C.; et al. Clinical Characteristics of Coronavirus Disease 2019 in China. *N. Engl. J. Med.* **2020**, *382*, 1708–1720. [CrossRef] [PubMed]
104. Gupta, A.; Madhavan, M.V.; Sehgal, K.; Nair, N.; Mahajan, S.; Sehrawat, T.S.; Bikdeli, B.; Ahluwalia, N.; Ausiello, J.C.; Wan, E.Y.; et al. Extrapulmonary Manifestations of COVID-19. *Nat. Med.* **2020**, *26*, 1017–1032. [CrossRef]
105. Ackermann, M.; Verleden, S.E.; Kuehnel, M.; Haverich, A.; Welte, T.; Laenger, F.; Vanstapel, A.; Werlein, C.; Stark, H.; Tzankov, A.; et al. Pulmonary Vascular Endothelialitis, Thrombosis, and Angiogenesis in COVID-19. *N. Engl. J. Med.* **2020**, *383*, 120–128. [CrossRef] [PubMed]
106. Henderson, L.A.; Canna, S.W.; Schulert, G.S.; Volpi, S.; Lee, P.Y.; Kernan, K.F.; Caricchio, R.; Mahmud, S.; Hazen, M.M.; Halyabar, O.; et al. On the Alert for Cytokine Storm: Immunopathology in COVID-19. *Arthritis Rheumatol.* **2020**, *72*, 1059–1063. [CrossRef]
107. Ballering, A.V.; van Zon, S.K.R.; olde Hartman, T.C.; Rosmalen, J.G.M. Persistence of Somatic Symptoms after COVID-19 in the Netherlands: An Observational Cohort Study. *Lancet* **2022**, *400*, 452–461. [CrossRef]
108. Soriano, J.B.; Murthy, S.; Marshall, J.C.; Relan, P.; Diaz, J.V. A Clinical Case Definition of Post-COVID-19 Condition by a Delphi Consensus. *Lancet Infect. Dis.* **2022**, *22*, e102–e107. [CrossRef]
109. Iqbal, F.M.; Lam, K.; Sounderajah, V.; Clarke, J.M.; Ashrafian, H.; Darzi, A. Characteristics and Predictors of Acute and Chronic Post-COVID Syndrome: A Systematic Review and Meta-Analysis. *eClinicalMedicine* **2021**, *36*, 100899. [CrossRef]
110. Davis, H.E.; Assaf, G.S.; McCorkell, L.; Wei, H.; Low, R.J.; Re'em, Y.; Redfield, S.; Austin, J.P.; Akrami, A. Characterizing Long COVID in an International Cohort: 7 Months of Symptoms and Their Impact. *eClinicalMedicine* **2021**, *38*, 101019. [CrossRef]
111. Giszas, B.; Trommer, S.; Schüßler, N.; Rodewald, A.; Besteher, B.; Bleidorn, J.; Dickmann, P.; Finke, K.; Katzer, K.; Lehmann-Pohl, K.; et al. Post-COVID-19 Condition Is Not Only a Question of Persistent Symptoms: Structured Screening Including Health-Related Quality of Life Reveals Two Separate Clusters of Post-COVID. *Infection* **2022**. [CrossRef]
112. Merad, M.; Blish, C.A.; Sallusto, F.; Iwasaki, A. The Immunology and Immunopathology of COVID-19. *Science* **2022**, *375*, 1122–1127. [CrossRef] [PubMed]
113. Sun, B.; Tang, N.; Peluso, M.J.; Iyer, N.S.; Torres, L.; Donatelli, J.L.; Munter, S.E.; Nixon, C.C.; Rutishauser, R.L.; Rodriguez-Barraquer, I.; et al. Characterization and Biomarker Analyses of Post-COVID-19 Complications and Neurological Manifestations. *Cells* **2021**, *10*, 386. [CrossRef] [PubMed]
114. Peluso, M.J.; Lu, S.; Tang, A.F.; Durstenfeld, M.S.; Ho, H.; Goldberg, S.A.; Forman, C.A.; Munter, S.E.; Hoh, R.; Tai, V.; et al. Markers of Immune Activation and Inflammation in Individuals With Postacute Sequelae of Severe Acute Respiratory Syndrome Coronavirus 2 Infection. *J. Infect. Dis.* **2021**, *224*, 1839–1848. [CrossRef] [PubMed]
115. Galán, M.; Vigón, L.; Fuertes, D.; Murciano-Antón, M.A.; Casado-Fernández, G.; Domínguez-Mateos, S.; Mateos, E.; Ramos-Martín, F.; Planelles, V.; Torres, M.; et al. Persistent Overactive Cytotoxic Immune Response in a Spanish Cohort of Individuals With Long-COVID: Identification of Diagnostic Biomarkers. *Front. Immunol.* **2022**, *13*, 848886. [CrossRef]
116. Patterson, B.K.; Guevara-Coto, J.; Yogendra, R.; Francisco, E.B.; Long, E.; Pise, A.; Rodrigues, H.; Parikh, P.; Mora, J.; Mora-Rodríguez, R.A. Immune-Based Prediction of COVID-19 Severity and Chronicity Decoded Using Machine Learning. *Front. Immunol.* **2021**, *12*, 700782. [CrossRef] [PubMed]
117. Utrero-Rico, A.; Ruiz-Ruigómez, M.; Laguna-Goya, R.; Arrieta-Ortubay, E.; Chivite-Lacaba, M.; González-Cuadrado, C.; Lalueza, A.; Almendro-Vazquez, P.; Serrano, A.; Aguado, J.M.; et al. A Short Corticosteroid Course Reduces Symptoms and Immunological Alterations Underlying Long-COVID. *Biomedicines* **2021**, *9*, 1540. [CrossRef]
118. Petrara, M.R.; Bonfante, F.; Costenaro, P.; Cantarutti, A.; Carmona, F.; Ruffoni, E.; Di Chiara, C.; Zanchetta, M.; Barzon, L.; Donà, D.; et al. Asymptomatic and Mild SARS-CoV-2 Infections Elicit Lower Immune Activation and Higher Specific Neutralizing Antibodies in Children Than in Adults. *Front. Immunol.* **2021**, *12*, 741796. [CrossRef] [PubMed]
119. Ryan, F.J.; Hope, C.M.; Masavuli, M.G.; Lynn, M.A.; Mekonnen, Z.A.; Yeow, A.E.L.; Garcia-Valtanen, P.; Al-Delfi, Z.; Gummow, J.; Ferguson, C.; et al. Long-Term Perturbation of the Peripheral Immune System Months after SARS-CoV-2 Infection. *BMC Med.* **2022**, *20*, 26. [CrossRef]

120. Wiech, M.; Chroscicki, P.; Swatler, J.; Stepnik, D.; De Biasi, S.; Hampel, M.; Brewinska-Olchowik, M.; Maliszewska, A.; Sklinda, K.; Durlik, M.; et al. Remodeling of T Cell Dynamics During Long COVID Is Dependent on Severity of SARS-CoV-2 Infection. *Front. Immunol.* **2022**, *13*, 886431. [CrossRef]
121. Garcia-Gasalla, M.; Berman-Riu, M.; Pons, J.; Rodríguez, A.; Iglesias, A.; Martínez-Pomar, N.; Llompart-Alabern, I.; Riera, M.; Ferré Beltrán, A.; Figueras-Castilla, A.; et al. Hyperinflammatory State and Low T1 Adaptive Immune Response in Severe and Critical Acute COVID-19 Patients. *Front. Med.* **2022**, *9*, 828678. [CrossRef]
122. Suvvari, T.K.; Kutikuppala, L.V.S.; Tsagkaris, C.; Corriero, A.C.; Kandi, V. Post-COVID-19 Complications: Multisystemic Approach. *J. Med. Virol.* **2021**, *93*, 6451–6455. [CrossRef]
123. Ståhlberg, M.; Reistam, U.; Fedorowski, A.; Villacorta, H.; Horiuchi, Y.; Bax, J.; Pitt, B.; Matskeplishvili, S.; Lüscher, T.F.; Weichert, I.; et al. Post-COVID-19 Tachycardia Syndrome: A Distinct Phenotype of Post-Acute COVID-19 Syndrome. *Am. J. Med.* **2021**, *134*, 1451–1456. [CrossRef]
124. Afrin, L.B.; Weinstock, L.B.; Molderings, G.J. COVID–19 Hyperinflammation and Post-COVID–19 Illness May Be Rooted in Mast Cell Activation Syndrome. *Int. J. Infect. Dis.* **2020**, *100*, 327–332. [CrossRef] [PubMed]
125. Whitaker, M.; Elliott, J.; Chadeau-Hyam, M.; Riley, S.; Darzi, A.; Cooke, G.; Ward, H.; Elliott, P. Persistent COVID-19 Symptoms in a Community Study of 606,434 People in England. *Nat. Commun.* **2022**, *13*, 1957. [CrossRef]
126. Hefazi, M.; Bolivar-Wagers, S.; Blazar, B.R. Regulatory T Cell Therapy of Graft-versus-Host Disease: Advances and Challenges. *Int. J. Mol. Sci.* **2021**, *22*, 9676. [CrossRef]
127. Sun, J.; Han, Z.-B.; Liao, W.; Yang, S.G.; Yang, Z.; Yu, J.; Meng, L.; Wu, R.; Han, Z.C. Intrapulmonary Delivery of Human Umbilical Cord Mesenchymal Stem Cells Attenuates Acute Lung Injury by Expanding $CD4^+CD25^+$ Forkhead Boxp3 (FOXP3) $^+$ Regulatory T Cells and Balancing Anti- and Pro-Inflammatory Factors. *Cell. Physiol. Biochem.* **2011**, *27*, 587–596. [CrossRef] [PubMed]
128. Cao, Y.; Xu, W.; Xiong, S. Adoptive Transfer of Regulatory T Cells Protects against Coxsackievirus B3-Induced Cardiac Fibrosis. *PLoS ONE* **2013**, *8*, e74955. [CrossRef] [PubMed]
129. Gladstone, D.E.; Kim, B.S.; Mooney, K.; Karaba, A.H.; D'Alessio, F.R. Regulatory T Cells for Treating Patients With COVID-19 and Acute Respiratory Distress Syndrome: Two Case Reports. *Ann. Intern. Med.* **2020**, *173*, 852–853. [CrossRef]
130. Hossein-khannazer, N.; Shokoohian, B.; Shpichka, A.; Aghdaei, H.A.; Timashev, P.; Vosough, M. An Update to "Novel Therapeutic Approaches for Treatment of COVID-19". *J. Mol. Med.* **2021**, *99*, 303–310. [CrossRef]
131. Zhang, Y.; Wang, X.; Li, X.; Xi, D.; Mao, R.; Wu, X.; Cheng, S.; Sun, X.; Yi, C.; Ling, Z.; et al. Potential Contribution of Increased Soluble IL-2R to Lymphopenia in COVID-19 Patients. *Cell. Mol. Immunol.* **2020**, *17*, 878–880. [CrossRef] [PubMed]
132. Rabaan, A.A.; Al-Ahmed, S.H.; Muhammad, J.; Khan, A.; Sule, A.A.; Tirupathi, R.; Mutair, A.A.; Alhumaid, S.; Al-Omari, A.; Dhawan, M.; et al. Role of Inflammatory Cytokines in COVID-19 Patients: A Review on Molecular Mechanisms, Immune Functions, Immunopathology and Immunomodulatory Drugs to Counter Cytokine Storm. *Vaccines* **2021**, *9*, 436. [CrossRef] [PubMed]
133. Hartemann, A.; Bensimon, G.; Payan, C.A.; Jacqueminet, S.; Bourron, O.; Nicolas, N.; Fonfrede, M.; Rosenzwajg, M.; Bernard, C.; Klatzmann, D. Low-Dose Interleukin 2 in Patients with Type 1 Diabetes: A Phase 1/2 Randomised, Double-Blind, Placebo-Controlled Trial. *Lancet Diabetes Endocrinol.* **2013**, *1*, 295–305. [CrossRef]
134. Kennedy-Nasser, A.A.; Ku, S.; Castillo-Caro, P.; Hazrat, Y.; Wu, M.-F.; Liu, H.; Melenhorst, J.; Barrett, A.J.; Ito, S.; Foster, A.; et al. Ultra Low-Dose IL-2 for GVHD Prophylaxis after Allogeneic Hematopoietic Stem Cell Transplantation Mediates Expansion of Regulatory T Cells without Diminishing Antiviral and Antileukemic Activity. *Clin. Cancer Res.* **2014**, *20*, 2215–2225. [CrossRef] [PubMed]
135. Zhu, M.-E.; Wang, Q.; Zhou, S.; Wang, B.; Ke, L.; He, P. Recombinant Interleukin-2 Stimulates Lymphocyte Recovery in Patients with Severe COVID-19. *Exp. Ther. Med.* **2021**, *21*, 227. [CrossRef]
136. Hou, H.; Zhang, B.; Huang, H.; Luo, Y.; Wu, S.; Tang, G.; Liu, W.; Mao, L.; Mao, L.; Wang, F.; et al. Using IL-2R/Lymphocytes for Predicting the Clinical Progression of Patients with COVID-19. *Clin. Exp. Immunol.* **2020**, *201*, 76–84. [CrossRef]
137. Jang, H.J.; Leem, A.Y.; Chung, K.S.; Ahn, J.Y.; Jung, J.Y.; Kang, Y.A.; Park, M.S.; Kim, Y.S.; Lee, S.H. Soluble IL-2R Levels Predict in-Hospital Mortality in COVID-19 Patients with Respiratory Failure. *J. Clin. Med.* **2021**, *10*, 4242. [CrossRef]
138. Stephen-Victor, E.; Das, M.; Karnam, A.; Pitard, B.; Gautier, J.-F.; Bayry, J. Potential of Regulatory T-Cell-Based Therapies in the Management of Severe COVID-19. *Eur. Respir. J.* **2020**, *56*, 2002182. [CrossRef]
139. Trotta, E.; Bessette, P.H.; Silveria, S.L.; Ely, L.K.; Jude, K.M.; Le, D.T.; Holst, C.R.; Coyle, A.; Potempa, M.; Lanier, L.L.; et al. A Human Anti-IL-2 Antibody That Potentiates Regulatory T Cells by a Structure-Based Mechanism. *Nat. Med.* **2018**, *24*, 1005–1014. [CrossRef]
140. Webster, K.E.; Walters, S.; Kohler, R.E.; Mrkvan, T.; Boyman, O.; Surh, C.D.; Grey, S.T.; Sprent, J. In Vivo Expansion of T Reg Cells with IL-2–mAb Complexes: Induction of Resistance to EAE and Long-Term Acceptance of Islet Allografts without Immunosuppression. *J. Exp. Med.* **2009**, *206*, 751–760. [CrossRef] [PubMed]
141. Hosseini, A.; Gharibi, T.; Mohammadzadeh, A.; Ebrahimi-kalan, A.; Jadidi-niaragh, F.; Babaloo, Z.; Shanehbandi, D.; Baghbani, E.; Baradaran, B. Ruxolitinib Attenuates Experimental Autoimmune Encephalomyelitis (EAE) Development as Animal Models of Multiple Sclerosis (MS). *Life Sci.* **2021**, *276*, 119395. [CrossRef]
142. Uraki, R.; Imai, M.; Ito, M.; Shime, H.; Odanaka, M.; Okuda, M.; Kawaoka, Y.; Yamazaki, S. $Foxp3^+$ $CD4^+$ Regulatory T Cells Control Dendritic Cells in Inducing Antigen-Specific Immunity to Emerging SARS-CoV-2 Antigens. *PLOS Pathog.* **2021**, *17*, e1010085. [CrossRef] [PubMed]

143. Cheng, H.; Wang, L.; Yang, B.; Li, D.; Wang, X.; Liu, X.; Tian, N.; Huang, Q.; Feng, R.; Wang, Z.; et al. Cutting Edge: Inhibition of Glycogen Synthase Kinase 3 Activity Induces the Generation and Enhanced Suppressive Function of Human IL-10$^+$ FOXP3$^+$–Induced Regulatory T Cells. *J. Immunol.* **2020**, *205*, 1497–1502. [CrossRef] [PubMed]
144. Rudd, C.E. GSK-3 Inhibition as a Therapeutic Approach Against SARs CoV2: Dual Benefit of Inhibiting Viral Replication While Potentiating the Immune Response. *Front. Immunol.* **2020**, *11*, 1638. [CrossRef] [PubMed]
145. Sauer, S.; Bruno, L.; Hertweck, A.; Finlay, D.; Leleu, M.; Spivakov, M.; Knight, Z.A.; Cobb, B.S.; Cantrell, D.; O'Connor, E.; et al. T Cell Receptor Signaling Controls Foxp3 Expression via PI3K, Akt, and mTOR. *Proc. Natl. Acad. Sci. USA* **2008**, *105*, 7797–7802. [CrossRef] [PubMed]
146. Zeiser, R.; Leveson-Gower, D.B.; Zambricki, E.A.; Kambham, N.; Beilhack, A.; Loh, J.; Hou, J.-Z.; Negrin, R.S. Differential Impact of Mammalian Target of Rapamycin Inhibition on CD4$^+$CD25$^+$Foxp3$^+$ Regulatory T Cells Compared with Conventional CD4$^+$ T Cells. *Blood* **2008**, *111*, 453–462. [CrossRef]
147. Battaglia, M.; Stabilini, A.; Migliavacca, B.; Horejs-Hoeck, J.; Kaupper, T.; Roncarolo, M.-G. Rapamycin Promotes Expansion of Functional CD4$^+$CD25$^+$FOXP3$^+$ Regulatory T Cells of Both Healthy Subjects and Type 1 Diabetic Patients. *J. Immunol.* **2006**, *177*, 8338–8347. [CrossRef]
148. Bischof, E.; Siow, R.C.; Zhavoronkov, A.; Kaeberlein, M. The Potential of Rapalogs to Enhance Resilience against SARS-CoV-2 Infection and Reduce the Severity of COVID-19. *Lancet Healthy Longev.* **2021**, *2*, e105–e111. [CrossRef]
149. Lu, L.; Lan, Q.; Li, Z.; Zhou, X.; Gu, J.; Li, Q.; Wang, J.; Chen, M.; Liu, Y.; Shen, Y.; et al. Critical Role of All—Trans Retinoic Acid in Stabilizing Human Natural Regulatory T Cells under Inflammatory Conditions. *Proc. Natl. Acad. Sci. USA* **2014**, *111*, E3432–E3440. [CrossRef]
150. Elias, K.M.; Laurence, A.; Davidson, T.S.; Stephens, G.; Kanno, Y.; Shevach, E.M.; O'Shea, J.J. Retinoic Acid Inhibits Th17 Polarization and Enhances FoxP3 Expression through a Stat-3/Stat-5 Independent Signaling Pathway. *Blood* **2008**, *111*, 1013–1020. [CrossRef]
151. Zhou, X.; Kong, N.; Wang, J.; Fan, H.; Zou, H.; Horwitz, D.; Brand, D.; Liu, Z.; Zheng, S.G. Cutting Edge: All-Trans Retinoic Acid Sustains the Stability and Function of Natural Regulatory T Cells in an Inflammatory Milieu. *J. Immunol.* **2010**, *185*, 2675–2679. [CrossRef] [PubMed]
152. Morita, T.; Miyakawa, K.; Jeremiah, S.S.; Yamaoka, Y.; Sada, M.; Kuniyoshi, T.; Yang, J.; Kimura, H.; Ryo, A. All-Trans Retinoic Acid Exhibits Antiviral Effect against SARS-CoV-2 by Inhibiting 3CLpro Activity. *Viruses* **2021**, *13*, 1669. [CrossRef] [PubMed]
153. Eggenhuizen, P.J.; Ng, B.H.; Ooi, J.D. Treg Enhancing Therapies to Treat Autoimmune Diseases. *Int. J. Mol. Sci.* **2020**, *21*, 7015. [CrossRef] [PubMed]
154. Tang, Q.; Henriksen, K.J.; Bi, M.; Finger, E.B.; Szot, G.; Ye, J.; Masteller, E.L.; McDevitt, H.; Bonyhadi, M.; Bluestone, J.A. In Vitro–Expanded Antigen-Specific Regulatory T Cells Suppress Autoimmune Diabetes. *J. Exp. Med.* **2004**, *199*, 1455–1465. [CrossRef] [PubMed]
155. Wright, G.P.; Notley, C.A.; Xue, S.-A.; Bendle, G.M.; Holler, A.; Schumacher, T.N.; Ehrenstein, M.R.; Stauss, H.J. Adoptive Therapy with Redirected Primary Regulatory T Cells Results in Antigen-Specific Suppression of Arthritis. *Proc. Natl. Acad. Sci. USA* **2009**, *106*, 19078–19083. [CrossRef]
156. Tsang, J.Y.-S.; Tanriver, Y.; Jiang, S.; Xue, S.-A.; Ratnasothy, K.; Chen, D.; Stauss, H.J.; Bucy, R.P.; Lombardi, G.; Lechler, R. Conferring Indirect Allospecificity on CD4$^+$CD25$^+$ Tregs by TCR Gene Transfer Favors Transplantation Tolerance in Mice. *J. Clin. Investig.* **2008**, *118*, 3619–3628. [CrossRef]
157. Zhang, Q.; Lu, W.; Liang, C.-L.; Chen, Y.; Liu, H.; Qiu, F.; Dai, Z. Chimeric Antigen Receptor (CAR) Treg: A Promising Approach to Inducing Immunological Tolerance. *Front. Immunol.* **2018**, *9*, 2359. [CrossRef]
158. Fransson, M.; Piras, E.; Burman, J.; Nilsson, B.; Essand, M.; Lu, B.; Harris, R.A.; Magnusson, P.U.; Brittebo, E.; Loskog, A.S. CAR/FoxP3-Engineered T Regulatory Cells Target the CNS and Suppress EAE upon Intranasal Delivery. *J. Neuroinflammation* **2012**, *9*, 112. [CrossRef]
159. Blat, D.; Zigmond, E.; Alteber, Z.; Waks, T.; Eshhar, Z. Suppression of Murine Colitis and Its Associated Cancer by Carcinoembryonic Antigen-Specific Regulatory T Cells. *Mol. Ther.* **2014**, *22*, 1018–1028. [CrossRef]
160. Skuljec, J.; Chmielewski, M.; Happle, C.; Habener, A.; Busse, M.; Abken, H.; Hansen, G. Chimeric Antigen Receptor-Redirected Regulatory T Cells Suppress Experimental Allergic Airway Inflammation, a Model of Asthma. *Front. Immunol.* **2017**, *8*, 1125. [CrossRef]
161. Michelena, X.; Borrell, H.; López-Corbeto, M.; López-Lasanta, M.; Moreno, E.; Pascual-Pastor, M.; Erra, A.; Serrat, M.; Espartal, E.; Antón, S.; et al. Incidence of COVID-19 in a Cohort of Adult and Paediatric Patients with Rheumatic Diseases Treated with Targeted Biologic and Synthetic Disease-Modifying Anti-Rheumatic Drugs. *Semin. Arthritis Rheum.* **2020**, *50*, 564–570. [CrossRef]
162. Vaz de Paula, C.B.; Nagashima, S.; Liberalesso, V.; Collete, M.; da Silva, F.P.G.; Oricil, A.G.G.; Barbosa, G.S.; da Silva, G.V.C.; Wiedmer, D.B.; da Silva Dezidério, F.; et al. COVID-19: Immunohistochemical Analysis of TGF-β Signaling Pathways in Pulmonary Fibrosis. *Int. J. Mol. Sci.* **2021**, *23*, 168. [CrossRef]
163. Chen, W. A Potential Treatment of COVID-19 with TGF-β Blockade. *Int. J. Biol. Sci.* **2020**, *16*, 1954–1955. [CrossRef]
164. He, J.; Zhang, R.; Shao, M.; Zhao, X.; Miao, M.; Chen, J.; Liu, J.; Zhang, X.; Zhang, X.; Jin, Y.; et al. Efficacy and Safety of Low-Dose IL-2 in the Treatment of Systemic Lupus Erythematosus: A Randomised, Double-Blind, Placebo-Controlled Trial. *Ann. Rheum. Dis.* **2019**, *79*, 141–149. [CrossRef]

165. Chaudhary, B.; Elkord, E. Regulatory T Cells in the Tumor Microenvironment and Cancer Progression: Role and Therapeutic Targeting. *Vaccines* **2016**, *4*, 28. [CrossRef]
166. Gliwiński, M.; Iwaszkiewicz-Grześ, D.; Trzonkowski, P. Cell-Based Therapies with T Regulatory Cells. *BioDrugs* **2017**, *31*, 335–347. [CrossRef] [PubMed]
167. Ting, H.-A.; de Almeida Nagata, D.; Rasky, A.J.; Malinczak, C.-A.; Maillard, I.P.; Schaller, M.A.; Lukacs, N.W. Notch Ligand Delta-like 4 Induces Epigenetic Regulation of Treg Cell Differentiation and Function in Viral Infection. *Mucosal Immunol.* **2018**, *11*, 1524–1536. [CrossRef]
168. Batah, S.S.; Fabro, A.T. Pulmonary Pathology of ARDS in COVID-19: A Pathological Review for Clinicians. *Respir. Med.* **2021**, *176*, 106239. [CrossRef]
169. Xu, G.; Qi, F.; Li, H.; Yang, Q.; Wang, H.; Wang, X.; Liu, X.; Zhao, J.; Liao, X.; Liu, Y.; et al. The Differential Immune Responses to COVID-19 in Peripheral and Lung Revealed by Single-Cell RNA Sequencing. *Cell Discov.* **2020**, *6*, 73. [CrossRef] [PubMed]
170. Alahyari, S.; Rajaeinejad, M.; Jalaeikhoo, H.; Amani, D. Regulatory T Cells in Immunopathogenesis and Severity of COVID-19: A Systematic Review. *Arch. Iran. Med.* **2022**, *25*, 127–132. [CrossRef] [PubMed]

MDPI AG
Grosspeteranlage 5
4052 Basel
Switzerland
Tel.: +41 61 683 77 34

Vaccines Editorial Office
E-mail: vaccines@mdpi.com
www.mdpi.com/journal/vaccines

www.ingramcontent.com/pod-product-compliance
Lightning Source LLC
Chambersburg PA
CBHW061449210926
51850CB00008B/1664
* 9 7 8 3 7 2 5 8 5 9 6 7 2 *